PREFACE

This is a textbook for a one-term course whose goal is to ease the transition from lower-division calculus courses to upper-division courses in linear and abstract algebra, real and complex analysis, number theory, topology, combinatorics, and so on. Without such a "bridge" course, most upper-division instructors feel the need to start their courses with the rudiments of logic, set theory, equivalence relations, and other basic mathematical raw materials before getting on with the subject at hand. Students who are new to higher mathematics are often startled to discover that mathematics is a subject of *ideas*, and not just formulaic rituals, and that they are now expected to understand and create mathematical proofs. Mastery of an assortment of technical tricks may have carried the students through calculus, but it is no longer a guarantee of academic success.

Students need experience in working with abstract ideas at a nontrivial level if they are to achieve the sophisticated blend of knowledge, discipline, and creativity that we call "mathematical maturity." I don't believe that "theorem-proving" can be taught any more than "question-answering" can be taught. Nevertheless, I have found that it is possible to guide students gently into the process of mathematical proof in such a way that they become comfortable with the experience and begin asking themselves questions that will lead them in the right direction. As with learning to swim or ride a bicycle, there are usually anxieties to be overcome; and, especially in view of the "cookbook" experience of many calculus courses, it takes a while for students to come to believe that they may be capable of solving a problem even when no *instantaneous* solution presents itself.

But in time students become familiar with the process by which we prove most theorems: a thoughtful oscillation between what we know to be true and what we want to *show* to be true, until the gap between the two has been closed. Sometimes this involves a gradual buildup of knowledge, coupled with a breakup of the objective into more manageable parts. Sometimes computational experiments lead to new understanding of the structures under investigation. Sometimes sudden insights come after a period of quiet reflection. There is no section in the book called "How to Prove a Theorem," because it would be dishonest to pretend that mechanical rituals can replace creative thinking when we are doing substantial mathematics. However, after going through the material in this book, the student who is asked to prove something will not feel like a stranger in a hostile land.

Part of the transition to mathematical maturity involves learning to use the *language* of mathematics. Having convinced ourselves that we have solved a difficult problem, we need to write up the solution in a way that will convince the possibly skeptical reader. This task can be made easier by the judicious use of the notation and terminology that have been developed for the purpose of presenting mathematics in a clear and efficient fashion. We will spend a good deal of time exploring this mode of expression, because mastery of language is an important step toward the mastery of ideas.

In writing this book, beyond introducing fundamental mathematical structures and exploring techniques of proof, I have tried to convey some of the excitement and delightful confusion that a professional mathematician experiences when confronting the unknown. It is important that students develop an awareness of mathematics as an independent science, and not just as a collection of tools. Like any science, mathematics is a thriving wonderland of research, with many mysteries to keep us humble despite the subject's many remarkable achievements. The final chapter, on number theory, includes the statement of several problems whose solutions have so far eluded mathematicians, in some cases for centuries.

Strictly speaking, there are no college-level prerequisites for the material to be found here; indeed, this book could be used as a source of special topics for talented high school students. But in fact I have assumed that this is *not* the student's first encounter with college mathematics, and that some "seasoning" from, say, a year of calculus has already occurred (though calculus is not a prerequisite for anything here). I have also assumed that the student is prepared to pursue ideas with considerable intensity.

Because this is an introductory text, I have made every effort to give students a broad view of the mathematical experience. Accordingly, the

INTRODUCTION·TO MATHEMATICAL STRUCTURES AND·PROOFS

Springer
Berlin
Heidelberg
New York
Barcelona
Budapest
Hong Kong
London
Milan
Paris
Santa Clara
Singapore
Tokyo

INTRODUCTION·TO MATHEMATICAL STRUCTURES AND·PROOFS

LARRY J. GERSTEIN

UNIVERSITY OF CALIFORNIA,
SANTA BARBARA

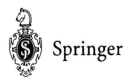
Springer

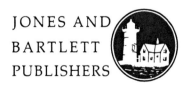
JONES AND
BARTLETT
PUBLISHERS

Textbooks in Mathematical Sciences

Series Editors:

Thomas F. Banchoff
Brown University

Jerrold Marsden
California Institute of Technology

Keith Devlin
St. Mary's College

Stan Wagon
Macalester College

Gaston Gonnet
ETH Zentrum, Zürich

COVER: Francisco de Zurbaran (Spanish, 1598–1664), *Still Life with Lemons, Oranges, and a Rose*, 1633. Oil on canvas, 24 ½ × 43 ⅛ in. Used by permission of The Norton Simon Foundation, Pasadena, CA.

Library of Congress Cataloging-in-Publication Data
Gerstein, Larry J.
    Introduction to mathematical structures and proofs / Larry J.
Gerstein.
        p.   cm. — (Textbooks in mathematical sciences)
    Includes bibliographical references and index.
    ISBN 0-387-97997-2 (hardcover : alk. paper)
    1. Logic, Symbolic and mathematical.   I. Title.   II. Series.
QA9.G358   1996
511.3—dc20   95-44881
                                                   CIP

Under the co-publishing agreement between Springer-Verlag and Jones and Bartlett Publishers, the text is available in North America exclusively from Jones and Bartlett Publishers and outside North America exclusively from Springer-Verlag.

ISBN 0-387-97997-2 Springer-Verlag New York Berlin Heidelberg SPIN 10425367
ISBN 0-7637-0203-X Jones and Bartlett Publishers Sudbury, MA

book includes a wide-ranging assortment of examples and imagery to motivate the material and to enhance the underlying intuitions. I have tried to strike a balance between rigor and informality, not by operating in some middle region but by using both styles in what I think is a reasonably balanced way. Also, I have not hesitated to consider a given topic from more than one perspective or at more than one level of rigor.

Most exercise sets include at least some routine exercises that check whether the student has mastered the meaning of terminology and notation. But the majority of the exercises are more substantial and will require some cogitation, experimentation, review of definitions, clarification of goals ("What do I have to show?" "What am I after?"), and perhaps some struggle. While re-reading some or all of the section (and especially the *definitions*) may be helpful in solving an exercise, it will usually be futile to search for a worked example in a section that is identical to the exercise except for a trivial change. My goal throughout has been to encourage the flexible and original thinking that characterizes creative mathematical activity, not to serve as a drill sergeant. In some cases a complicating issue will arise in an exercise that will not be completely resolved until later in the book, though that later material will not be needed in order to solve the exercise.

I want to thank my publisher, Jerry Lyons, for accepting this book for Springer-Verlag's Textbooks in Mathematical Sciences series, and for his calm and intelligent guidance; and I thank the book production and manufacturing staff for ably steering the book through the production process. Throughout my work on this project I have been sustained by the cheerful affection I have received from my family. I thank my sons, Ben and David, for the inspiration I have derived from their creativity; and I think David again for his drawings (on pages 103, 153, and 194). Finally, I want to express my unbounded appreciation to my wife Susan, the Lone Ranger of mathematics copyediting, who has come to the rescue again and again, her red pencils ablaze in the moonlight. Where she has found confusion she has brought clarity; where she has found despair she has brought hope; where she has found sadness she has brought joy.

I dedicate this book to my remarkable family.

LARRY J. GERSTEIN

CONTENTS

LOGIC

1.1 Statements, Propositions, and Theorems

Mathematics, like ice cream and politics, is discussed in sentences. This is not always immediately apparent, because mathematical sentences may be presented in eccentric formats. For example,

$$\begin{array}{r} 2 \\ +3 \\ \hline 5 \end{array} \quad \text{and} \quad \int_0^{2\pi} \sin x \, dx = 0$$

are sentences. We will not give a precise definition of *sentence* or *statement* (the terms will be used interchangeably), or of the adjectives *true* and *false* used in classifying sentences. But we will adopt the convention that some sentences are true, others are false, no sentence is simultaneously true and false, and some are neither true nor false.

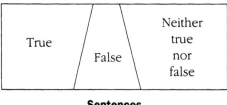

Sentences

Care is essential if we are to make sense out of this scheme of sentence classification. For example, consider the simple statement, "Charles snores." Does this mean "Charles snores every night," "Charles has been known to snore," "Charles is presently snoring," or what? To which "Charles" does the sentence refer? We cannot label the statement true or false until we have further clarification.

Distinguishing what is true from what is not true is fundamental in mathematics, and, if we are to proceed without confusion, we must first establish the rules of the game. We begin our activities in a mathematical system by agreeing to recognize certain kinds of expressions as statements in our mathematical language. For example, these might be ordinary English sentences, or statements in a particular computer language, or strings of newly created symbols assembled according to some given guidelines. Next we agree to classify a given collection of one or more mathematical statements as *true*; these statements are called **axioms**. (The word "true" here will not always relate to our ordinary notions of truth, especially since the expressions we accept as statements might not resemble statements in our natural language.) Last, we adopt a system of rules by which we can label certain new statements as "true"; these statements will be related in carefully specified ways to statements that we already accept as true. These rules of truth assignment are called our laws of **logic**, **deduction**, **inference**, or **proof**. A proof is a chain of statements leading, implicitly or explicitly, from the axioms to a statement under consideration, compelling us to declare that *that* statement, too, is true. Once we have assumed a system of axioms and logical laws, we become concerned with the consequences of those assumptions, rather than with a more absolute level of truth. A statement that is an axiom or that has been proved is called a **theorem**.

Swallowing a list of axioms as an initial mathematical act may not be easy; the axioms may be in conflict with our intuitions, if "true" has its usual meaning. Consider the following excerpt from Bertrand Russell's autobiography, describing Russell's first encounter with Euclidean geometry. [Russell (1872–1970) was a great mathematical philosopher.]

> At the age of eleven, I began Euclid, with my brother as my tutor. This was one of the great events of my life, as dazzling as first love. I had not imagined that there was anything so delicious in the world. From that moment until Whitehead and I finished *Principia Mathematica*, when I was thirty-eight, mathematics was my chief interest, and my chief source of happiness. Like all happiness, however, it was not unalloyed. I had been told that Euclid proved things, and was much disappointed that he started with axioms. At first I refused to accept them unless my brother could offer me some reason for doing so, but he said: "If you don't accept them we cannot go on," and as I wished to go on, I reluctantly admitted them pro tem. The doubt as to the premisses of mathematics which I felt at that moment remained with me, and determined the course of my subsequent work.

The axiom system in the following example is more abstract than that of Euclid's geometry, and this system runs no risk of unsettling our intuitions.

1.1 EXAMPLE. Consider a mathematical system in which a statement is a string of symbols from the list a, b, S. Some typical statements are

$$abaaS \qquad bSSaba \qquad baaaab \qquad SSS$$

Take as a system of axioms the statement

$$S$$

The logic consists of two rules: (1) a statement obtained from a true statement by replacing an S with aSb is also true; (2) a statement obtained from a true statement by deleting an S and closing up any resulting space is also true.

In this system the statement $aaabbb$ is a theorem, and here is a proof:

S	(axiom)
aSb	(rule 1)
$aaSbb$	(rule 1)
$aaaSbbb$	(rule 1)
$aaabbb$	(rule 2)

More generally, the theorems in this system are all the statements of the form

$$\underbrace{a \ldots a}_{n} S \underbrace{b \ldots b}_{n} \qquad \text{or} \qquad \underbrace{a \ldots a}_{n} \underbrace{b \ldots b}_{n}$$

where n is a nonnegative integer. We omit a formal proof.

In Example 1.1 we operated on the initial string S (the axiom system) using successive applications of certain production rules (the logic), and the result was a collection of symbol strings (the theorems) of a special form. This process is an example of what is called *language generation* in computer science. We will have more to say about languages later in the book.

In most mathematical systems, some or all of the statements that are not true are labelled "false," and there may be standard techniques for constructing false statements from true ones, and vice versa. For instance, the false statement $2 + 3 = 7$ has the true companion $2 + 3 \neq 7$. In a mathematical system, the true statements and false statements are the **propositions** of the system, and the label "true" or "false" associated with a given proposition is its **truth value**.

1.2 EXAMPLE.   We take the standard facts and procedures of elementary arithmetic as our axiom system and logic in this example.

(a) The statement "$x + 5 = 7$" is a theorem if it is understood from the context that $x = 2$; it is a false proposition if x represents another numerical value; and it is a statement but not a proposition if no value has been assigned to x.

(b) Recall that a **prime number** is an integer greater than 1 that cannot be expressed as a product of two smaller positive integers. Thus 2, 3, 5, 7, and 11 are primes, as are 17 and 103. [The prime numbers are a central topic of investigation in the study of *number theory*; we will have more to say about this mysterious and intriguing subject in Chapter 6.] Consider the mammoth integer

$$n = 2^{2^{24}} + 1 = 2^{16777216} + 1$$

(This number has 5,050,445 decimal digits!!) The statement "n is prime" is a proposition, since it is either true or false; but neither "n is prime" nor "n is not prime" is a theorem, because testing n for "primality" is beyond the present capability of our most sophisticated computer technology.

At any level of formality, the search for new truths leads us to link statements together in a variety of ways. To keep mathematical discussions from lapsing into incoherence, we have to standardize the procedures by which truth values are assigned to new propositions. We make these assignments in ways that are **truth functional**; that is, the truth value of a new proposition depends only on the truth values of its component propositions and on the way in which those components have been linked to form the new one.

1.3 EXAMPLE.   Consider the following three statements, and assume them all to be true.

P: This is a good day for a picnic.
W: The weather is beautiful today.
M: Measles is an illness.

We will probably agree that "P because W" is true and "W because M" is false. So when propositions are linked by "because," the truth value of the resulting statement is based on more than the truth values of the component propositions; that is, "because" is *not* truth functional.

Exercises

1. In each case say whether or not the given statement is a proposition. If it is a proposition, indicate its truth value. If it is not a proposition, explain *why* it is not, and then mold it into a proposition by suitable rewriting.
   (a) Lemuel Harrington, of Burbank, California, was President of the United States on July 18, 1897.
   (b) $x/x = 1$
   (c) $13 + 24 = 35$
   (d) "The Star Spangled Banner" was played on that occasion.
   (e) x is positive, negative, or zero.
   (f) If x is a real number, then x is positive, negative, or zero.

2. Jones says, "On election day I will vote for the Democratic candidate for President or for the Republican candidate for President."
   Smith says, "Tomorrow I will take you to the movies or I will take you out to dinner."
   (a) In each case, describe the circumstances under which the speaker can be said to be dishonest.
   (b) Example 1.3 showed that "because" is not truth functional. Does the answer to (a) suggest that "or" is not truth functional?

3. Consider a mathematical system with the following ingredients: A *statement* is a string of letters, where "letter" means either capital S or a lowercase member of our usual alphabet: $a, b, c, \ldots, z$. The only *axiom*: S; the *logic*: in any theorem, if an occurrence of the letter S is deleted or replaced by one of aSa, bSb, cSc, etc., or by a lowercase letter, the resulting statement will also be a theorem. Describe how to recognize theorems in this system, and write two theorems that are also ordinary English words. Include a proof of each of your theorems.

4. Consider a mathematical system in which a *statement* is a string of five letters from our usual alphabet. For example, zraav, ththw, and housg are statements. A *proposition* is a statement (as just defined) found in the latest edition of *Webster's Collegiate Dictionary* (that is, an ordinary five-letter English word); there is only on *axiom*: groan. The *logic* works like this: a proof of a proposition P is a list of propositions,

$P_1, P_2, P_3, \ldots, P_n$ in which P_1 is a theorem, P_n is just P itself, and for $i > 1$, each P_i is obtained from its immediate predecessor by changing exactly one letter and holding the others fixed. For example, here is a proof of the proposition "frail": groan, groin, grain, grail, frail. (Each word just listed is a now a theorem.) A proposition is false if no such proof is possible.

(a) Prove this proposition: cloth.

(b) Discuss the distinction between true propositions and false propositions in this system, and describe some procedure that would convince you that a particular proposition in this system is false. For instance, suppose you want to demonstrate that the proposition "xylem" is false. How could you proceed? (Describe what needs to be done, but you needn't actually carry out the procedure.)

5. A word that can be inserted between two ordinary English sentences to produce a new sentence is called a **connective**. Consider these connectives: and, hence, yet, unless, that. Give an example of each connective's use by placing it between two sentence in a way that makes sense. Discuss whether or not the connective is **truth functional**; that is, does the truth or falsity of a new sentence involving a connective depend only on the truth or falsity of the two smaller sentences? If the connective under discussion *is* truth functional, describe its truth-functional action. (That is, which conditions of truth and falsity for the two smaller sentences yield true results, and which yield false results?)

1.2 Logical Connectives and Truth Tables

We form the **negation** of a statement by using the logical term "not," symbolically denoted by $\sim$. If P is a statement, then $\sim P$ (verbalized as "not P") denotes its negation. In our ordinary language, $\sim P$ is usually obtained from P by attaching "not" in a grammatically appropriate way to the main verb. If P is "Rosco is smiling," then $\sim P$ is "Rosco is not smiling." ("Rosco is frowning" is *not* the negation of P, since the mere absence of a smile does not force a frown to appear.) There are variations on the ways to phrase a negation, due to the complexities of our language; for example, the negation of "No man is an island" is "At least one man is an island" or "Some man is an island." A safe way to negate P is to precede P by "It is not the case that," though this can lack in linguistic grace what it possesses in logical security. In mathematical contexts, negation is accomplished by a variety of symbolic devices: If P is $2 - 7 = 4$, then $\sim P$ is $2 - 7 \neq 4$. (Here P is a false proposition and $\sim P$ is true.)

The effect of negation on the truth values of propositions is summarized in the following table, called the **truth table** for $\sim$. Here the letter T in a column indicates that the proposition named at the top of the column is true, and F indicates that it is false. For example, the bottom row of Table 1.4 tells us that when P is true, $\sim P$ is false.

(1.4)

P	$\sim P$
F	T
T	F

Two statements P and Q can be joined together with "and" to make a new statement, verbalized as "P and Q," symbolically denoted as $P \wedge Q$, and called the **conjunction** of P and Q. If P and Q are propositions, then asserting that $P \wedge Q$ is true is the same as asserting that P and Q are *both* true. Thus the truth value of $P \wedge Q$ is given by Table 1.5.

(1.5)

P	Q	$P \wedge Q$
F	F	F
F	T	F
T	F	F
T	T	T

The truth value of $P \wedge Q$ depends only on the truth values of P and Q, and there need be no connection between the subject matter of P and that of Q. Thus the conjunction

$$\underbrace{\text{Most seals swim well}}_{P} \quad \text{and} \quad \underbrace{3 + 14 = 17}_{Q}$$

is a true proposition, although the occasion may seldom arise when we might wish to state it.

The symbolic expression $P \wedge Q$ is not in itself a statement, but it *becomes* a statement when the letters P and Q are replaced by statements. Expressions can be built up from letters (perhaps with numerical subscripts), logical connective symbols (so far we have seen only $\sim$ and $\wedge$), and parentheses (if necessary for clarity). Those expressions that become statements when the letters are replaced by explicit statements are called **statement forms** or **sentential forms**; the letters in such forms are called **statement letters** or **sentential variables**. (See Exercise 10 in the next exercise set for further discussion of sentential forms.)

1.6 EXAMPLE.   Here are a few statement forms using the connectives ~ and ∧ and the statement letters P, Q, and R:

$$(P\wedge(\sim Q))\wedge R, \quad \sim(\sim Q), \quad \sim P\wedge((\sim Q)\wedge R), \quad Q\wedge(\sim(\sim(\sim(\sim P))))$$

But the following are *not* statement forms:

$$\wedge\wedge P\wedge, \quad P\sim Q, \quad Q\wedge)\sim\sim(R$$

When the variables in a statement form are replaced by propositions, the result is a proposition. A truth table for the form displays its truth values in rows, with each row corresponding to a particular combination of truth values for the propositions. To ensure that the truth tables include all possible truth-value combinations, imagine replacing the symbols F and T by 0 and 1, respectively. Then a string of F's and T's takes the form of an integer in binary (base 2) notation: FTTFTFT becomes 0110101. To get all possible strings of length n using the digits 0 and 1, we just count from

$$\underbrace{000\ldots 0}_{n \text{ digits}} \quad \text{to} \quad \underbrace{111\ldots 1}_{n \text{ digits}}$$

in base 2. That is, we count from 0 to $2^n - 1$. Accordingly, the truth-value combinations in our table will range·from

$$\underbrace{FFF\ldots F}_{n \text{ digits}} \quad \text{to} \quad \underbrace{TTT\ldots T}_{n \text{ digits}}$$

giving 2^n rows in all.

1.7 EXAMPLE.   If a statement form S has three variables P_1, P_2, and P_3, then the left part of the truth table will look like this:

P_1	P_2	P_3
F	F	F
F	F	T
F	T	F
F	T	T
T	F	F
T	F	T
T	T	F
T	T	T

When we say "and" we think of the usual English conjunction if our statements are standard English sentences. But if statements have no intuitive meaning (as in Example 1.1), then what we are presently saying is just this: the expression obtained by inserting $\wedge$ between two statements (or statement forms) in our system will also be viewed as a statement (or statement form). If the two component statements are propositions, then so is the new one, and its truth value is dictated by Table 1.5. A similar observation carries over to the other logical symbols that will appear in this chapter.

The word "or" has at least two meanings in standard English, as the following examples illustrate: (1) At the airport while waiting to board our plane we hear, "Parties with young children or physically handicapped individuals will be seated first." (2) At the restaurant we learn that "the price of dinner includes soup or salad." In example (1) we understand that if our party satisfies *at least* one of the specified conditions, then we will be seated first; in particular, if our party includes both a physically handicapped person and a child, or if it includes a physically handicapped child, we will still qualify to be seated first. This "or" is called **inclusive**, since our fulfillment of one condition includes the possibility that we may also fulfill the other. In example (2) we understand that we are entitled to *exactly* one of the two possibilities; hence this "or" is called **exclusive**. In mathematics the convention is to use "or" in the inclusive sense unless we explicitly state otherwise; thus "P or Q" is true if P is true, Q is true, or both are true. For example,

$$\underbrace{\text{Lions are birds}}_{P} \quad \text{or} \quad \underbrace{6 = 2 + 4}_{Q}$$

and

$$\underbrace{3 + 2 = 5}_{P} \quad \text{or} \quad \underbrace{5 - 7 = 2}_{Q}$$

are both true propositions. And you should henceforth assume that a host who offers the ambiguous invitation, "We hope you or your sister will come to our party" will be pleased to have both of you attend if you can.

The proposition "P or Q" is called the **disjunction** of P and Q. It is denoted symbolically by $P \vee Q$; its truth table is

P	Q	P $\bigvee$ Q
F	F	F
F	T	T
T	F	T
T	T	T

(1.8)

Here is a mnemonic for distinguishing $\bigwedge$ from $\bigvee$: notice that $\bigwedge$ resembles the A in AND; also, classicists will be happy to learn that the symbol $\bigvee$ is derived from the Latin *vel* (or).

Now that we have negation, conjunction, and disjunction in hand, we can determine the truth value of more complicated propositions. The strategy is as follows: Decompose the given proposition into **atomic propositions** (that is, propositions that cannot themselves be broken into smaller propositions) linked by logical connectives. (This may require some judicious rephrasing of the original proposition.) Then label each atomic proposition with a sentential variable. The result will be a statement form that represents the given proposition. A truth table will complete the analysis.

1.9 EXAMPLE.   When is the following statement false?

I am either a polo player or the Queen of Zorbia.

The answer, obtained from pure thought (and without the use of truth tables or a logic chapter), is that the statement is false under exactly one pair of circumstances: I am not a polo player *and* I am not the Queen of Zorbia. Although this is clear upon reading the given statement, let's go through the formal analysis anyway to get a feeling for the technique. Introduce sentential variables for the atomic sentences as follows:

P: I am a polo player.
Q: I am the Queen of Zorbia.

The proposition is represented by $P \bigvee Q$, so Table 1.8 gives the asserted result. (The top row is the only row with "F" under $P \bigvee Q$, and in that row both P and Q are false.)

1.10 EXAMPLE.   Represent the statement

I will go to the movies on Monday or Tuesday, but not on both days.

by a sentential form.

SOLUTION. Make the assignments

P: I will go to the movies on Monday.

Q: I will go to the movies on Tuesday.

The first clause of the given statement is represented by $P \lor Q$, and the last by $\sim(P \land Q)$, so the complete answer is

$$(P \lor Q) \land \sim(P \land Q)$$

Here parentheses guide us in our use of the logical connectives. Notice that the effect of the phrase "but not on both days" is to make the "or" exclusive. Thus the essence of "exclusive or" has been captured by a conspiracy of $\lor$, $\land$, and $\sim$. Also notice that in terms of the logical structure of the sentence, the word "but" is synonymous with "and" here.

1.11 EXAMPLE. Let K be the following sentential form:

$$\sim(P \land Q) \land \underbrace{\left(P \land \left(\sim Q \lor (\sim P \lor Q)\right)\right)}_{J}$$

Under what truth values for propositions P and Q is the proposition represented by K true?

SOLUTION. Construct a truth table for K:

P	Q	$P \land Q$	$\sim Q$	$\sim P$	$\sim P \lor Q$	$\sim Q \lor (\sim P \lor Q)$	J	$\sim(P \land Q)$	K
F	F	F	T	T	T	T	F	T	F
F	T	F	F	T	T	T	F	T	F
T	F	F	T	F	F	T	T	T	T
T	T	T	F	F	T	T	T	F	F

Here the two columns on the left display all possible truth-value combinations for the sentential variables, and each subsequent column corresponds to a sentential form built from one or two of its predecessors by applying $\sim$, $\land$, or $\lor$ and invoking Table 1.4, 1.5, or 1.8, respectively. We conclude that K is true only when P is true and Q is simultaneously false.

1.12 Remark. Another sentential form that is true precisely when P is true and Q is simultaneously false is $P \land \sim Q$. So it would be reasonable to say that statement form K in Example 1.11 is "logically equivalent" to $P \land \sim Q$. We will return to this point later.

Exercises for this section are included in the exercise set at the end of Section 1.3.

1.3 Conditional Statements

"All your troubles are due to those 'ifs'," declared the Wizard.

L. FRANK BAUM
The Emerald City of Oz

If P and Q are propositions (whose truth values may or may not be known), we may wish to assert this:

(1.13)   Truth of P and falsity of Q do not coexist.

1.14 EXAMPLE.   Your mother tells you

If $\underbrace{\text{yesterday's weather was nice in Boise,}}_{P}$

then $\underbrace{\text{Uncle Harry went fishing yesterday.}}_{Q}$

In other words, nice weather in Boise didn't coexist with a nonfishing day for Uncle Harry. There is only one combination of circumstances under which Mom would be wrong: Boise's weather was nice, yet Uncle Harry failed to fish. In particular, if the weather was poor, your mother spoke the truth (that is, her statement was not false) whether or not your uncle went fishing.

Assertion 1.13 is represented by the sentential form $\sim(P \wedge \sim Q)$ (stated formally: it is not the case that P and not Q), which we now abbreviate by

$$P \Rightarrow Q$$

(Other common notations are $P \rightarrow Q$, $P \supset Q$, $Q \Leftarrow P$.) The effect of the new logical connective $\Rightarrow$ can be summarized by Table 1.15:

(1.15)

P	Q	$P \Rightarrow Q$
F	F	T
F	T	T
T	F	F
T	T	T

A proposition of the form $P \Rightarrow Q$ is called a **conditional proposition** or a **material implication**. The proposition P is the **antecedent** or **hypothesis** of the conditional proposition, and Q is the **consequent** or **conclusion**. We usually verbalize "$P \Rightarrow Q$" as "If P then Q" or "P implies Q," although these usages can lead to confusion by suggesting a relationship (perhaps of obscure origin) between the contents of P and Q that goes beyond their truth values. (See Example 1.16.)

To avoid monotony it is common practice to have several English statements corresponding to one mathematical one. For example, the conditional $P \Rightarrow Q$ can also be read "P is **sufficient** (or a **sufficient condition**) for Q," and "Q is **necessary** (or a **necessary condition**) for P." Other phrasings are "P only if Q," and "Q if P."

1.16 EXAMPLE. Consider the following conditional statements:

(a) If Utah is a state then $2 + 2 = 4$.

(b) If the moon is made of cheese, then an average duck weighs 3 tons.

(c) $23 \cdot 6 = 17$ implies $1 + 23 \cdot 6 = 18$.

(d) $23 \cdot 6 = 17$ implies $1 + 23 \cdot 6 = 2$.

(e) If common digits in the numerator and denominator of a fraction can be cancelled, then $\frac{16}{64} = \frac{1}{4}$.

(f) If $2 + 2 = 4$ then $6 \cdot 3 = 19$.

Statement (a) has the form T $\Rightarrow$ T. (We are abbreviating furiously by replacing each component proposition by its truth value, since that is our only concern here.) Hence statement (a) is true, though there is no evident natural pathway from P to Q. Statements (b) through (e) all have false antecedents and are therefore true conditionals; of these only statement (e) has a true consequent. Also note that in statements (c) and (e) the antecedent appears to lead "naturally" to the consequent, whereas in statements (b) and (d) no such connection is evident. Statement (f) has the form T $\Rightarrow$ F and is therefore the only false proposition on the list.

1.17 EXAMPLE. Construct a truth table for the following propositional form J:

$$P \Rightarrow \underbrace{\left((\sim Q \Rightarrow P) \wedge (Q \vee \sim P)\right)}_{K}$$

SOLUTION.

P	Q	$\sim P$	$\sim Q$	$\sim Q \Rightarrow P$	$Q \vee \sim P$	K	J
F	F	T	T	F	T	F	T
F	T	T	F	T	T	T	T
T	F	F	T	T	F	F	F
T	T	F	F	T	T	T	T

Thus J is true unless P and Q have truth values T and F, respectively. Suggestion: now reread Remark 1.12.

Conditional statements are an important feature of most computer programming languages. They are used in choosing among two or more procedures at some stage in a program's execution, and they can prevent a program from going into spasm when confronted with an impossible task. For example, suppose an integer n has been defined and a program that handles only real numbers demands "Let $m = \sqrt{n}$." Should it turn out that $n < 0$, the program will tie up. But a conditional statement of the form "If $n \geq 0$, then let $m = \sqrt{n}$, else ... [insert some other appropriate procedure]" allows the program to proceed regardless of the truth value of the hypothesis $n \geq 0$. Thus a computer program accepts a conditional statement whose hypothesis is false, just as we label as "true" a conditional statement whose hypothesis is false.

If P and Q are propositions, we abbreviate the proposition

$$(P \Leftarrow Q) \wedge (P \Rightarrow Q)$$

$$(P \text{ if } Q) \quad \text{and} \quad (P \text{ only if } Q)$$

by

$$P \Leftrightarrow Q$$

$$(P \text{ if and only if } Q)$$

(The implication $P \Leftarrow Q$ is called the **converse** of $P \Rightarrow Q$.) Such a statement is called a **biconditional proposition** or a **material equivalence**; we say that P and Q are **equivalent propositions** if $P \Leftrightarrow Q$ is true. From the truth table

(1.18)

P	Q	$P \Rightarrow Q$	$P \Leftarrow Q$	$P \Leftrightarrow Q$
F	F	T	T	T
F	T	T	F	F
T	F	F	T	F
T	T	T	T	T

we see that the statement $P \Leftrightarrow Q$ is true only when P and Q have the same truth value. Thus

$$\text{George Washington was a President} \quad \Leftrightarrow \quad 3 + 5 = 8$$

and

$$2 + 2 = 5 \quad \Leftrightarrow \quad 2 + 2 = 6$$

are both true.

Our intuitive notion of equivalent statements in ordinary language is concerned with *meaning*, which is a philosophical concept, and not just with truth value. Two statements that are equivalent in that philosophical sense are also equivalent in the sense that has been defined here. (That is, both are true or both are false.) But our equivalence is a simpler concept, since if P and Q are propositions, then a statement of the form $P \Leftrightarrow Q$ is either true or false; whereas outside the strictly logical realm, two statements whose meanings have no evident bearing on one another are regarded as incomparable.

We have defined $P \Rightarrow Q$ as an abbreviation for $\sim(P \wedge \sim Q)$, so everything we can express with $\Rightarrow$ can also be expressed with $\sim$, $\wedge$, and parentheses. But conditional statements are ubiquitous in mathematics, and whatever we write is likely to be read (otherwise why write it?), so we retain the connective $\Rightarrow$ in order to avoid the vertigo that can result from fusillades of symbols.

Exercises

1. Let P be the statement "Howard fell" and let Q be the statement "Howard broke his leg."

   (a) Write English statements corresponding to each of these:

   $$P \wedge Q, \quad \sim P \wedge \sim Q, \quad \sim(P \wedge Q), \quad Q \vee \sim P$$

   When is one of the last two of these statements true and the other one false?

   (b) With P and Q as given, under what conditions is the statement "P or Q" true when "or" is *exclusive*? *Inclusive*?

2. One Tuesday morning your friend says, "If today is Wednesday, then today is Thursday." Discuss the truth value of your friend's statement.

3. Let $\veebar$ denote "exclusive or," and exhibit a truth table for the sentential form $P \veebar Q$.

4. The connective "unless" can be ambiguous, and this exercise will pinpoint the ambiguity.

   We awake at dawn, and we are told

   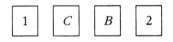

   $$\underbrace{\textit{We will have a picnic today}}_{P} \textit{ unless } \underbrace{\textit{it is raining at 10 A.M.}}_{Q}$$

   Let PuQ denote "P unless Q." (This is not a standard notation.) Complete as much of a truth table as possible for PuQ, and discuss any ambiguous lines.

5. Suppose four cards are given, each of which has a letter on one side and a number on the other. They are displayed as follows:

   | 1 | | C | | B | | 2 |

   Which card(s) need *not* be turned over in order to determine the truth value of the following statement: If a card has B on one side, then it has 2 on the other side. (This is a standard problem on psychological tests.)

6. Your uncle tells you, "Next Sunday if the weather is nice we will either go on a picnic or go fishing, unless my car needs repair." Represent this statement symbolically and determine those conditions under which you will declare your uncle a liar. (You may wish to refer to Exercise 4.)

7. Represent the following two statements as statement forms (they are both implications) and discuss their truth values.

   (a) I go to the movies in the afternoon if it is rainy.

   (b) I go to the movies in the afternoon only if it is rainy.

8. Represent each of the following as a statement form.

   (a) Claudia will run in the marathon if she has trained properly or is injury-free at race time.

   (b) Claudia will run in the marathon only if she is injury-free at race time.

   (c) Claudia will run in the marathon if and only if she has trained properly and is injury-free at race time.

9. (a) Exhibit a truth table that shows the truth values for the sentential form $P \Rightarrow Q$ and its converse.

   (b) Replace the variables P and Q by English sentences so that $P \Rightarrow Q$ becomes a true proposition and $P \Leftarrow Q$ a false one.

10. The notion of *statement form* (also called *well-formed formula*) can be described more carefully than in the text. Start with a collection of symbols that we agree to call **statement letters**. [Do not allow the symbols), (, ∼, $\vee$, $\wedge$, $\Rightarrow$, $\Leftrightarrow$ to be in this collection.] A statement letter is a statement form of the simplest kind; and if S_1 and S_2 are statement forms, then so are $\sim(S_1)$, $(S_1) \vee (S_2)$, $(S_1) \wedge (S_2)$, $(S_1) \Rightarrow (S_2)$, and $(S_1) \Leftrightarrow (S_2)$. Parentheses may be omitted when confusion is unlikely. [But they are sometimes essential; if S_1 is $P \Rightarrow Q$ and S_2 is $Q \Rightarrow R$, then $S_1 \Rightarrow S_2$ is written $(P \Rightarrow Q) \Rightarrow (Q \Rightarrow R)$.] Taking our usual alphabet as the collection of statement letters, determine which of the following

:ase when the given expression is *not* a

ieses so that it becomes such a form.

› Q)

Use Print Block

$\dagger$

·$(P \vee Q))$

'$(P \wedge R)) \Rightarrow (S \vee \sim P))$

f the following statement forms:

/ P))

ough seventeen in binary notation.

ile for a statement form that has seven

six rows by mistake. How many rows

s in the truth table for the form

$$(((\sim P) \vee R) \Leftrightarrow (R \Rightarrow S))$$

15. Let S be a statement form in which the sentential variables P, Q, R do not occur. Consider the new statement form

$$S \vee (P \Rightarrow ((\sim Q) \wedge R))$$

How does the number of rows in the truth table for the new form compare with the number of rows in the table for S?

16. Suppose S is a statement form with n variables $P_1, P_2, \ldots, P_n$, where $n \geq 3$. In exactly how many rows of the truth table for S is P_1 false? In how many rows is P_1 false while P_2 is true?

17. We have defined $P \Rightarrow Q$ as an abbreviation for $\sim(P \wedge \sim Q)$. Express the sentential form

$$P \Rightarrow (Q \Rightarrow (R \Rightarrow S))$$

using $\sim$ and $\wedge$ as the only logical connectives. (That is, pretend the symbol "$\Rightarrow$" has not been introduced.)

18. A **tautology** is a sentential form that becomes a true proposition whenever the letters in the expression are replaced by actual propositions. For example, the expressions $P \vee \sim P$ and $(P \vee Q) \Leftrightarrow (Q \vee P)$ are both tautologies. Use truth tables to determine which of the following are tautologies:

    (a) $P \Rightarrow ((\sim P) \Rightarrow Q)$
    (b) $(P \wedge Q) \Rightarrow (P \vee R)$
    (c) $((P \Rightarrow Q) \Leftrightarrow Q) \Rightarrow P$
    (d) $P \Rightarrow (Q \Rightarrow (Q \Rightarrow P))$

    If a given form is *not* a tautology, display a line of the truth table corresponding to one instance in which the form becomes a false proposition.

19. Are the statements $32 - 5 = 18$ and $32 + 5 = 34$ equivalent propositions? Explain briefly.

1.4 Proofs: Structures and Strategies

Truth tables can be applied systematically to determine the truth values of certain new propositions constructed from old ones. For example, if P_1 and P_2 are theorems (that is, propositions known to be true), then $\sim P_2$ is false and $(\sim P_2) \vee P_1$ is true. But mathematics extends far beyond the uninspired linking of one randomly chosen proposition to another. Mathematics also involves enlightened speculation about what *might* be true, given what is already known to be true; the creation of interesting new propositions on the basis of the calculations, hunches, and fantasies that constitute that speculation; and the proving or disproving of those propositions. In this section some techniques of mathematical proof are discussed, but nowhere will it be suggested that creating and proving interesting new theorems is an automatic consequence of certain rules of procedure. Consider the following remarks on proof technique.

(The quotation is from *The Mathematical Experience*, by P. J. Davis and R. Hersh;[*] it refers to a proof of the Pythagorean theorem in which the key to the argument is the supplementation of an initial diagram with certain "construction lines.")

> Now, how does one know where to draw these lines so as to reason with them? It would seem that these lines are accidental or fortuitous. In a sense this is true and constitutes the genius or the trick of the thing. Finding the lines is part of finding a proof, and this may be no easy matter. With experience come insight and skill at finding proper construction lines. One person may be more skillful at it than another. There is no guaranteed way to arrive at a proof. This sad truth is equally rankling to schoolchildren and to skillful professionals. Mathematics as a whole may be regarded as a systemization of just those questions which have been pursued successfully.

Once again: *There is no guaranteed way to arrive at a proof.*

What are the criteria for validity and goodness of a proof? This is not a simple issue. In an interesting mathematical system, the formal requirements of the laws of deduction are likely to be so awesome in their complexity and rigidity that it is a common practice to adopt a less formal style of discussion, consisting of a palatable mixture of mathematical expressions and ordinary sentences in our natural language. We will follow that practice here. So what we customarily call a proof is usually only an outline of the genuine article, and we must be on guard for irrational leaps that cannot be justified by the available body of axioms, theorems, and logical rules. The alternative to the informal approach is strict adherence to the formal laws, and this can involve intuition-free arguments of colossal length and complexity; any resulting gains in accuracy can easily be offset by losses in insight. For instance, consider this story from mathematician John Kemeny (excerpted from his article "Rigor versus intuition in mathematics"):[†]

> There was an advanced seminar . . . in which the lecturer devoted the entire hour to writing out a proof with complete rigor. After having filled all the blackboards, he had everyone in the room completely lost, including one of his own colleagues, who jumped up and said, "Look, I just don't understand this proof at all. I tried to follow you, but I got lost somewhere. I just didn't get it at all." The lecturer stopped for a moment, looked at him, and said, "Oh, didn't you see it? You see, it's just that the two spaces connect like this," intertwining his two arms in a picturesque fashion. And then his colleague exclaimed, "Oh, now I get the whole proof."

[*]Boston: Houghton Mifflin, 1981.
[†]In Douglas Campbell and John C. Higgens (eds.), *Mathematics: People. Problems. Results.* (Belmont, Calif.: Wadsworth, 1984).

The notion of proof is discussed with charm and eloquence by Yu. I. Manin in his book, *A Course in Mathematical Logic,*[*] and here is an excerpt:

> A proof only becomes a proof after the social act of "accepting it as a proof." This is as true for mathematics as it is for physics, linguistics, or biology. The evolution of commonly accepted criteria for an argument's being a proof is an almost untouched theme in the history of science. In any case, the ideal for what constitutes a mathematical demonstration of a "nonobvious truth" has remained unchanged since the time of Euclid: we must arrive a such a truth from "obvious" hypotheses, or assertions which have already been proved, by means of a series of explicitly described, "obviously valid" elementary deductions.

Manin points out that the "ideal" mentioned in the preceding paragraph is rarely achieved:

> The absence of errors in a mathematical paper (assuming that none are discovered), as in other natural sciences, is often established indirectly: how well the results correspond to what was generally expected, the use of similar arguments in other papers, examination of small sections of the proof "under the microscope," even the reputation of the author.

The history of mathematics includes many instances in which propositions that were widely believed (sometimes for years) to have been proved were later found to be false. We now ask: can we relay on *computers* to lead us safely through the Valley of the Shadow of Falsehood and thereby let us know with certainty what is true and what is not? In considering the role of computers in mathematical proofs, Manin supplies this quotation from a research article by H. P. F. Swinnerton-Dyer:

> When a theorem has been proved with the help of a computer, it is impossible to give an exposition of the proof which meets the traditional test—that a sufficiently patient reader should be able to work through the proof and verify that it is correct. Even if one were to print all the programs and all the sets of data used (which in this case would occupy some forty very dull pages) there can be no assurance that a data tape has not been mispunched or misread. Moreover, every modern computer has obscure faults in its software and hardware—which so seldom cause errors that they go undetected for years—and every computer is liable to transient faults. Such errors are rare, but a few of them have probably occurred in the course of the calculations reported here.

After further discussion, Manin concludes with this moral:

> A good proof is one that makes us wiser.

End of philosophy.

Now, suppose we have at hand a proposition Q that we want to prove. We ask ourselves: Does it seem *likely* to be true? Why? If we suspect that Q is true, we are probably aware (perhaps subconsciously) of a theorem P whose truth seems to be incompatible with the falsity of Q. By explicitly recalling P and establishing that incompatibility, we will have proved Q (this will be shown). After some reflection, if no such P presents itself, we can consider as *candidates* for P some known truths intuitively related to the subject matter of Q. Perhaps one of these or a combination of several will, when subjected to suitable logical maneuvers, lead to a proof of Q.

Let's take a closer look at the logic. We claim that to prove a proposition Q it suffices to isolate a true proposition P such that the implication $P \Rightarrow Q$ is also true. To see this, consider the first three columns of Table 1.19.

(1.19)

P	Q	$P \Rightarrow Q$	$\sim P$	$\sim Q$	$\sim Q \Rightarrow \sim P$	$Q \Rightarrow P$
F	F	T	T	T	T	T
F	T	T	T	F	T	F
T	F	F	F	T	F	T
T	T	T	F	F	T	T

Notice that only on the bottom line are both P and $P \Rightarrow Q$ true, and in this situation Q is also true. Therefore, to prove Q it is enough to prove $P \wedge (P \Rightarrow Q)$, as claimed. In words: if P is true and if it is also true that P implies Q, then Q is true. This fundamental logical principle is called the **rule of *modus ponens*** or the **law of detachment**, and it dates back at least to Aristotle (384–322 B.C.). An argument of the pattern described here is called a **direct proof** of Q.

1.20 EXAMPLE. Let $\triangle$ denote a triangle with one vertex at the center of a circle C and the other two vertices on C itself. Consider the following proposition Q: Triangle $\triangle$ has two equal angles. Let's quickly sketch a proof and then analyze its logical structure. Let O denote the vertex at the center of C, and let A and B be the other two vertices.

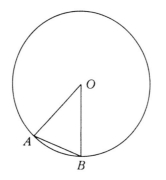

Lines *OA* and *OB* have the same length, since they are both radii of *C*. Therefore △ is isosceles. However, base angles of an isosceles triangle are equal, hence △ has two equal angles, and we're done.

The heart of the argument is that base angles of an isosceles triangle are equal, which we can rewrite as an implication:

$$\underbrace{\triangle \text{ is an isosceles triangle}}_{P} \quad \Rightarrow \quad \underbrace{\triangle \text{ has two equal angles}}_{Q}$$

The proof assumes that the truth of $P \Rightarrow Q$ is known; then we use the definition of *circle* to deduce the truth of P for our triangle △, and finally *modus ponens* yields the truth of Q.

In "real life" the thinking leading to the preceding proof might go like this: "Let's see, what do I have to do to show that a triangle has two equal sides? Hmmm…showing it's *isosceles* would do the job. Hey, but two of this triangle's sides are radii of the same circle, so they *automatically* have the same length. I'm done!" We need to distinguish the *process* of coming up with a proof from the proof itself. The *process* can involve hunches, speculation, memory, intuition, cleverness, surprises, luck, and assorted psychological and intellectual skills. The final written proof is unlikely to exhibit these elements of mental drama, although the skilled reader may still detect crucial points where the argument takes a startling turn in a new direction. The discoverer of a proof is under no moral or scientific obligation to display to the reader the false starts, aimless meanderings, fruitless speculations, and outright blunders experienced while searching for a proof. It's the final argument that matters. An unfortunate consequence of all this is that the reader studying a proof may think, "This complicated argument flows along so smoothly and so cleverly. I could never do something like this." But actually the theorem prover, like the theorem reader, is (or was) a human being, probably with the standard number of anxieties and complexes. It's just that the argument has been organized, cleaned up, and manicured before going to the printer.

1.21 EXAMPLE.   Take the facts of elementary arithmetic as our body of "known truths," and consider a proof of this proposition: The square of an odd integer has the form $8k + 1$ for some integer k.

PROOF *(Rambling Style).*   Consider an odd integer n. Our task involves the close scrutiny of n^2 without knowing anything about n except for its oddness. However, "odd" means "not divisible by 2"; so when we attempt to divide n by 2, we get a quotient q and a remainder 1. That is, $n = 2q + 1$. Notice a consequence of what we have done so far: every integer has the property that either it or its successor (the next largest integer) is even. (*Why* is this a consequence?) We now have

$$n^2 = (2q + 1)^2 = 4q^2 + 4q + 1 = 4q(q + 1) + 1$$

Either q or $q + 1$ is even, as we noted a moment ago, so $q(q + 1)$ is even and $4q(q + 1)$ is therefore divisible by 8, say $4q(q + 1) = 8k$. Thus $n^2 = 8k + 1$, as desired. □

Let's be frank. In practice, printed proofs are almost never as expansive as this one. First, space is generally limited; second, there is much to be said for the reader's pushing through the details independently; and, last, a mountain of details can bury the central ideas beyond excavation. A textbook version of the above proof is more likely to read as follows:

PROOF (*Compact Style*).   An odd integer can be written $n = 2q + 1$ for some integer q. Thus $n^2 = 4q(q + 1) + 1$, and putting $q(q + 1) = 2k$ gives $n^2 = 8k + 1$, as desired. □

The underlying logic is the same in both proofs. Elementary arithmetic provides the axiomatic foundation. The proof opens when we choose the symbol n for "an odd integer." The key to the proof lies in using arithmetic to translate the statement "n is odd" (taken as true) into its equational formula, $n = 2q + 1$, then proving the implication

$$\underbrace{(n = 2q + 1)}_{P} \implies \underbrace{(n^2 = 8k + 1)}_{Q}$$

by showing that truth of P must inevitably be accompanied by truth of Q. Finally we apply *modus ponens* (without saying so explicitly) to conclude that Q is true.

It would be comforting to know that any proposition that can be stated can be proved or disproved (a *disproof* of P is a proof of $\sim P$), but in the 1930s the logician Kurt Gödel showed that certain kinds of mathematical systems in which we can do ordinary arithmetic must inevitably contain propositions that can be neither proved nor disproved. Determining exactly which propositions fall into this murky category is a subject of continuing mystery.

There are some general psychological guidelines that can be useful in the search for proofs. Imagine that you are standing at the foot of a mountain and you want to reach the top. Perhaps you will be lucky and see a path in front of you that seems to be headed in the right direction; so you take the path and you reach the top. Great. But you may see no immediate path, or you may see several and have to choose one. What then? By looking through binoculars you may see that the top is accessible only from a few directions, and this may help you eliminate certain paths at the start, or it may encourage you to look for a path in a location you haven't yet fully checked. You may succeed by being continually aware of your location, of the directions in which you can travel from your location, and of the places near the mountaintop from which the top is accessible. If you are prepared to move forward along many different paths from the starting point, and if you can imagine backing down from the top in many different ways, you may discover a route from the bottom to the top. Of course, once you know the way you can draw a map, and then the next person can follow your path directly.

Now suppose you want to prove proposition Q, and you think you know all that is needed for the job; say you know that a proposition P is true. Think: If I know P, what *else* do I know as a consequence? (This corresponds to looking for a path to start up the mountain.) Also, what does it mean to say that Q is true? Are there one or more statements, perhaps simpler than Q, and perhaps separately provable, from which Q will follow readily? (This is like looking for locations near the mountaintop from which the top is accessible.)

In mathematical proofs, definitions are often crucial. A **definition** is a statement introducing a new symbol or word that abbreviates a package of statements or expressions (or both) whose meanings or uses are already understood. Asserting that an object "satisfies" a definition asserts that the statements in the package are true for that object. For instance, saying that an object T "satisfies the definition of trapezoid" says that T is a closed polygon, that it has four sides, and that two of its sides are parallel. In the proofs we have already discussed, the definitions of "odd integer" and "isosceles triangle" play a central role. If a proposition P claims that an object has a certain property then, in the absence of inspiration, try playing with one or more of the properties that characterize the object under consideration; also toy with the definitions of the terms in the desired conclusion.

Strive for flexibility: if an argument leads you in the wrong direction, and if you have been careful with the details, abandon your dedication to it and try another approach. (If a path toward the mountain dead-ends at a swamp, will you take it again and again?) An interesting proposition might not have a proof that comes easily, but if you get it you will rejoice. As you struggle with a proof, these two questions should dominate the proceedings at all times: *What do I know? What do I want to show?*

We will now consider a proof technique called **indirect proof** (also called **proof by contradiction**, or *reductio ad absurdum*). The technique involves proving a proposition Q by showing that the negation $\sim Q$ implies a statement that we know to be false (that is, $\sim Q$ leads to a contradiction of a known truth). Thus $\sim Q$ must itself be false, and therefore Q is true. The logician W. Quine described the method this way: "It consists in assuming the contradictory of what is to be proved and then looking for trouble." As we did with direct proofs, we can justify this procedure by means of Table 1.19. Only on the bottom line of the table are $\sim P$ false and $\sim Q \Rightarrow \sim P$ true; and also on this line Q is true, which is what we want to show.

1.22 EXAMPLE. Let's give an indirect proof of proposition Q in Example 1.20 using the notation introduced in our first proof. If $\triangle$ does *not* have two equal angles, then $\triangle$ cannot be isosceles (by what we know about isosceles triangles); thus OA and OB must have different lengths. This contradicts the fact that all radii of the same circle have equal length, and the argument is finished. Symbolically, let P be the true proposition, "All radii of a given circle have equal length." We have just verified the statement $\sim Q \Rightarrow \sim P$, so by our earlier discussion Q is true.

The basic strategy in proofs by contradiction is to ask this question: What would go wrong if the proposition I am trying to prove were actually *false*?

You may ask: For a given proposition Q, what is better, a direct proof or an indirect proof? The answer varies with the proposition, but in specific cases the information provided by the two kinds of proofs can differ substantially. For example, suppose Q asserts the existence of a number with a certain property. A direct proof of Q may actually produce the number or lead to its discovery, but an indirect proof will merely rule out the possibility that there is *no* such number and leave untouched the problem of actually finding it. Why would anyone *ever* choose to construct an indirect proof? Because we do what we can do. The facts at hand may lack the clout required for a direct proof of a proposition Q, whereas adding $\sim Q$ to our arsenal of assumptions *may* lead to the negation of a known theorem. In this event we know that $\sim Q$ must be false, hence Q is true.

A special form of indirect proof for a proposition Q consists of proving an implication $P \Rightarrow Q$, in which P is known to be true, by proving the implication $\sim Q \Rightarrow \sim P$ instead. As in the general case for indirect proofs, we assume $\sim Q$ and seek a false consequence; however, here we specifically work to deduce $\sim P$ as that false consequence. The sentential form $\sim Q \Rightarrow \sim P$ is called the **contrapositive** of the form $P \Rightarrow Q$.

1.23 EXAMPLE.   Let n denote an integer. Prove the implication

$$\text{If } \underbrace{n^2 \text{ is even}}_{P} \text{ then } \underbrace{n \text{ is even}}_{Q}.$$

SOLUTION.   We prove the contrapositive, assuming the facts of elementary arithmetic. Suppose n is odd (this is $\sim Q$), say $n = 2k + 1$. (Glance back at the proof of Example 1.21 for justification.) Then

$$n^2 = (2k + 1)^2 = 4k^2 + 4k + 1 = \underbrace{4(k^2 + k)}_{\text{even}} + 1$$

This number is odd, so we have proved $\sim Q \Rightarrow \sim P$, and we are through.

The reader is advised to construct a truth table displaying the truth values of both $P \Rightarrow Q$ and $\sim Q \Rightarrow \sim P$. Having done that, observe that in every row of the table the truth values of $P \Rightarrow Q$ and $\sim Q \Rightarrow \sim P$ are the same. For this reason, the forms $P \Rightarrow Q$ and $\sim Q \Rightarrow \sim P$ are said to be *logically equivalent*. We'll return to this idea in the next section.

Exercises

1. Suppose the following propositions are known to be true:

> If Dracula seizes power then democracy is lost.
> If democracy is lost then the use of food additives increases.
> If the use of food additives increases, then mutations can be expected.
> Dracula seizes power.

Represent each proposition by a sentential form, then show that repeated application of *modus ponens* proves the truth of "mutations can be expected."

2. Use ordinary English to write sentences representing the (i) converse, (ii) contrapositive, and (iii) negation of the following sentence: *If all cats meow then some dogs bark.* Do not use the phrases "it is not the case" or "it is false" or "it is not true" in what you write.

3. For each of the following propositions, answer the question, "What must I prove?" To do this, use the definition of each mathematical term to rephrase the given proposition. In each case assume that a planar geometrical configuration G has been presented to you. (That is, G is a collection of points or lines or both in a given plane.)

   (a) G is a rectangle.

   (b) G is a circle.

   (c) G is a parabola.

4. Prove that the sum of two odd numbers or two even numbers is even, and that the sum of an odd number and an even number is odd. (You are really being asked to prove three propositions here.)

5. Prove that 5 is a prime number.

6. In Section 1.4 the process of proving a theorem is compared to the process of climbing to the top of a mountain. Compare the notions of direct and indirect proof from this "mountain-theoretic" point of view.

7. A diamond is inscribed in a rectangle that is inscribed in a circle, as pictured here:

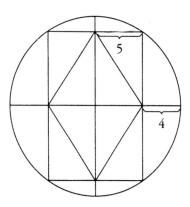

Determine the length of a side of the diamond, and then write a proof of your claim. (In the figure, the point that looks like the center *is* the center; and you may assume that lines that look perpendicular *are* perpendicular.)

1.5 Logical Equivalence

Imagine someone with the bizarre habit of stating all his atomic sentences twice, with "and" wedged in between. Thus his days are filled with the likes of "the toast is hot and the toast is hot," "$2+3 = 5$ and $2+3 = 5$," and so on. In response to this, your instinct tells you that if P is a proposition, the statement symbolized by $P \wedge P$ carries the same information as P alone; in particular, P and $P \wedge P$ have the same truth value. You may even develop the urge to say that P and $P \wedge P$ are "logically equivalent." Giving a precise definition of this concept is our goal here. In the next section we will see a useful application to electronic circuit design.

1.24 Definition. A statement form is said to be a **tautology** if every substitution of propositions for its sentential variables yields a true proposition.

The truth value of a proposition depends only on the *truth values* of its atomic components, not on the *meaning* of those components. So to check whether or not a given statement form is a tautology, we inspect the form's truth table: the column under the form itself must be an unbroken column of T's.

1.25 EXAMPLE. Each of the following statement forms is a tautology:

$$P \Leftrightarrow \sim(\sim P) \qquad (P \wedge Q) \Rightarrow P \qquad \sim(P \wedge \sim P) \qquad ((P \Rightarrow Q) \wedge P) \Rightarrow Q$$

When we replace the variables in tautologies by propositions, the new propositions thus obtained are true as a consequence of their form, not because of their specific content. For example, here are some incarnations of the tautologies in Example 1.25:

Jones likes waffles if and only if it is not the case that Jones dislikes waffles.
If Smith is dead and Doe likes melon, then Smith is dead.
It is not the case that today is Tuesday and not Tuesday.
If Washington is President implies Disney is Vice President, and Washington *is* President, then Disney is Vice President.

None of these statements creates major excitement, because in each case the truth values of the components have no bearing on the truth value of the complete statement.

Now (before reading the next definition) would be a good time to reread the last paragraph of Section 1.4.

1.26 Definition. Suppose S_1 and S_2 are sentential forms. We say that S_1 and S_2 are **logically equivalent** if the sentential form $S_1 \Leftrightarrow S_2$ is a tautology; the form $S_1 \Leftrightarrow S_2$ is then called a **logical equivalence**. Thus a logical equivalence is a sentential form that becomes a true material equivalence whenever its variables are replaced by specific propositions.

1.27 EXAMPLE. Let S_1 be the sentential form $\sim(P \wedge Q)$, and let S_2 denote the form $\sim P \vee \sim Q$. We claim that S_1 and S_2 are logically equivalent. To see this, consider the truth table for $S_1 \Leftrightarrow S_2$:

P	Q	$\sim P$	$\sim Q$	$P \wedge Q$	S_1	S_2	$S_1 \Leftrightarrow S_2$
F	F	T	T	F	T	T	T
F	T	T	F	F	T	T	T
T	F	F	T	F	T	T	T
T	T	F	F	T	F	F	T

The T's in the right-hand column show that $S_1 \Leftrightarrow S_2$ is a tautology, and this proves the claim. A similar argument will show that $\sim(P \vee Q)$ is logically equivalent to $\sim P \wedge \sim Q$. The two logical equivalences in this example are called **De Morgan's laws**.

Example 1.27 illustrates the standard test for logical equivalence of two forms S_1 and S_2: construct a truth table for the form $S_1 \Leftrightarrow S_2$ and ask, "Are the truth values of $S_1 \Leftrightarrow S_2$ all T's?"

For two statement forms S_1 and S_2, the assertion "S_1 is logically equivalent to S_2" is sometimes abbreviated

$$S_1 \equiv S_2$$

For instance, in this notation De Morgan's laws look like this:

(1.28)
$$\sim(P \wedge Q) \equiv \sim P \vee \sim Q$$
$$\sim(P \vee Q) \equiv \sim P \wedge \sim Q$$

In elementary arithmetic we are accustomed to replacing part of an algebraic expression by something equal to it, thereby getting a new expression equal to the original. Thus the equality $3 + 10 = 13$ enables us to write $5 - \sqrt{3 + 10} = 5 - \sqrt{13}$. A similar principle holds in our present context:

Replacement Principle. If $S_1 \equiv S_2$ and if in some sentential form S an occurrence of S_1 is replaced by S_2, the resulting sentential form is logically equivalent to S.

1.29 EXAMPLE. The statement form $A \Leftrightarrow A \wedge (A \vee B)$ is a tautology (check this!); hence the logical equivalence $A \equiv A \wedge (A \vee B)$ holds. The replacement principle then says that replacement of $A \wedge (A \vee B)$ by A in any sentential form yields a logically equivalent form. For instance,

$$\sim\big((A \wedge (A \vee B)) \Rightarrow C\big) \equiv \sim(A \Rightarrow C)$$

A formal proof of the replacement principle will not be given here, but the principle is clearly reasonable. For suppose S' is the sentential form resulting from the substitution of S_2 for S_1 in S, where $S_1 \equiv S_2$. Then, in the truth table for S', the column of truth values under S_2 is identical to the column under S_1 in the table for S. Thus, linking S_2 with the other components to get S' produces the same pattern of truth values that linking S_1 with those components produces in the construction of S.

Here is a list of some of the most basic logical equivalences, with their names. (Also see 1.28.) In each case it is left for you to verify the result with a truth table.

$$(1.30) \qquad \left.\begin{array}{l} P \wedge (Q \wedge R) \equiv (P \wedge Q) \wedge R \\ P \vee (Q \vee R) \equiv (P \vee Q) \vee R \end{array}\right\} \qquad \textbf{associative laws}$$

$$(1.31) \qquad \left.\begin{array}{l} P \Leftrightarrow Q \equiv Q \Leftrightarrow P \\ P \wedge Q \equiv Q \wedge P \\ P \vee Q \equiv Q \vee P \end{array}\right\} \qquad \textbf{commutative laws}$$

$$(1.32) \qquad \left.\begin{array}{l} P \wedge P \equiv P \\ P \vee P \equiv P \end{array}\right\} \qquad \textbf{idempotency laws}$$

$$(1.33) \qquad \left.\begin{array}{l} P \wedge (P \vee Q) \equiv P \\ P \vee (P \wedge Q) \equiv P \end{array}\right\} \qquad \textbf{absorption laws}$$

$$(1.34) \qquad \left.\begin{array}{l} P \wedge (Q \vee R) \equiv (P \wedge Q) \vee (P \wedge R) \\ P \vee (Q \wedge R) \equiv (P \vee Q) \wedge (P \vee R) \end{array}\right\} \qquad \textbf{distributive laws}$$

$$(1.35) \qquad \sim(\sim P) \equiv P \qquad \textbf{law of double negation}$$

Our interest in a sentential form centers on its truth-functional behavior. That is, we view the truth values of inserted propositions as "inputs"; and then the outputs are the truth values of the resulting propositions after the insertions. The form's "behavior" is determined by the pattern of inputs and outputs. (So the leftmost columns of the truth table, in which truth values are assigned to the variables, and the rightmost column, in which the truth values of the entire form appear, are the "behavioral" columns.) Logically equivalent forms have the same behavior in this sense. Notice that in each of laws 1.32 through 1.35 and in De Morgan's laws (1.28), one of the two equivalent forms is shorter than the other. Our natural desire for notational economy will usually lead us to choose the shorter of two equivalent forms for our work, just as in numerical calculations we prefer to use the numeral 1 in place of $(\cos \pi)^3/(\sin \frac{3}{2}\pi)^{77}$. There are payoffs. Shortening the sentential forms that represent statements in a mathematical proof (or a computer program) may provide simplifications that lead to greater understanding (or greater efficiency) and therefore perhaps to further developments. Sentential forms can be used as symbolic representations of certain kinds of electronic circuits (we will have a brief look at this in the next section), and simpler forms can lead to simpler and less expensive circuits.

Exercises

1. Do Exercise 18 (if you have not already done so) in Section 1.4.

2. A statement form S is said to be a **contradiction** if every substitution of propositions for its sentential variables yields a false proposition. Rewrite this definition using the term "tautology."

3. (a) Write a sentential form logically equivalent to

$$P \Rightarrow (Q \Rightarrow R)$$

   in which the symbol "$\Rightarrow$" does not occur.

   (b) Write a sentential form logically equivalent to $P \vee Q$ in which the only logical connectives are $\sim$ and $\wedge$.

   (c) Deduce that the work of the connectives $\wedge, \vee, \sim, \Rightarrow$ can be done by $\wedge$ and $\sim$ alone. (We say, therefore, that $\wedge$ and $\sim$ together constitute an **adequate set of connectives**).

4. The purpose of this exercise is to improve upon Exercise 3(c) by introducing a *single* logical connective that can serve by itself as an adequate set of connectives. We write

$$P \uparrow Q$$

as an abbreviation for $\sim(P \wedge Q)$; this new connective $\uparrow$ is called the **Sheffer stroke**. Use truth tables to verify the following logical equivalences.

(a) $\sim P \equiv P \uparrow P$

(b) $P \vee Q \equiv (P \uparrow P) \uparrow (Q \uparrow Q)$

(c) $P \wedge Q \equiv (P \uparrow Q) \uparrow (P \uparrow Q)$

(d) $(P \Rightarrow Q) \equiv$ _____

(Fill the blank with a form having only $\uparrow$ as a connective, and verify.)

5. (Companion to Exercise 4) We write $P \downarrow Q$ as an abbreviation for $\sim(P \vee Q)$. The symbol $\downarrow$ is the **dagger**. Represent each of the sentential forms $\sim P$, $P \vee Q$, $P \wedge Q$, $P \Rightarrow Q$ by forms using $\downarrow$ as the only connective, and verify your results.

6. Let S_1 and S_2 be sentential forms. Briefly discuss the distinctions between the expressions $S_1 \Leftrightarrow S_2$ and $S_1 \equiv S_2$.

7. Show that the sentential form

$$\big((P \wedge Q) \vee (P \wedge \sim Q)\big) \wedge (R \vee \sim R)$$

is logically equivalent to a form consisting of just a single sentential variable.

8. Let S_1 and S_2 be sentential forms. The statement "S_1 **logically implies** S_2," written $S_1 \models S_2$, is defined to mean that the sentential form $S_1 \Rightarrow S_2$ is a tautology. (*Example:* $P \wedge Q \models P$. *Proof:* The truth table

P	Q	$P \wedge Q$	$(P \wedge Q) \Rightarrow P$
F	F	F	T
F	T	F	T
T	F	F	T
T	T	T	T

shows that $(P \wedge Q) \Rightarrow P$ is a tautology.) The terminology "logically implies" is modelled on common usage. A randomly chosen educated individual who has never studied logic will readily agree that "I like jam and Benjamin is charming" is a statement that "logically implies" that Benjamin is charming, even with no personal knowledge of Benjamin.

(a) How does logical implication relate to material implication? (See page 13.)

(b) How does logical implication relate to logical equivalence? (See page 29.)

1.6 Application: A Brief Introduction to Switching Circuits

Sentential forms are commonly used as mathematical representations of electronic switching circuits. Picture a collection of wires connected to independent electrical power sources; visualize these as lines coming in from the left side of a diagram. At any given moment some of these may be "alive" or "on," which means that they are supplying power to the system (that is, the voltage in those wires is positive), while others are dormant ("off"). These wires, and others not directly connected to the power sources, are linked together by an assortment of switching devices called *gates*, each of which has one or two wires entering it from the left side and one wire exiting it from the right. Ultimately only one wire exits the diagram on the right.

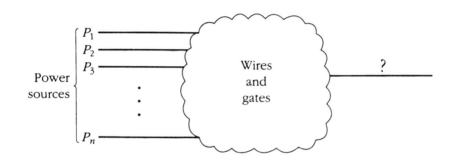

We will consider two basic problems:

(1) to determine, for a given pattern of power input from the given sources (typically some are "on" and some are "off") on the left side of the diagram, whether power will be flowing out of the diagram through the wire exiting the diagram on the right side.

(2) to try to design another network whose behavior perfectly mimics that of the original network, but which involves fewer gates. Such a network is likely to be cheaper and more compact than the original one; these are two major considerations in any design project.

The idea of this section (the clarifying details will come after this paragraph) is to represent a circuit (of the kind just described) by a sentential form, with each power source represented by a sentential variable and each gate represented by a suitable logical connective. Replacing a variable by a true proposition corresponds to that power source's being "on," and replacement by a false proposition corresponds to power "off." If we do it correctly, the truth values of the propositions resulting from such replacements will tell us when power will flow through the circuit (again, "true" corresponds to current flow and "false" corresponds to no flow); this will settle problem (1). And if we can replace our propositional form with a logically equivalent form with fewer connectives, then we will have solved problem (2).

Three of the most basic gates are pictured as follows:

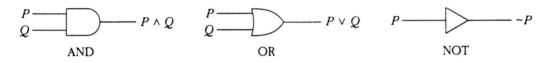

$P \wedge Q$ $P \vee Q$ $\sim P$

AND   OR   NOT

In each case, current (if any) is understood to flow through the gate from left to right. The AND gate is designed so that if the wires labelled P and Q are simultaneously "on," then the wire labelled $P \wedge Q$ is also "on"; otherwise $P \wedge Q$ is "off." This pattern can be read directly from the truth table for $P \wedge Q$ by reading "on" and "off" in place of T and F, respectively. Similarly, the actions for the OR and NOT gates can be read from the truth tables for $P \vee Q$ and $\sim P$, respectively.

1.36 EXAMPLE. A room light is to be connected to switches in two locations, and a flick of either switch should change the state of the light (turns it off when on, and vice versa). Design a circuit for this purpose, using gates of the kind that have been described here.

SOLUTION. Let P and Q denote wires leading from the two wall switches. Then, according to the circuit design specifications, a sentential form S with the following truth table will represent a satisfactory circuit:

P	Q	S
F	F	F
F	T	T
T	F	T
T	T	F

Thus S is true when either $\sim P \wedge Q$ is true (this is from line 2 of the truth table) or when $P \wedge \sim Q$ is true (from line 3); otherwise S is false. Thus S has the same truth-value assignments as $(\sim P \wedge Q) \vee (P \wedge \sim Q)$. That is,

$$S \equiv (\sim P \wedge Q) \vee (P \wedge \sim Q)$$

This solution to the problem has the following design:

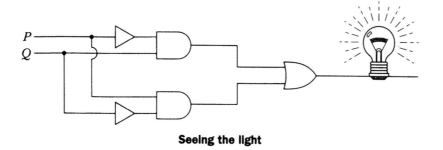

Seeing the light

We note that if an EXCLUSIVE OR gate

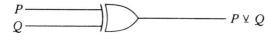

is available, it will achieve the same goal, because the forms $P \veebar Q$ and $(\sim P \wedge Q) \vee (P \wedge \sim Q)$ are logically equivalent.

1.37 EXAMPLE. A zoo has two special cages, each with its own power source, for endangered species. An alarm will be installed in the zoo office that will clang if either (or both) of the special cages is opened, assuming that the cage's power source and the alarm's power source are on. Give a diagram of an appropriate circuit.

SOLUTION. Let A, C_1, and C_2 denote the power supplies for the alarm and the two cages, respectively. We could proceed with a truth table, as in the previous example, but instead let's think it through informally.

For the alarm to sound, either A and C_1 must both be activated or A and C_2 must both be activated. Thus $(A \wedge C_1) \vee (A \wedge C_2)$ represents a solution, and this corresponds to the following circuit diagram.

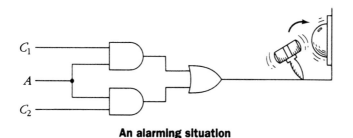

An alarming situation

Now notice the logical equivalence

$$(A \wedge C_1) \vee (A \wedge C_2) \equiv A \wedge (C_1 \vee C_2)$$

[This is one of the distributive laws; see (1.34).] That is, the alarm will sound if it is on and either C_1 or C_2 is activated. The shorter sentential form $A \wedge (C_1 \vee C_2)$ yields a simpler circuit:

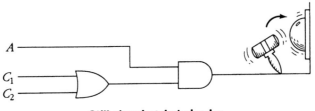

Still alarming, but simpler

The new circuit is said to be **equivalent** to the original.

If we were to proceed by studying a truth table, as we did in Example 1.36, we would arrive at the grotesque sentential form

$$((A \wedge (C_1 \wedge C_2)) \vee (A \wedge (C_1 \wedge \sim C_2))) \vee (A \wedge (\sim C_1 \wedge C_2))$$

whose corresponding circuit is a labyrinthine atrocity. (Draw it if you feel the compulsion.)

As Example 1.37 illustrates, the theory of switching circuits leads naturally to the *minimization problem* for sentential forms: given a sentential form S, determine the simplest sentential form among all those logically equivalent to S. The issue is of major importance in the design of complex electronic systems. We will not pursue this topic here. (An important first step would be to give a precise definition of "simple," and this may vary with the situation. For instance, in the design of the extraordinarily complex circuitry for a computer, reducing the amount of interchip communication can outweigh the benefits of reducing the total number of gates in the circuit.) Instead we refer the interested reader to the book *Boolean Algebra and Switching Circuits*, by Elliott Mendelson (New York: McGraw-Hill, 1970) for further discussion; in particular, see the extensive list of references given there. Also see *Introduction to Switching Theory & Logical Design*, by Frederick Hill and Gerald Peterson (New York: Wiley, 1981).

Exercises

1. A room light is to be connected to three wall switches, each of which has a "down" position and an "up" position. In each case, design a circuit satisfying the stated specifications.

   (a) The light will be on if *at least* one switch is up; otherwise it will be off.

   (b) The light will be on if *exactly* one switch is up; otherwise it will be off.

   (c) If all switches are down the light is off; and flicking any switch at any time changes the state of the light.

2. Replace the following circuit with an equivalent circuit having only four gates. (Use only the NOT, AND, and OR gates.)

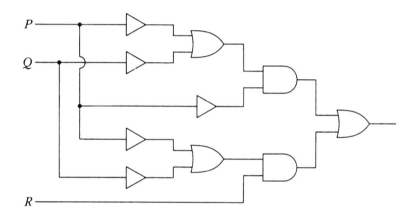

SETS

He had . . . twelve marbles, part of a jew's-harp, a piece of blue bottle glass to look through, a spool cannon, a key that wouldn't unlock anything, a fragment of chalk, a glass stopper of a decanter, a tin soldier, a couple of tadpoles, six firecrackers, a kitten with only one eye, a brass doorknob, a dog collar—but no dog—the handle of a knife, four pieces of orange peel, and a dilapidated old window sash.

MARK TWAIN
The Adventures of Tom Sawyer

"Gentlemen," returned Mr. Micawber, "do with me as you will! I am a straw upon the surface of the deep, and am tossed in all directions by the elephants—I beg your pardon; I should have said the elements."

CHARLES DICKENS
David Copperfield

2.1 Fundamentals

We learn the meaning of a word either by seeing it defined in terms of words already known to us or by experiencing examples of its use and sensing the common properties of the examples. For instance, consider these statements: "Snerd is a member of the country club," "This saucer belongs to my dinnerware set," "*Fromage* is one of the French nouns,"

"Points A and B are on the perpendicular bisector of angle α," "The assault on the western flank was a key element of Varnish's battle plan." In each of these assertions something is said to be a member or element of some collection or set of things. As the examples suggest, sets are of wildly different sorts and, accordingly, "membership" can have a variety of meanings. (Dictionaries provide no substantial help: a standard dictionary defines a set as a "collection of objects," a collection as an "aggregate," and an aggregate as a "collection"; and a member is "one of the elements of which an aggregate is composed." Check *your* dictionary.) But mathematics has to start somewhere, so we agree to accept the words **set** and **member** as undefined (or *primitive*) terms, though we take comfort from the meaningful interpretations we give the terms in our daily lives. For linguistic variety we sometimes use the words **family** and **collection** as synonyms for set, we use the word **element** for a member of a set, and we say that an element **belongs** to any set of which it is a member.

Our goals in this chapter are to learn to describe and manipulate sets and to develop techniques for the construction of new sets from given ones: we'll glue sets together, examine their overlap, take products and differences of them, and chop them up. Justification for our constructions is contained in the axioms of set theory, which we will usually not state formally; we prefer instead a more casual approach to the subject.

Set theory is at the foundation of mathematics, and nearly every mathematical object of interest is a set of some kind. Even the real numbers that we all grew up with (like 1, π, $-\frac{2}{3}$, and $\sqrt{5}$) have definitions as sets, but we will not go into the details here, and we will assume a familiarity with the basic arithmetic of real numbers.

If x is an element (that is, x is a member of *some* set) and A is a set, the expression $x \in A$ denotes the statement "x is a member of A," which is either true or false. (In the language of Chapter 1, the statement "$x \in A$" is a *proposition*.) The symbol $\in$ is called the **membership symbol**. The negation of $x \in A$ is usually written $x \notin A$ instead of $\sim(x \in A)$. Another common abbreviation: the statement "$a \in S$ and $b \in S$" is shortened to "$a, b \in S$," and similarly for longer expressions (such as "$x, y, z \in S$"). To minimize confusion in writing about sets and their elements, it is useful to use uppercase letters for sets and lowercase letters for their elements ($x \in X$ instead of $X \in x$). However, we cannot be consistent about this, since, as we will see, sets are themselves members of sets, and larger type is not always a possibility.

$$x \in X \quad \text{and} \quad X \in X \quad \text{and} \quad X \in X \quad \text{and} \ldots$$

An element of an element of an element of an element of . . .

2.1 Definition. Sets A and B are said to be **equal**, written $A = B$, if they have the same members, that is, if every member of A is a member of B and vice versa. More formally, the statement $A = B$ means that for every element x the following equivalence holds:

$$x \in A \Leftrightarrow x \in B$$

If A and B are not equal we write $A \neq B$.

2.2 EXAMPLE. Let A be the set of nonnegative real numbers, and let B be the set of all real numbers that are squares of real numbers. Then by Definition 2.1 we have $A = B$, even though the descriptions of A and B are quite different. The first describes the location of the set's elements on the real line, the second has to do with solvability of equations. Thus the first description is essentially geometric, while the second is algebraic.

Since a set is completely determined by its members, if we wish to define a set (that is, to specify it completely) it suffices to indicate what its members are, and there are several standard ways to do this. If a set is small we may be able to list its elements between braces: $\{1, \sqrt{2}\}$ has as its elements the numbers 1 and $\sqrt{2}$. When we use this notational device, it is understood that the order in which we list the terms is irrelevant, and also that symbol repetition has no effect on the set being described. Thus

$$\{1, \sqrt{2}\} = \{\sqrt{2}, 1, \sqrt{2}, 1, 1\} = \{\sqrt{2}, 1, \sqrt{2}\} = \{\sqrt{2}, 1\}$$

Sometimes it is more convenient to *suggest* a listing of the elements: the expression

$$\{0, 1, 2, \ldots, 1000\}$$

denotes the set whose members are the nonnegative integers from 0 through 1000. It is important that we be on guard for ambiguities: does the expression

$$\{3, 5, 7, \ldots, 23\}$$

denote the set of eleven odd numbers from 3 through 23,

$$\{3, 5, 7, 9, 11, 13, 15, 17, 19, 21, 23\}$$

does it represent the set consisting of the first eight odd prime numbers,

$$\{3, 5, 7, 11, 13, 17, 19, 23\}$$

or does it represent some other set? We cannot know without more information.

Very often there is a property P that completely characterizes the elements of a set A, in which case we can write

$$A = \{x \mid P(x)\}$$

which reads, "A is equal to the set of all x such that property P holds for x." We will not explicitly define what a "property" is. But for any given element x, the statement $P(x)$ should be either true or false; that is, in the terminology of Chapter 1, $P(x)$ should be a *proposition*. (If this is not the case we say that a set has not been **well defined** by our statements.)

For example, the set $B = \{0, 1, 2, \ldots, 1000\}$ can be written

$$B = \{x \mid \underbrace{x \text{ is an integer and } 0 \leq x \leq 1000}_{P(x)}\}$$

In this format the letters chosen to represent elements are unimportant:

$$\{x \mid P(x)\} = \{y \mid P(y)\}$$

For example,

$$\{x \mid x \text{ is an integer and } 1 < x \leq 3\} = \{y \mid y \text{ is an integer and } 1 < y \leq 3\}$$
$$= \{2, 3\}$$

2.3 EXAMPLE. Consider the following three expressions.

$A = \{x \mid x \text{ is a left shoe }\}$

$B = \{y \mid y \text{ is a left sock }\}$

$C = \{z \mid z \text{ is a Tuesday before January 1983 and after February 1400 on which it rained at noon on what is now the site of the Washington Monument}\}$

Here A is a set, assuming that we have an unambiguous definition of "shoe" to work with. But B is not a set since the term "left sock" is ambiguous. Imagine this: you find a sock on the floor. Is the statement "x is a left sock" (call this $P(x)$) true or false? What makes a sock a "left" sock? Until this criterion has been clarified, B will not be well defined. For instance, if a left sock is defined to be a sock that is actually on someone's left foot at the moment you read the last word of this sentence, then for each element x the statement $P(x)$ will be a proposition, and therefore B will be a well-defined set. Finally, C *is* a well defined set, since on any Tuesday in the given time interval it either did or did not rain at the indicated time and place. (So if x is an element, the statement $x \in C$ is a proposition.) But we have no way to determine all the members of C. For example, is the second Tuesday of the year 1417 a member of C?

Once again let us note the distinction between B and C. No set B has been defined because the criterion for membership is unclear. On the other hand, C *is* a set because there is no ambiguity in the membership requirement; yet in practice there is no way of actually determining its members. Thus B fails to be a set because the statement that seems to define it is not a proposition; C *achieves* set-hood, but C is unlikely to be useful because we cannot reliably determine the truth value of its defining statement for all membership candidates.

Certain sets are used so often that they have been given standard names, and here are a few of them:

$\mathbb{N} = \{1, 2, 3, 4, 5, \ldots\}$, the **natural numbers** or **positive integers**

$\mathbb{Z} = \{\ldots, -3, -2, -1, 0, 1, 2, 3, \ldots\}$, the **integers** or **whole numbers**

$\mathbb{Q} = \{x \mid x = a/b \text{ for some } a, b \in \mathbb{Z}, b \neq 0\}$, the **rational numbers**

$\mathbb{R}$,   the **real numbers**

We won't attempt a definition of the real numbers. Let's say only that they are often expressed as decimals (possibly of infinite length), and it is convenient to think of them as points on a line (called, accordingly, the *real line*).

These number collections are familiar to everyone who has done arithmetic, and we will use them freely. Carefully justifying the assertion that these are sets is not an elementary matter, and we will leave this task for more advanced courses. (Consider this: if terrorists were to demand that you give a precise definition of "positive integer," would you be able to satisfy their demand?)

We have seen that some sets can be defined with a characterizing property $P(x)$. We do *not* mean to suggest that there is always a sort of camaraderie among the members of a given set that enables us to view them all as variations on a single theme. For instance, if

$$S = \{\pi, \text{Franklin Delano Roosevelt}, -\sqrt{53}, \text{spaghetti}, 12, 0\}$$

then we would be hard put to specify a property characterizing the elements of S other than the property of being on the given list. Similar considerations hold for the set of Tom Sawyer's goods listed at the start of this chapter.

The axioms of set theory tell us that sets exist. These axioms also provide us with some explicit examples, and they guide us in the formation of new sets from given ones by a variety of abstract cutting-and-pasting maneuvers. The axiom that follows is the set-theoretic version of this common kitchen wisdom: an individual is not obliged to consume an entire roast turkey at one sitting; instead, the diner can extract an appropriate portion with skillful carving.

Axiom of Separation. Given a set X and a property P, there is a set whose elements are the elements of X that have property P. That is, $\{x \mid x \in X \text{ and } P(x)\}$ is a set.

A convenient abbreviation: if S is a set and P is a property, the set

$$\{x \mid x \in S \text{ and } P(x)\}$$

is usually written

$$\{x \in S \mid P(x)\}$$

2.4 EXAMPLE.   We have already introduced the set of integers, $\mathbb{Z} = \{0, \pm 1, \pm 2, \pm 3, \ldots\}$. Therefore, by the axiom of separation, the following are also sets:

$\{x \in \mathbb{Z} \mid x = 2y \text{ for some } y \in \mathbb{Z}\}$, the set of even integers
$\{x \in \mathbb{Z} \mid x = 2y + 1 \text{ for some } y \in \mathbb{Z}\}$, the set of odd integers
$\{n \in \mathbb{Z} \mid n > 0 \text{ and } x^n + y^n = z^n \text{ is solvable for some } x, y, z, \in \mathbb{Z} \text{ with } xyz \neq 0\}$

The numbers 1 and 2 are members of this last set. The French mathematician Pierre de Fermat claimed (apparently in the 1630s) in the margin of a book that these were the *only* members. In detail, he stated: "To divide a cube into two other cubes, a fourth power, or in general any power whatever into two powers of the same denomination above the second is impossible, and I have assuredly found an admirable proof of this, but the margin is too narrow to contain it."[*] This assertion is commonly known as "Fermat's Last Theorem," although most mathematicians doubt that Fermat really had a proof (so it wasn't really a theorem); moreover, he subsequently proved many other results (so it would not have been his last theorem). As of this writing (in 1995), it appears that the proof of Fermat's Last Theorem has at last been completed, thanks to the effort of a great many mathematicians over the years, culminating in the recent work of Andrew Wiles.

In general, from now on we will feel free to discuss sets of real numbers that satisfy virtually any condition without officially announcing our dependence on the axiom of separation. We will refer, for instance, to the set of prime numbers, the set of irrational numbers, the set of negative real numbers, and so on.

Just as it is useful to have the number zero available to indicate the absence of items to count, it is useful to have the concept of a set that has no elements. Thus we view a stamp collector as having a collection even if he has just declared himself a collector and as yet has acquired no stamps; we say this collection is *empty*. We can formally justify this idea by appealing to the axiom of separation, which assures us that the following object is a set:

$$\emptyset = \{x \in \mathbb{Z} \mid x \neq x\}$$

This set clearly has no elements, since no integer has the property $x \neq x$; we call $\emptyset$ an **empty set**.[†]

We can use the axiom of separation in other ways to define empty sets; for example, these are also empty sets:

$$\{x \in \mathbb{Z} \mid x^2 = 2\} \quad \text{and} \quad \{x \in \mathbb{R} \mid x^2 = -1\}$$

---

[*]See D. J. Struik, *A Concise History of Mathematics*, 4th ed. (New York: Dover Publications, 1987), pp. 102–103.

[†]In formal studies of the foundations of mathematics, the existence of an empty set is asserted at or near the very beginning of set theory, and this set is a fundamental building block in the subsequent development of number sets. In our less formal approach we have taken the number sets for granted and deduced the existence of an empty set as a consequence.

We claim: *all empty sets are equal.* To prove this, suppose $\emptyset$ and $\emptyset'$ are both empty sets; we must prove $\emptyset = \emptyset'$. (That is, if Joe collects stamps and has no stamps, and Pat collects coins and has no coins, then their collections are equal.) By definition of set equality (2.1), we must verify the equivalence $x \in \emptyset \Leftrightarrow x \in \emptyset'$ for every element x. But for every x the statements $x \in \emptyset$ and $x \in \emptyset'$ are both false, since $\emptyset$ and $\emptyset'$ have no elements; therefore the desired equivalence is true for every x. (Recall Table 1.18.) To sum up, we have proved the following:

2.5 Theorem. There is exactly one empty set.

We will continue to use the symbol $\emptyset$ for the empty set.

The complete set of photographs of ninth-century life
(alias $\emptyset$)

2.6 EXAMPLE. We assert:

$$\emptyset \neq \{\emptyset\}$$

PROOF. The set on the left has no members. The set on the right has $\emptyset$ as a member. Therefore the inequality holds. □

Notice that in stating Example 2.6 we have used an unannounced axiom of set theory: If S is a set then so is $\{S\}$; that is, there is a set that has S as its only member. Thus every set is itself an element of some set, so we cannot say that elements and sets are fundamentally different kinds of entities. For example, let B denote the Boston Red Sox baseball team. Then B can be viewed as a set of ball players. On the other hand, if M denotes the set of all major league baseball teams, then $B \in M$; and if T is the set of all major league baseball teams based in New England, then $T = \{B\}$. Finally, we remark that if Jones plays for the Red Sox, then

$$\text{Jones} \in B \quad \text{and} \quad B \in T, \quad \text{yet} \quad \text{Jones} \notin T$$

because Jones is not a team.

Exercises

1. At Ace Elementary School the basketball team consists of Martha, Chet, Fred, Mervin, and Peggy. The softball team has exactly the same members. Are they the same set?

2. Describe each of the following sets in the format $\{x \mid P(x)\}$.
   (a) $A = \{0, 2, 4, 6, 8, 10, 12, 14, 16, 18, \ldots\}$
   (b) $B = \{1, 2, 5, 10, 17, 26, 37, 50, \ldots\}$
   (c) $C = \{1, 5, 9, 13, 17, 21, \ldots\}$
   (d) $D = \{1, \frac{1}{2}, \frac{1}{3}, \frac{1}{4}, \frac{1}{5}, \ldots\}$
   (e) $E = \{\text{lemon}, 1, 2, 3, 4, 5, \ldots\}$

3. Describe each of the following sets by listing all its elements between a pair of brackets.
   (a) $\{x \in \mathbb{N} \mid x \text{ is prime and } x^2 < 30\}$
   (b) $\{x \in \mathbb{Z} \mid x \text{ is prime and } (x \text{ is even or } 3 \le x \le 10)\}$
   (c) $\{x \in \mathbb{Q} \mid x \in \mathbb{N} \text{ and } 1 \le x \le 3\}$
   (d) $\{x \in \mathbb{Z} \mid \text{There is an element } y \in \mathbb{N} \text{ such that } x^2 + y^2 \le 25\}$

4. Which of the following are well-defined sets? Explain briefly.
   (a) The set of large real numbers.
   (b) The set of all integers that are not integer multiples of 7.
   (c) The set of all four-digit strings that appear in the decimal expansion of π to the right of the decimal point. (Example: Since $\pi = 3.1415926535\ldots$, the first four strings of this kind are 1415, 4159, 1592, and 5926.)

5. Label each statement *true* or *false*.
   (a) $\{1, 2, 3\} = \{3, 1, 2\}$
   (b) $\{1, 2, 3\} = \{2, 1, 3, 3, 2\}$
   (c) $\{5, \emptyset\} = \{5\}$
   (d) $\{5\} \in \{2, 5\}$
   (e) $\emptyset \in \{1, 2\}$
   (f) $\{1, 2\} \in \{1, 2\}$
   (g) $\{1, 2\} \in \{3, \{1, 2\}\}$
   (h) $2 \in \{\{1, 2\}\}$
   (i) $\{x \in \mathbb{R} \mid x^2 = -2\} = \emptyset$
   (j) $\emptyset \in \emptyset$

6. Is it true that if $\{a, b, c\} = \{a, b, d\}$ then $c = d$? (Here assume that a, b, c, and d represent numbers.)

7. In each part give an example of sets A, B, C that simultaneously satisfy the stated conditions.

   (a) $A \in B$, $B \in C$, $A \notin C$

   (b) $A \in B$, $B \in C$, $A \in C$

   (c) $A \notin B$, $B \in C$, $A \in C$

8. Take the following statement as an axiom: No set is a member of itself.

   (a) Show that if A is any set then $A \neq \{A\}$.

   (b) Argue convincingly that if A is a set and $n \in \mathbb{N}$ then

$$\underbrace{\{\{\{\cdots\{\{A\}\}\cdots\}\}\}}_{n \text{ braces}} \neq \underbrace{\{\{\{\cdots\{\{A\}\}\cdots\}\}\}}_{n+1 \text{ braces}},$$

(A precise proof requires *mathematical induction*, a technique to be considered later.)

2.2 Russell's Paradox

We may find it reasonable to expect that every property P defines a set, namely, the set of all objects that satisfy the property: $\{x \mid P(x)\}$. Let us assume for the moment that this is the case. Consider the set

$$S = \{A \mid A \text{ is a set and } A \notin A\}$$

For instance, if A is a set of pencils, then A is not itself a pencil, so $A \notin A$, and therefore $A \in S$. On the other hand, the collection B of all abstract ideas is itself an abstract idea, hence $B \in B$, and so $B \notin S$.

Question: Is the set S under discussion a member of itself? If $S \in S$, then the description of the elements of S tells us that $S \notin S$. On the other hand, if $S \notin S$, then S satisfies the property required of elements of S, and so $S \in S$. We have therefore verified the equivalence

$$S \in S \Leftrightarrow S \notin S.$$

This is lunacy, because the statement $S \in S$ is a proposition and therefore has *opposite* truth value from that of its negation, $S \notin S$. What has gone wrong? Answer: **The assumption that S is a set has led to a contradiction.** Therefore *we must abandon the notion that S is a set,—and also the wider assumption that for every property P the expression $\{x \mid P(x)\}$ defines a set.*

Bertrand Russell presented this disheartening news to the mathematical world in 1901, and Russell's paradox (the apparent set that is and is not a member of itself) caused widespread fear that the foundations of mathematics were built in quicksand. The axiom of separation, which we discussed earlier, enables us to avoid Russell's paradox by limiting our expectations: instead of asserting that every property determines a set, the axiom says that *inside a given set whose existence has already been guaranteed*, the elements satisfying a given property constitute a set. For example, once we have accepted the existence of the set $\mathbb{R}$ of real numbers, we are then free to define sets of real numbers that satisfy whatever further property our hearts desire. (Of course, if the property is outrageous the resulting set may be empty.)

2.7 EXAMPLE. Assume that X is a set. Then

$$S = \{A \in X \mid A \text{ is a set and } A \notin A\}$$

is a set, by the axiom of separation. At first glance this set resembles the subject of Russell's paradox. Again we ask: Is S a member of itself? If $S \in S$ then our description of elements of S tells us these facts: $S \in X$, and S is a set, and $S \notin S$. But the last of these facts contradicts the statement $S \in S$. Therefore the hypothesis $S \in S$ is false, so we have $S \notin S$. Thus S must fail to satisfy some criterion for membership in S. But S is a set and $S \notin S$, so S must fail the only other requirement for membership in S; that is, we conclude that $S \notin X$. *This is no paradox; nowhere did we assume that $S \in X$.*

Example 2.7 shows that given any set X, there is something (in the example it is S) that is not a member of X. So:

There is no set that contains everything.

2.3 Quantifiers

The statement $x^2 + 8 = 17$ is not a proposition, because until we know what x is, we cannot assign a truth value to the statement. But it becomes a proposition when x is replaced by a number: $5^2 + 8 = 17$ is false, $(-3)^2 + 8 = 17$ is true. Here we say that x is a **variable**: it is a symbol used in a statement P in such a way that P becomes a proposition when the symbol is replaced by a specific element, whereas in its original form P is not a proposition.

Sometimes we may want to say that a given statement P with a variable x is true for *at least one* substitution of an element x. For this purpose we introduce the notation

$$(\exists x)P$$

which we verbalize as "There exists an x such that P" or "For some x, P" or "There is at least one x for which P is true." On the other hand, to say that *every* element has property P amounts to saying that it is not the case that some element has property $\sim P$; symbolically: $\sim(\exists x)(\sim P)$. We abbreviate this by the notation

$$(\forall x)P$$

which is verbalized "for every x, P" or "for all x, P." The symbol $\exists$ is called the **existential quantifier**, and $\forall$ is the **universal qualifier**.

2.8 EXAMPLES.   (a) The statement

$$(\exists x)(x \in \mathbb{R} \text{ and } x^2 + \pi x - 2\pi^2 = 0)$$

is a true proposition since the substitution of π for x yields a true equation. In practice, abbreviations are common. For instance we may shorten the preceding statement to

$$(\exists x \in \mathbb{R})(x^2 + \pi x - 2\pi^2 = 0)$$

or, if we understand that $\mathbb{R}$ is the underlying set of interest, to

$$(\exists x)(x^2 + \pi x - 2\pi^2 = 0)$$

Notice that if the set $\mathbb{Z}$ of integers were under discussion (instead of $\mathbb{R}$), then the proposition $(\exists x)(x^2 + \pi x - 2\pi^2 = 0)$ would be false, since the only roots of the equation $x^2 + \pi x - 2\pi^2 = 0$ are π and -2π, neither of which is in $\mathbb{Z}$. So the truth value of a quantified proposition may depend on the prior specification of a set from which all elements are understood to come. Such a set is called the **universe** or **universal set** or **domain of interpretation** for the proposition.

(b) A remarkable theorem in number theory known as **Bertrand's Postulate** states that for every integer $n > 1$ there is a prime number p strictly between n and $2n$. With the set of integers greater than

1 as our universal set, Bertrand's Postulate can be represented using quantifiers as follows:

$$(\forall n)(\exists p)(p \text{ is prime and } n < p < 2n)$$

(c) A well-known theorem states that every nonnegative real number has a square root; this statement is represented by the two-variable proposition

$$(\forall x)\left(x \in \mathbb{R} \wedge x \geq 0 \Rightarrow (\exists y)(y \in \mathbb{R} \wedge y^2 = x)\right)$$

if $\mathbb{R}$ is fixed as the domain of interpretation, this expression shortens to

$$(\forall x)\left(x \geq 0 \Rightarrow (\exists y)(y^2 = x)\right)$$

More informally (mixing words and symbols), we can write

$$\forall x \geq 0, \quad \exists y \text{ such that } y^2 = x$$

which in turn has the compactification

$$(\forall x \geq 0)(\exists y)(y^2 = x)$$

Notice that the order in which the quantifying phrases occur is crucial. The present example has the form, "For every nonnegative x something happens"; accordingly, $\forall x$ starts off the symbolic representation. The "something" that happens is that "there is an element with a certain property," and therefore the next part of the symbolic representation starts with $\exists y$. By contrast, the expression

$$(\exists y)(\forall x \geq 0)(y^2 = x)$$

translates into "There is a number y that serves as a simultaneous square root for all nonnegative real numbers," clearly a falsehood.

(d) For variety, sometimes instead of $(\forall x)P$ we write $P, \forall x$. For example in analytic geometry we assert that every point (x, y) in a given set A lies outside the unit circle (the circle with center $(0, 0)$ and radius 1) as follows:

$$x^2 + y^2 > 1, \quad \forall (x, y) \in A$$

Now let's consider the negation of quantified statements, using the notation of logical equivalence from Section 1.5. Since $(\forall x)P$ is an abbreviation for $\sim(\exists x)(\sim P)$, we have

$$\sim(\forall x)P \equiv \sim\sim(\exists x)(\sim P) \equiv (\exists x)(\sim P)$$

In the same vein we have

$$\sim(\exists x)P \equiv \sim(\exists x)\big(\sim(\sim P)\big) \equiv (\forall x)(\sim P)$$

Thus we have obtained the following two basic logical equivalences for negating quantified statements:

(2.9) $$\sim(\exists x)P \equiv (\forall x)(\sim P)$$

(2.10) $$\sim(\forall x)P \equiv (\exists x)(\sim P)$$

2.11 EXAMPLES. The purpose of this example is to familiarize you quickly and informally with quantifier manipulation, without getting entangled in substantive mathematical issues. Here are some standard English sentences and their negations in the quantification format. Each variable is named with the initial of the word it represents.

(a) "There is a cat in that house" can be represented

$$(\exists c)(c \text{ is in that house})$$

By 2.9 the negation is

$$(\forall c)(c \text{ is outside that house})$$

which means, "Every cat is outside that house."

(b) "Every animal eats some food" is written

$$(\forall a)(\exists f)(a \text{ eats } f)$$

By 2.10 the negation can be written

$$(\exists a)\big(\sim(\exists f)(a \text{ eats } f)\big)$$

By 2.9 this in turn is equivalent to

$$(\exists a)(\forall f)(a \text{ does not eat } f)$$

meaning "There is an animal that eats no food."

(c) "There is an animal that eats every food" becomes

$$(\exists a)(\forall f)(a \text{ eats } f)$$

By 2.9 and 2.10, this negates to

$$(\forall a)(\exists f)(a \text{ does not eat } f)$$

which we may interpret as "Associated with every animal is some food it doesn't eat."

(d) As we saw in Example 2.8(c), the order in which variables are quantified can affect the meaning. For example, if instead of (b) we write

$$(\exists f)(\forall a)(a \text{ eats } f)$$

we get "There is a food that every animal eats." Thus, statement (b) is a statement about each animal; and we would presumably label it "true," assuming that "eats" is interpreted to mean "consumes as a part of its natural diet." But the present statement asserts the existence of a certain extraordinary food, and we must clearly label the statement "false" (if we interpret "eats" in the same way). Is there any food eaten by both lobsters and giant pandas?

Similarly, modifying (c) to

$$(\forall f)(\exists a)(a \text{ eats } f)$$

yields "Every food is eaten by some animal." The negations of these two statements are left for you to consider.

(e) "You can fool all of the people all of the time" is represented

$$(\forall p)(\forall t)(\text{You can fool } p \text{ at time } t)$$

By a double application of 2.10, this has the negation

$$(\exists p)(\exists t)(\text{You can't fool } p \text{ at time } t)$$

which translates to "There is a person who sometimes can't be fooled." Alternatively, we could have started with the representation

$$(\forall t)(\forall p)(\text{You can fool } p \text{ at time } t)$$

This negates to

$$(\exists t)(\exists p)(\text{You can't fool } p \text{ at time } t)$$

which means, "There is a time when at least one person can't be fooled."

The analysis of examples of the kind we have been considering here illustrates the vagueness that permeates our usual language. "There is a song that everyone is singing" and "Everyone is singing a song" have different intended meanings that can be captured by different quantifications, whereas in ordinary conversation we may require further discussion for clarification. Ambiguities like this will keep lawyers in business forever.

It is appropriate to pause for a moment to appreciate the benefits of our notation. If we are given a statement of staggering complexity, of the form

$$(\forall x_1)(\exists x_2)(\exists x_3)(\forall x_4)\cdots(\exists x_n)P$$

(where P is a proposition), we can now negate it mechanically to

$$(\exists x_1)(\forall x_2)(\forall x_3)(\exists x_4)\cdots(\forall x_n)(\sim P)$$

by repeated application of rules 2.9 and 2.10, without struggling to grasp the meaning of the given statement. Indeed, a computer can be programmed to carry out the symbol manipulation. Here is a commentary by Alfred North Whitehead, a distinguished mathematical philosopher (and a colleague of Bertrand Russell, our friend from an earlier section), in response to a similar notational triumph:

> This example shows that, by the aid of symbolism, we can make transitions in reasoning almost mechanically by the eye, which otherwise would call into play the higher faculties of the brain.
>
> It is a profoundly erroneous truism, repeated by all copybooks and by eminent people when they are making speeches, that we should cultivate the habit of thinking of what we are doing. The precise opposite is the case. Civilization advances by extending the number of important operations which we can perform without thinking about them. Operations of thought are like cavalry charges in a battle—they are strictly limited in number, they require fresh horses, and must only be made at decisive moments.[*]

[*]From A. N. Whitehead, *An Introduction to Mathematics* (Oxford: Oxford University Press, 1958).

There is one more useful quantifier, really a souped-up existential quantifier: the prefix

$$(\exists! x)$$

means "There is exactly one x" or "There is a unique x." A proof of a statement of the form $(\exists! x)P$ has two parts: the *existence* part, in which we prove $(\exists x)P$; and the *uniqueness* part, in which we prove that if statement P is true for both x and y then necessarily $x = y$.

Exercises

1. Express the following statements symbolically, using quantifiers, logical connectives [$\wedge$ (and), $\vee$ (or), $\sim$ (not), $\Rightarrow$ (implies)], and standard mathematical symbols from arithmetic, but using no English words. [Example: The false proposition "every real number's square is less than 8" can be written $(\forall x)(x \in \mathbb{R} \Rightarrow x^2 < 8)$, or in this shorter and less formal way (without all the parentheses separating parts of the statement from each other): $\forall x \in \mathbb{R},\ x^2 < 8$.]

   (a) There is a positive integer whose cube, when added to 15, yields a sum of 22.

   (b) Every positive integer has the property that when its cube is added to 15, the result is 22.

   (c) It is not the case that every real number is a square of a real number.

   (d) There is a real number that is not the square of a real number.

   (e) Every real number has a unique cube root.

2. Let $A = \{1, 2, \pi\}$, and let P be the statement "$x \in A$ and $x \in \mathbb{Z}$." Determine the truth value of each of the following implications, and justify briefly. Take the set $\mathbb{R}$ of real numbers as the universal set.

   (a) $(\exists x)P \Rightarrow (\forall x)P$

   (b) $(\forall x)P \Rightarrow (\exists x)P$

3. (a) Redo Exercise 2, using $A = \emptyset$ instead.

   (b) Is there a set A for which the truth value of statement (b) of Exercise 2 is *false*? Explain.

4. Write the following statements in more abbreviated form, using quantifiers. Here the short phrases "is prime" and "is a line" are allowed, and the symbol Π may be used for "the plane."

   (a) 17 is not the largest prime number.

   (b) There is no largest prime number.

(c) Every real number has a fifth root.

(d) Every pair of distinct points in the plane lies on a unique line.

5. The following definition can be found in most calculus books. A function f is **continuous** at $x \in \mathbb{R}$ if the following condition holds:

For every $\epsilon > 0$ there is a number $\delta > 0$ such that
$|f(x') - f(x)| < \epsilon$ whenever $|x' - x| < \delta$

(a) Write the condition in abbreviated form, using quantifiers.

(b) Write the negation of this condition in a quantified form, using no negation symbols.

(c) Write out part (b) mostly in words: "A function f is not continuous if . . . ."

6. A **prime number** is an integer greater than 1 that cannot be written as a product of smaller positive integers. Write the definition of prime number using symbols and no words. That is, complete the statement

p is a prime number $\Leftrightarrow$ _____

with a suitable symbolic expression.

7. Suppose you are working with real numbers. Devise equations P and Q, in which x appears as the only variable, such that the propositions

$$(\exists x)(P \wedge Q) \quad \text{and} \quad (\exists x)P \wedge (\exists x)Q$$

have opposite truth values.

8. Show the ambiguity of the statement "All men are not liars" by giving two reasonable interpretations that have different meanings. Use quantifiers, as in Example 2.11; and to convince the reader that your two interpretations are different, give a condition under which one is true while the other is false.

9. Label each of the following statements *true* or *false*. All statements here have $\mathbb{R}$ as the underlying universal set.

(a) $(x \geq 0) \Rightarrow (\exists y)(y^2 = x)$

(b) $(x \geq 0) \Rightarrow (\exists! y)(y^2 = x)$

(c) $(\forall x)(\exists! y)(y^3 = x)$

(d) $(\exists! x)(\forall y)(xy = y)$

(e) $(\forall x)(\exists! y)(xy = 0)$

(f) $(\exists x)(\exists! y)(xy = 0)$

(g) $(\forall x)(\exists! y)(x + y = 0)$

(h) $\sim(\exists x)(\forall y)(x \leq y)$

2.4 Set Inclusion

We often recognize that a given collection of objects is part of a broader class of things: my books are among my prized possessions; owls are nocturnal creatures; the integers are real numbers.

2.12 Definition. Let A and B be sets. We say A is a **subset** of B (or A is **contained** in B, or B **contains** A, or B **includes** A), written $A \subseteq B$ (or $B \supseteq A$) if every member of A is a member of B. More formally,

$$A \subseteq B \Leftrightarrow (\forall x)(x \in A \Rightarrow x \in B)$$

The symbol "$\subseteq$" is called the **set inclusion** symbol. If A is not a subset of B we write $A \nsubseteq B$ instead of the longer statement $\sim(A \subseteq B)$.

2.13 EXAMPLES. (a) $\{1,3\} \subseteq \{1, \pi, 3\}$

(b) $\{\emptyset\} \subseteq \{\emptyset, 5\}$

(c) $\mathbb{N} \subseteq \mathbb{Z} \subseteq \mathbb{Q} \subseteq \mathbb{R}$

Suppose we wish to prove $A \subseteq B$ for some given sets A and B. We first recall that an implication $P \Rightarrow Q$ is always true if P is false. In particular, the statement $x \in A \Rightarrow x \in B$ is automatically a true proposition whenever x is replaced by an element that is not a member of A. Therefore we need only be concerned with the truth value when x is replaced by a member of A. So we start a *direct* proof of the statement $A \subseteq B$ with "Let $x \in A$. Then ..." or "If $x \in A$, then ..." and we show that it follows that x must be a member of B. Or we could exhibit a chain of true implications of the form

$$x \in A \Rightarrow \cdots \Rightarrow x \in B$$

giving reasons whenever the justification is not obvious. We begin an *indirect* proof of $A \subseteq B$ by supposing that $x \notin B$ and showing that consequently $x \notin A$. [Reason: $(x \notin B \Rightarrow x \notin A)$ is the contrapositive of $(x \in A \Rightarrow x \in B)$.]

Suppose we want to prove $A \nsubseteq B$. We have

$$\begin{aligned}
A \nsubseteq B &\Leftrightarrow \sim(\forall x)(x \in A \Rightarrow x \in B) &&\text{(by 2.12)} \\
&\Leftrightarrow (\exists x) \sim (x \in A \Rightarrow x \in B) &&\text{(by 2.10)} \\
&\Leftrightarrow (\exists x)(x \in A \text{ and } x \notin B) &&\text{(use a truth table)}
\end{aligned}$$

Thus, *to prove $A \nsubseteq B$ it suffices to show that A contains an element that is not in B.*

2.14 Theorem.   Let A be a set. Then $A \subseteq A$ and $\emptyset \subseteq A$.

PROOF.   The inclusion $A \subseteq A$ follows from the truth of the insultingly trivial implication

$$x \in A \Rightarrow x \in A$$

To see that $\emptyset \subseteq A$, notice that the implication

$$x \in \emptyset \Rightarrow x \in A$$

is always true, since its hypothesis is false no matter how x is chosen.* $\square$

EXERCISE.   Give an *indirect* proof of the inclusion $\emptyset \subseteq A$.

2.15 Theorem.   If $A \subseteq B$ and $B \subseteq C$ then $A \subseteq C$.

PROOF 1. *(Detailed, with reasoning exposed)*   We follow the strategy described in the paragraph after Examples 2.13. From the definition of $\subseteq$ (see 2.12), to prove $A \subseteq C$ we must show that every element of A is an element of C. Equivalently, we must verify the conditional statement

$$x \in A \Rightarrow x \in C$$

For this purpose, let $x \in A$. That is, assume that the statement "$x \in A$" is true. Now we consult the hypothesis (that is, what the statement of the theorem tells us to assume is true) for assistance. Since $A \subseteq B$, the conditional statement "$x \in A \Rightarrow x \in B$" is true; so, since $x \in A$ is true, also $x \in B$ must be true. (In the language of Chapter 1, this is *modus ponens* in action.) Then, by exactly the same reasoning, since $B \subseteq C$, we conclude that $x \in C$. But all we assumed about x is that it is an element of A, and from this we have deduced (using the hypothesis) that $x \in C$. Therefore we have proved $A \subseteq C$, as desired. $\square$

PROOF 2. *(Really, this is the same as Proof 1, but the chattiness has been suppressed.)*   Let $x \in A$. Then, since $A \subseteq B$, we have $x \in B$. From this and the hypothesis $B \subseteq C$ we conclude that $x \in C$. Thus $A \subseteq C$. $\square$

---

*From now on, we will use the symbol $\square$ to mark the end of a proof or partial proof.

2.16 EXAMPLE. We can use the symbolism of Theorem 2.15 to express many standard logical arguments. For example, consider the sentence

All cats eat fish, and every fish-eater sings; therefore cats sing.

Translation: Let C, E, and S denote (respectively) the sets of cats, fish-eaters, and singers. Then $C \subseteq E \subseteq S$, and so $C \subseteq S$; that is, all cats sing.

2.17 Theorem. $A = B \Leftrightarrow A \subseteq B$ and $B \subseteq A$.

PROOF OUTLINE. Compare Definitions 2.1 and 2.12. □

2.18 EXAMPLE. In the set T of all triangles, define

$$S = \{\triangle \in T \mid \triangle \text{ has two sides of equal length}\}$$
$$A = \{\triangle \in T \mid \triangle \text{ has two equal angles}\}$$

Show that $S = A$. (Here assume that the standard criteria for triangle congruence are known.)

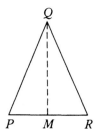

SEMISOLUTION. By Theorem 2.17, it suffices to show that $S \subseteq A$ and $A \subseteq S$. Let $\triangle \in S$, and let P, Q, R denote the vertices of $\triangle$, labeled so that $\overline{PQ} = \overline{QR}$. Construct a line from Q to the midpoint of M of PR. Then there is a congruence $\triangle PMQ \cong \triangle RMQ$, since these two triangles have sides of the same lengths. Therefore $\angle MPQ = \angle MRQ$ (why?), and $\triangle \in A$. This shows that $S \subseteq A$. Exercise: Prove that $A \subseteq S$ to finish the solution. □

2.19 Definition. For sets A and B we define the **proper** (or **strict**) **inclusion** relation, denoted $\subset$, as follows:

$$A \subset B \Leftrightarrow A \subseteq B \text{ and } A \neq B$$

We say that A is a **proper subset** of B (or **properly contained** in B) if this condition holds. In view of 2.12 and 2.17, we can reformulate this definition as follows:

$$A \subset B \Leftrightarrow A \subseteq B \text{ and } (\exists x)(x \in B \text{ and } x \notin A)$$

In words: A is a proper subset of B when A is a subset of B and B contains some element not in A.

If A is not a proper subset of B we write $A \not\subset B$.

Many authors use "$\subset$" for ordinary set inclusion instead of our "$\subseteq$." Therefore check the notation carefully when reading material on set theory in other sources.

2.20 EXAMPLES.   (a) $\{1, 7\} \not\subset \{1, 7\} \subset \{1, 2, 7\}$

(b) If A is any nonempty set then $\emptyset \subset A$.

PROOF.   The implication

$$x \in \emptyset \Rightarrow x \in A$$

is true, since its hypothesis is false for every x; therefore $\emptyset \subseteq A$. Also, the statement $\emptyset \neq A$ is true by the assumption that A is not empty. Therefore $\emptyset \subset A$.   □

(c) If $A \subset B$ and $B \subset C$ then $A \subset C$. (Check this!)

(d) Define $A = \{1, 2\}$, $B = \{1, 2, 3\}$, $C = \{3, \{1, 2\}\}$, $D = \{1, 2, \{1, 2\}\}$. Then the following assertions are true, and they should be verified by the reader.

$$A \subset B, \qquad A \notin B, \qquad A \in C, \qquad A \not\subseteq C, \qquad A \in D, \qquad A \subset D$$

Notice that A and C each have two elements, while B and D each have three elements.

(e) The set $S = \{$Boston Red Sox, New York Yankees$\}$ is a set with two members, each of which is itself a set. Thus if Jones is a member of the Boston Red Sox then

$$\text{Jones} \in \text{Boston Red Sox}$$

is true, while

$$\text{Jones} \in S$$

is false.

Exercises

1. (a) List the subsets of the set $A = \{1, 2, 3\}$.
   (b) List the subsets of the set $B = \{1, \{2, 3\}\}$.
   (c) List the subsets of the set $C = \{\{1, 2, 3\}\}$.

2. Can a set be a proper subset of itself? Explain.

3. Let $A = \{1, 2, -1, 5\}$, $B = \mathbb{N}$, $C = \{-2, -1, 0, 1, 2\}$, $D = \{1, \{1, 2\}, 2\}$, $E = \{-2, -1, 0, 2, 7\}$. In each case find a set S satisfying all the stated conditions and having the property that no set properly containing S also satisfies the conditions. (The set S is then said to be *maximal* with respect to the conditions.)

   (a) $S \subseteq A$ and $S \subseteq E$
   (b) $S \subseteq A$ and $S \subseteq D$
   (c) $S \subseteq B$ and $S \subseteq E$
   (d) $S \subseteq E$ and $S \not\subseteq C$
   (e) The statement

$$x \in C \quad \text{or} \quad x \in D$$

   is true for each $x \in S$.

   (f) The statement

$$x \in C \quad \text{and} \quad x \in D$$

   is true for each $x \in S$.

4. Prove the following implications.
   (a) $A \subset B \Rightarrow B \not\subset A$
   (b) $A \subseteq \emptyset \Rightarrow A = \emptyset$

5. Let S be a set. Prove the statement

$$a \in S \Leftrightarrow \{a\} \subseteq S$$

6. Prove that if $A \subset B$ and $B \subseteq C$ then $A \subset C$.

7. Prove the following two propositions.
   (a) $\{x \in \mathbb{N} \mid x^2 \leq 6\} \subseteq \{x \in \mathbb{Z} \mid x = 2^n \text{ for some } n \in \mathbb{Z}\}$
   (b) $(A \subseteq B \text{ and } B \subseteq C \text{ and } C \subseteq A) \Rightarrow A = B = C$

8. Let A and B be sets. Show that $A \subseteq B$ if and only if every subset of A is a subset of B.

9. Give sets A and B such that the statements $A \in B$ and $A \subseteq B$ are both true.

10. Prove or disprove: $\{\{\{5\}\}\} = \{\{5\}\}$.

2.5 Union, Intersection, and Complement

Throughout this section, capital letters $A, B, C, \ldots$ will denote sets. Our goal here is to begin to compare sets with each other and to see how sets can interact to produce offspring: a process known informally as "the joy of sets."

Given sets A and B, it is natural to consider the subset of A that consists of precisely those elements of A that don't belong to B.

2.21 Definition. If A and B are sets, we define their **difference**

$$A - B = \{x \in A \mid x \notin B\}$$

also called the **complement of B in A**. In the event that all sets under consideration in a particular discussion are subsets of a given set U (referred to as the **universal set** throughout that discussion), the compliment of any set A in U is called the **complement of A**, denoted A'.

2.22 Examples. (a) Let $A = \{1, 2, 3\}$ and $B = \{2, 3, 4\}$. Then $A - B = \{1\}$ and $B - A = \{4\}$.

(b) $\{\emptyset, \{\emptyset\}\} - \{\emptyset\} = \{\{\emptyset\}\}$

Proof of (b). The set $A = \{\emptyset, \{\emptyset\}\}$ has two elements, namely, $\emptyset$ and $\{\emptyset\}$; and $B = \{\emptyset\}$ is a set with $\emptyset$ as its only element. So the only element that belongs to A and not to B is $\{\emptyset\}$. That is, $A - B = \{\{\emptyset\}\}$. □

2.23 Exercises. Verify each of the following assertions.

(a) $A - A = \emptyset = \emptyset - a$

(b) $A - \emptyset = A$

(c) $A - B = B - A \Leftrightarrow A = B$

(d) If U is the universal set, then

$$(A')' = A, \qquad \emptyset' = U, \qquad U' = \emptyset$$

Our next constructions build sets either by uniting two sets into one or by restricting our attention to the elements two sets share.

2.24 Definition. The **union** of A and B is the set

$$A \cup B = \{x \mid x \in A \text{ or } x \in B\}$$

(Remember, our "or" is *inclusive*; recall Table 1.10.) The **intersection** of A and B is the set

$$A \cap B = \{x \mid x \in A \text{ and } x \in B\}$$

2.25 EXAMPLE. Let $A = \{1, 2, 3, 4\}$, $B = \{0, 1, 3, 5, 7\}$, and $C = \{2, 4, 6, 8\}$. Then

$$A \cup B = \{0, 1, 2, 3, 4, 5, 7\}$$
$$A \cap B = \{1, 3\} \qquad B \cap C = \emptyset$$
$$(A \cup B) \cap C = \{2, 4\} = A \cap C$$

We sometimes find it useful to represent sets pictorially by disks or blobs, shading appropriate regions to correspond to the subsets of interest. Such pictures are called *Venn diagrams* (after John Venn, who is credited with originating the procedure in the 1880s.) For instance, we can represent difference, union, and intersection by

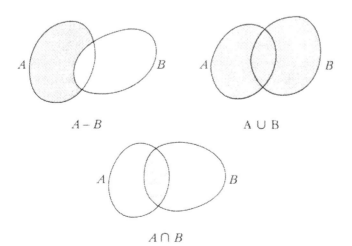

$A - B$ A $\cup$ B

$A \cap B$

and the complement by

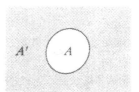

Here the universal set _U_ is represented by the entire rectangle.

Venn diagrams are a useful visual aid in the search for theorems about set equality. For example, if in the diagram

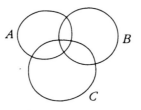

we shade the region corresponding to $A \cap (B \cup C)$, and in another copy of the diagram we shade the region for $(A \cap B) \cup (A \cap C)$, the result in each case looks like

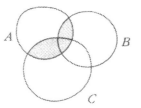

This similarity suggests the equality $A \cap (B \cup C) = (A \cap B) \cup (A \cap C)$. It does not _prove_ the equality, it _suggests_ it. Pictorial arguments can be misleading, and their worship should be avoided. To illustrate: if $A \cap B = \emptyset$ (in which case we say A and B are **disjoint**), an intersection portrait like

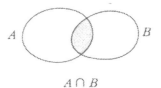

$A \cap B$

suggests that A and B have common elements, contrary to the hypothesis.

The equalities in the following theorem all follow from logical manipulations (justifiable by truth tables) and the definitions of union and intersection. The proof strategy goes back to the definition of set equality in 2.1. Should you feel the urge to draw Venn diagrams to supplement the proofs, go ahead.

2.26 Theorem.

(a) $A \cap (B \cap C) = (A \cap B) \cap C$
(b) $A \cup (B \cup C) = (A \cup B) \cup C$ ⎫ **associative laws**

(c) $A \cap (B \cup C) = (A \cap B) \cup (A \cap C)$
(d) $A \cup (B \cap C) = (A \cup B) \cap (A \cup C)$ ⎫ **distributive laws**

(e) $A - (B \cup C) = (A - B) \cap (A - C)$
(f) $A - (B \cap C) = (A - B) \cup (A - C)$
(g) $(A \cup B)' = A' \cap B'$
(h) $(A \cap B)' = A' \cup B'$ ⎫ **De Morgan's laws**

PARTIAL PROOF.

(a)
$$x \in A \cap (B \cap C) \Leftrightarrow x \in A \text{ and } x \in (B \cap C)$$
$$\Leftrightarrow x \in A \text{ and } (x \in B \text{ and } x \in C)$$
$$\Leftrightarrow (x \in A \text{ and } x \in B) \text{ and } x \in C$$
$$\Leftrightarrow x \in (A \cap B) \cap C$$

Therefore the definition of set equality yields the series conclusion. [Basically the argument is a consequence of the logical equivalence $P \wedge (Q \wedge R) \equiv (P \wedge Q) \wedge R$.]

(b) This proof is essentially the same as the proof of (a), merely replacing "∩" by "∪" and "and" by "or."

(c)–(h) Exercises.   □

2.27 Theorem.   (a) If $X \subseteq Z$ and $Y \subseteq Z$ then $X \cup Y \subseteq Z$.

(b) If $Z \subseteq X$ and $Z \subseteq Y$ then $Z \subseteq X \cap Y$.

PROOF.   (a) If $w \in X \cup Y$ then either $w \in X$ or $w \in Y$. In either case $w \in Z$, since $X \subseteq Z$ and $Y \subseteq Z$. Therefore $X \cup Y \subseteq Z$.

(b) This is left as an exercise.   □

Exercises

1. Let $A = \{1, 2, 3, 4, 5\}$, $B = \{3, 4, 5, 6\}$, $C = \{x \in \mathbb{Z} \mid x \text{ is even}\}$. Determine each of the following sets.

   (a) $A - B$ (d) $A \cup B$ (g) $(A \cap B) \cup C$

   (b) $B - A$ (e) $C - B$ (h) $B \cup \emptyset$

   (c) $B \cap A$ (f) $(A \cap B) \cap C$ (i) $\emptyset \cap C$

2. Take $\mathbb{Z}$ as the universal set. Using the sets A and C defined in Exercise 1, determine the sets A', C', and $(A \cap C)'$.

3. In each case indicate whether the given statement is true or false, and briefly justify your answer.

   (a) $\emptyset \in \{1, 2\} \cup \emptyset$

   (b) $\emptyset \subseteq \{1, 2, 3\} \cap \{3, 4, 5\}$

4. (a) Prove the following statements.

    (i) $A \cap B' \subseteq (A \cap B)'$

    (ii) If $B \subseteq A$ then $A \cap B' \subseteq (A \cap B)'$.

    (iii) If $B \not\subseteq A$ then $A \cap B' \not\subseteq (A \cap B)'$.

   (b) Under what condition involving the universal set does "=" hold in statement (ii) of part (a) in place of "$\subseteq$"? Explain.

5. Verify the following propositions. (Here A is any set.)

   (a) $A \cup \emptyset = A$

   (b) $A \cap \emptyset = \emptyset$

   (c) $(A - A) - A = \emptyset$

   (d) $A - (A - A) = A$

   (e) $A \cup A = A$

6. On one copy of the following diagram, shade the region corresponding to $A - (B - C)$; on another copy shade $(A - B) - C$. If the results are the same, prove the proposition $(A - B) - C = A - (B - C)$. If the results are different, give an explicit counterexample to the proposition.

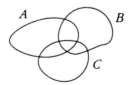

7. Prove each of the following.
   (a) $(A - B) \cap (B - A) = \emptyset$
   (b) $(A \cap B) \cap (A - B) = \emptyset$
   (c) $A = (A \cap B) \cup (A - B)$
8. Prove parts (c), (e), and (g) of Theorem 2.26.
9. Prove part (b) of Theorem 2.27.
10. Let A and B be sets. Define the **symmetric difference** to be

$$A \oplus B = (A - B) \cup (B - A)$$

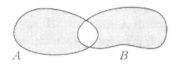

For example, if $A = \{-3, 0, 1, 2\}$ and $B = \{1, 2, 3, 4\}$, then

$$A \oplus B = \underbrace{\{-3, 0\}}_{A - B} \cup \underbrace{\{3, 4\}}_{B - A} = \{-3, 0, 3, 4\}$$

The set $A \oplus B$ consists of those elements of $A \cup B$ that belong to exactly one of the sets A, B. Prove the following statements. (Assume only that A and B are sets. Do not assume that we know what their elements are.)
   (a) $A \oplus A = \emptyset$
   (b) $A \oplus \emptyset = A$
   (c) $(A \oplus B) - (A - B) = B - A$
   (d) $A \oplus B = \emptyset \Rightarrow A = B$ (Therefore, combining parts (a) and (d) gives the equivalence $A \oplus B = \emptyset \Leftrightarrow A = B$.)
   (e) $(A \oplus B) \oplus C = A \oplus (B \oplus C)$ (Start with a Venn diagram.)
11. Let S be a nonempty set. All capital letters in this problem will denote subsets of S; and throughout this problem we will write $A + B$ instead of $A \cup B$, and AB instead of $A \cap B$.
   (a) Verify the following three assertions.

$$A + B = B + A \text{ and } AB = BA$$

$$A(B + C) = AB + AC$$

$$A + BC = (A + B)(A + C) \quad \text{(unfortunate!)}$$

   (b) Given A, for which sets B is it true that $A + B = A$? (Find them all.)

(c) Given A, for which sets B is it true that $AB = A$? (Find them all.)

(d) Show that $AX = A$ for all A if and only if $X = S$.

(e) Show that $A + X = A$ for all A if and only if $X = \emptyset$.

(f) Show that $A(B - A) = \emptyset$.

(g) Show that $A + (B - A) = A + B$. (Here "$-$" is the usual set difference.)

2.6 Indexed Sets

Imagine that a dog barks four times. How can we denote the set of barks? An easy (and quiet) answer: write $B = \{b_1, b_2, b_3, b_4\}$, where b_1 stands for the first bark, b_2 stands for the second bark, etc. Here we have used the members of a set $I = \{1, 2, 3, 4\}$ as labels or **indexes** for the members of B; I is therefore called the **index set**. Once the indexes have been assigned we can write $B = \{b_i \mid i \in I\}$. There may be more than one reasonable way to index the members of the set and, if the set is large, choosing an optimal indexing scheme is not an inconsequential matter. For instance, if someone is concerned with the problem of storing large amounts of data in such a way that information can easily be retrieved and manipulated, the way in which the data has been indexed can be crucial.

2.28 EXAMPLES. (a) Suppose you own many books on a wide variety of subjects, and you want to arrange them on your bookshelves in an optimal way. If you position them alphabetically by author, and books by the same author alphabetically by title, then it will be a triviality for you to locate a book with a given author and title; but, should the need arise to survey all your books that deal with a particular subject, you may have some trouble. On the other hand, if the books are filed by subject, you may have difficulty locating a book with a given author and title if the book's subject area is unknown to you.

(b) Each account file in a savings bank is a set of information about the account holder (name, address, employer, etc.) together with a listing of the amount of money in the account. If electronic access to the money could be had by anyone knowing the name of the account holder, then no depositor's money would be safe. So access is available only to someone knowing a secret number assigned to the account holder. That is, account files are indexed by code numbers and not by people's names.

(c) Analytic geometry grew out of René Decartes's insight (in 1637) that the points in a plane Π can be indexed with ordered pairs of real numbers by superimposing a pair of axes on Π and labeling each point according to its position with respect to the axes.

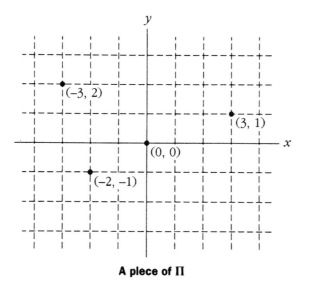

A piece of Π

When the set $I = \{(a, b) \mid a, b \in \mathbb{R}\}$ is the index set for Π, a typical point $P \in Π$ can be completely identified by using its full indexed name $P_{(a,b)}$. In practice we simplify the notation by suppressing the letter P, and we speak of "the point (a, b)." It is not essential that the axes be perpendicular or that the same units of distance be used on both. For example, in the mathematics of crystallography it is often more reasonable to use axes that suggest the geometry of the crystalline structure under consideration.

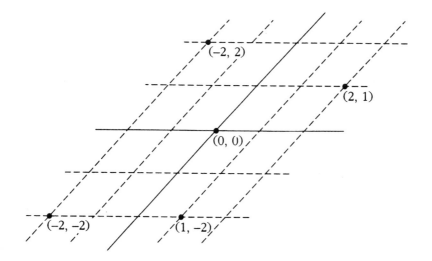

In this case the index set I is the same as it was for Descartes, but the scheme for assigning elements of I to elements of Π is different from his. There are also **polar coordinates** for Π: We choose a point in Π, label it O, and call it the **origin** or **pole**. Then we choose a ray (the **polar axis**) originating at O, and a unit distance. We index a point $P \in \Pi$ by its distance r from O and the angle α that the ray OP makes with the polar axis:

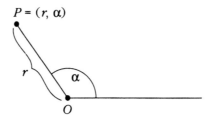

$$P = (r, \alpha)$$

The three indexing procedures just described provide dramatically different descriptions of the elements of Π.

(d) Consider the family $\mathcal{L}$ of all the vertical lines in the usual xy-plane. Each such line intersects the x-axis at exactly one point $(i, 0)$, and we can use the real number i to index the line. Thus for each $i \in \mathbb{R}$ we let L_i denote the vertical line through $(i, 0)$.

Now let's see another way to index the family $\mathcal{L}$. Each vertical line has exactly one point with y-coordinate 1. The line through the origin and that point makes an angle α (say in radians) with the x-axis, and α can be used to label the line: call the line L_α. In this way the open interval $I_0^\pi = \{\alpha \mid 0 < \alpha < \pi\}$ can serve as the index set for $\mathcal{L}$.

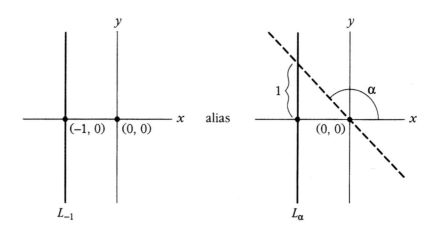

The notation $S = \{x_i \mid i \in I\}$ for an indexed set is often compactified to $S = \{x_i\}_{i \in I}$. Thus in Example 2.28(d), the two indexing procedures for the set $\mathcal{L}$ of vertical lines yield these notations for $\mathcal{L}$: $\{L_i\}_{i \in \mathbb{R}}$ and $\{L_\alpha\}_{\alpha \in I_0^\pi}$.

2.29 Examples. (a) A collection of sixteen sets

$$\{A, B, C, D, E, F, G, H, I, J, K, L, M, N, O, P\}$$

can be relabeled and written more compactly as the indexed family $\{A_i\}_{i \in I}$ with index set $I = \{i \in \mathbb{Z} \mid 1 \le i \le 16\}$.

(b) In the usual xy-plane, we associate the following sets with a real number r:

$$H_r = \{(x, y) \mid x \ge r\}, \qquad \text{a } right\ half\text{-}plane$$

and, if $r \ge 0$,

$$C_r = \{(x, y) \mid \sqrt{x^2 + y^2} = r\}, \qquad \text{the } circle \text{ with radius } r \text{ and center } (0, 0)$$

$$D_r = \{(x, y) \mid \sqrt{x^2 + y^2} \le r\}, \qquad \text{the } closed\ disk \text{ with radius } r \text{ and center } (0, 0)$$

This gives three indexed families:

$$\{H_r\}_{r \in \mathbb{R}} \qquad \{C_r\}_{r \ge 0} \qquad \{D_r\}_{r \ge 0}$$

In all three families, each object has been indexed with a number that is important in the object's definition.

Now we extend our notions of union and intersection, defined earlier for two sets (2.24), to arbitrary indexed families of sets.

2.30 Definition. Let $\{A_i\}_{i \in I}$ be an indexed family of sets. We define the

$$\textbf{union} \quad \bigcup_{i \in I} A_i$$

as the set of elements that belong to *at least one* A_i, and the

$$\textbf{intersection} \quad \bigcap_{i \in I} A_i$$

as the set of elements that belong to *all* A_i. More compactly:

$$\bigcup_{i \in I} A_i = \{x \mid x \in A_i \text{ for some } i \in I\},$$

$$\bigcap_{i \in I} A_i = \{x \mid x \in A_i \text{ for all } I \in I\}$$

With quantifiers:

$$\bigcup_{i \in I} A_i = \{x \mid (\exists i \in I)(x \in A_i)\}, \qquad \bigcap_{i \in I} A_i = \{x \mid (\forall i \in I)(x \in A_i)\}$$

To ease the printer's burden and simplify the notation, if no ambiguity is likely we sometimes write the union as $\cup_{i \in I} A_i$ or even $\cup A_i$, and we treat intersections similarly.

REMARK. From the definition of $\cap_{i \in I} A_i$ it follows that the statement $x \notin \cap_{i \in I} A_i$ is equivalent to $\sim (\forall i \in I)(x \in A_i)$, which in turn is equivalent to $(\exists i \in I)(x \notin A_I)$, by our rules for negating quantified statements. In words: if x is not simultaneously in all A_i, then there is some A_i that does not have x as a member. Similar considerations hold for $\cup_{i \in I} A_i$. (Check this.)

2.31 EXAMPLES. (a) Two given sets can be represented as an indexed family $\{A_1, A_2\}$ with index set $I = \{1, 2\}$. Having done that, we have $\cup_{i \in I} A_i = A_1 \cup A_2$ and $\cap_{i \in I} A_i = A_1 \cap A_2$. So the concepts defined in 2.30 include those in 2.24 as special cases.

(b) Consider the family $\mathcal{L} = \{L_i\}_{i \in \mathbb{R}}$ defined in 2.28(d). We claim that $\cup_{i \in \mathbb{R}} L_i$ is the entire plane, while $\cap_{i \in \mathbb{R}} L_i = \emptyset$. Let's verify the first of these assertions in detail. (The second is left as an exercise.) Denote the plane by E: we must show $E = \cup L_i$. Recall that to do this it suffices to show that $E \subseteq \cup L_i$ and $\cup L_i \subseteq E$. Conversationally: Each point in E is on some vertical line, hence each point is in the union of all the vertical lines, so $E \subseteq \cup L_i$. Conversely, every point in $\cup L_i$ is on some L_i; but L_i is contained in E, so $\cup L_i \subseteq E$. Here is a more detailed proof. If $P \in E$, then $P = (a, b)$ for some $a, b \in \mathbb{R}$. But then $P \in L_a$, since L_a is the vertical line through $(a, 0)$ [that is, $L_a = \{(a, y) \mid y \in \mathbb{R}\}$], and so $P \in \cup L_i$. Conversely, if $P \in \cup L_i$ then $P \in L_i$ for some i, by Definition 2.30. But $L_i \subseteq E$, and therefore $P \in E$.

(c) Let's briefly discuss the unions and intersections of the families defined in Example 2.29(b). As in part (b) of this example, we use E for the plane. We assert that $\cup H_r = E$. Every point in the union is in some H_r, and $H_r \subseteq E$, proving "$\subseteq$." Conversely, every point $(a, b) \in E$ is in the half-plane H_{a-1}, for example, hence in $\cup H_r$. Also, $\cap H_r = \emptyset$ because no point is in every half-plane; for instance, $(a, b) \notin H_{a+1}$. Next, $\cup C_r = E$, essentially because every point in the plane is on a circle centered at the origin, namely, (a, b) is on $C_{\sqrt{a^2+b^2}}$. (Really this only shows "$\supseteq$.") But $\cap C_r = \emptyset$ since no point is on more than one such circle. Finally, $\cup D_r = E$ since every point of E is in some disk (in fact many disks). We claim $\cap D_r = \{(0,0)\}$. Clearly, $(0,0)$ is an element of every disk centered at $(0,0)$. Moreover, any point $(a, b) \neq (0,0)$ is excluded from small enough disks (for example, from $D_{\sqrt{(a_2+b^2)/2}}$) and therefore from the intersection $\cap D_r$.

2.32 Theorem. Let A be a set and let $\{B_i\}_{i\in I}$ be an indexed family of sets. Then the following is true:

(a) $A - \cap_{i\in I} B_i = \cup_{i\in I}(A - B_i)$

(b) $A - \cup_{i\in I} B_i = \cap_{i\in I}(A - B_i)$

(c) $(\cap_{i\in I} B_i)' = \cup_{i\in I} B_i'$

(d) $(\cup_{i\in I} B_i)' = \cap_{i\in I} B_i'$

(This theorem extends Theorem 2.26, and is therefore also known as *De Morgan's laws*.)

PROOF OF (a).

$$x \in A - \bigcap_{i\in I} B_i \Leftrightarrow x \in A \text{ and } x \notin \bigcap_{i\in I} B_i$$

$$\Leftrightarrow x \in A \text{ and } (\exists i \in I)(x \notin B_i) \quad \text{(recall 2.30)}$$

$$\Leftrightarrow (\exists i \in I)(x \in A \text{ and } x \notin B_i)$$

$$\Leftrightarrow (\exists i \in I)(x \in A - B_i)$$

$$\Leftrightarrow x \in \bigcup_{i\in I}(A - B_i)$$

The proof of part (b) is left as an exercise.

In parts (c) and (d), all B_i are understood to be subsets of some unspecified universal set. If we call that universal set A, the proofs of (c) and (d) are immediate from (a) and (b), respectively, using the definition of complement. □

Exercises

1. Let $A_1 = \{1, 2, 3, 4\}$, $A_2 = \{0, 1, 2\}$, $A_3 = \{-1, 0, 1\}$, and let $I = \{1, 2, 3\}$. Determine the following sets.

   (a) $\bigcup_{i \in I} A_i$

   (b) $\bigcap_{i \in I} A_i$

   Take the set of integers, $\mathbb{Z}$, as the universal set. Determine the following sets.

   (c) $\bigcup_{i \in I} A_i'$

   (d) $\bigcap_{i \in I} A_i'$

2. Take the set of all living people as the universal set. Define

$$A_i = \{x \mid x \text{ was born on the } i\text{th day of his/her birth year}\}$$

$$B_j = \{x \mid x \text{ was born during the } j\text{th month of the year}\}$$

$$C_k = \{x \mid x \text{ was born on the } k\text{th day of the week}\}$$

   (start counting with Sunday). Use words to describe the elements of each of the following sets.

   (a) $B_1 \cap (\bigcup_{1 \le k \le 3} C_k)$

   (b) $(\bigcap_{1 \le j \le 5} B_j) \cup (\bigcup_{12 \le i \le 15} A_i)$

   (c) $C_6 \cap (\bigcup_{1 \le j \le 4} B_j)$

   (d) $(\bigcup_{1 \le k \le 5} C_k)'$

   (e) $\bigcup_{1 \le k \le 5} C_k'$

   (f) $\bigcap_{1 \le j \le 4} B_j'$

3. Let n be a positive integer, and suppose a set A_i is given for each $i \in I = \{1, 2, 3, \ldots n\}$, with $A_i \subseteq A_j$ whenever $i \le j$. Show that $\bigcup_{i \in I} A_i = A_n$ and $\bigcap_{i \in I} A_i = A_1$.

4. An indexed family of sets $\{A_i\}_{i \in I}$ is said to be **disjoint** if $\bigcap_{i \in I} A_i = \emptyset$, and the family is said to be **pairwise disjoint** if $A_i \cap A_j = \emptyset$ whenever $i \ne j$. In words: a family of sets is disjoint if there is no element shared by all sets in the family; a family is pairwise disjoint if no two sets with different indexes share a common element. The following pictures may help to clarify these ideas.

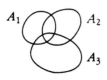

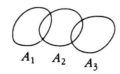

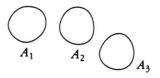

| Not disjoint | Disjoint but not pairwise disjoint | Pairwise disjoint |

(a) Let $A_1 = \{1, 2, 3, 4\}$, $A_2 = \{3, 4, 5, 6\}$, $A_3 = \{1, 6, 7\}$. Show that the family $\{A_1, A_2, A_3\}$ is disjoint but not pairwise disjoint.

(b) Show that if $\{B_1, B_2, B_3\}$ is a pairwise disjoint family of sets then it is disjoint.

5. Recall the closed interval notation $[-\alpha, \alpha] = \{x \in \mathbb{R} \mid -\alpha \le x \le \alpha\}$. Determine each of the following sets.

(a) $\bigcup_{\alpha > 0} [-\alpha, \alpha]$

(b) $\bigcap_{\alpha > 0} [-\alpha, \alpha]$

(c) $\bigcap_{\alpha \ge 5} [-\alpha, \alpha]$

6. For each integer n, let $M(n)$ be the set of all integer multiples of n. Thus, for example,

$$M_0 = \{0\}$$
$$M_1 = M_{-1} = \mathbb{Z}$$
$$M_2 = M_{-2} = \{0, \pm 2, \pm 4, \pm 6, \ldots\}$$
$$M_3 = M_{-3} = \{0, \pm 3, \pm 6, \pm 9, \ldots\}$$

Determine each of the following sets.

(a) $\bigcup_{n \in \mathbb{N}} M_n$

(b) $\bigcap_{n \in \mathbb{N}} M_n$

(c) $\bigcup_{p \text{ prime}} M_p$

(d) $\bigcap_{p \text{ prime}} M_p$

(e) $\bigcup_{n \ge 6} M_n$

(f) $\bigcup_{n \in M_5} M_n$

7. Prove Theorem 2.32(b).

8. Describe each of the following as an indexed family of sets. Here Π denotes the coordinatized xy-plane.

(a) The family of closed intervals of length 1 on the real line.

(b) The family of all circles in Π of radius 1 whose center is on the y-axis.

(c) The family of all circles in Π of radius 1.

(d) The family of all lines in Π with slope 6.

(e) The family of all lines in Π with y-intercept 5.

9. Find $\bigcup_{i \in I} A_i$ and $\bigcap_{i \in I} A_i$ for each family $\{A_i\}_{i \in I}$ in Exercise 8. That is, describe the union and intersection in each case, and briefly justify your claims. A complete proof is not required.

2.7 The Power Set

Mathematicians, surgeons, nuclear physicists, and ax murderers achieve many of their objectives by dissecting complicated structures and manipulating their pieces. In this section we begin such a dissection by considering the set of all subsets of a given set.

2.33 Definition.   The **power set** $P(A)$ of a set A is the collection of all subsets of A:

$$P(A) = \{X \mid X \subseteq A\}$$

So for any set X the statements "$X \subseteq A$" and "$X \in P(A)$" are equivalent. (We'll see that many proofs about power sets amount to remembering this equivalence.) Thus a subset of $P(A)$ is a set whose members are subsets of A. If A is small we can describe $P(A)$ by listing the subsets of A between a pair of braces.

2.34 EXAMPLES.   (a) $P(\{3\}) = \{\emptyset, \{3\}\}$
(b) $P(\{1, 2\}) = \{\emptyset, \{1\}, \{2\}, \{1, 2\}\}$
(c) $P(\emptyset) = \{\emptyset\}$

PROOF OF (c).   We have $\emptyset \subseteq \emptyset$ (recall Theorem 2.14), so $\emptyset \in P(\emptyset)$, and therefore $\{\emptyset\} \subseteq P(\emptyset)$. Conversely,

$$A \in P(\emptyset) \Rightarrow A \subseteq \emptyset$$

$$\Rightarrow A = \emptyset \quad \text{(If } A \neq \emptyset \text{ then } A \text{ has a member}$$
$$x, \text{ and the inclusion } A \subseteq \emptyset \text{ would}$$
$$\text{force } x \in \emptyset, \text{ an absurdity.)}$$

$$\Rightarrow A \in \{\emptyset\}$$

Hence, $P(\emptyset) \subseteq \{\emptyset\}$. When we combine this with the first part of the proof, we deduce $P(\emptyset) = \{\emptyset\}$, as claimed.   □

(d) $P(\{1, 2, 3\}) = \{\emptyset, \{1\}, \{2\}, \{3\}, \{1, 2\}, \{1, 3\}, \{2, 3\}, \{1, 2, 3\}\}$

Examples 2.34 lead us naturally to this conjecture:

If A has n elements then $P(A)$ has 2^n elements.

In other words:

A set with n elements has 2^n subsets.

We'll prove the conjecture toward the end of the chapter, but for now, a proof sketch goes like this: If $A = \{a_1, \ldots, a_n\}$, we can associate each subset of X and A with an n-digit binary expression $b_1 b_2 \ldots b_n$ (that is, a string of 0s and 1s) given by

$$b_i = \begin{cases} 1 & \text{if } a_i \in X \\ 0 & \text{if } a_i \notin X \end{cases}$$

(For example, $\emptyset$ is associated with $00\ldots0$, and A is associated with $11\ldots1$.) There are 2^n such expressions because there are two possible choices for the first digit on the left and, for each of these possibilities, two choices for the next digit to its right, and so on. Altogether, since there are n decisions in all, there are 2^n possible results.

It is helpful to represent the decision process graphically by a figure called a **decision tree**, which is pictured in 2.35.

(2.35)

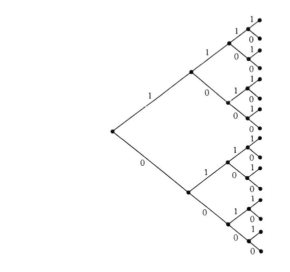

Here the marked points are called **vertices** (singular: **vertex**), and the line segments that connect two vertices are called **edges**. [There is also biological terminology for all this: the edges in a tree are often called **branches**, and a vertex at the end of exactly one branch (in the diagram, one of the far right vertices) is called—you guessed it—a **leaf**.] Each vertex at which a branching takes place (moving from left to right) represents a moment of decision, and an edge emanating to the right from a vertex represents a possible choice at that moment. In our pictured tree, we have labeled the edges to indicate the corresponding choices. Thus a path from the first vertex on the left (called the **root** of this tree) to the fifth vertex from the bottom on the far right of the tree corresponds to the four-digit binary string 0100. There are exactly $16 = 2^4$ left-to-right paths, one for each possible four-digit binary string. Accordingly, a set with four elements has 16 subsets. More generally, a tree associated with the choice of an n-digit binary string will have 2^n left-to-right paths, and a set with n elements has 2^n subsets.

Once we have accepted the concepts of the power set and the empty set, we are forced to admit the existence of very large sets. To see this, watch what happens upon repeatedly taking power sets:

$$P(\emptyset) = \{\emptyset\} \qquad P(P(\emptyset)) = \{\emptyset, \{\emptyset\}\}$$

$$P(P(P(\emptyset))) = \{\emptyset, \{\emptyset\}, \{\{\emptyset\}\}, \{\emptyset, \{\emptyset\}\}\}$$

$$\underbrace{P(P\cdots(P(P(\emptyset))\cdots))}_{n\ Ps} \text{ has } \left. 2^{2^{\cdot^{\cdot^{\cdot^{2^0}}}}} \right\} \text{ elements with } n \text{ 2s in the tower.}$$

2.36 ˙Theorem.   Let A and B be sets. Then

(a) $\{\emptyset, A\} \subseteq P(A)$;

(b) $A \subseteq B \Leftrightarrow P(A) \subseteq P(B)$;

(c) $P(A) \cup P(B) \subseteq P(A \cup B)$;

(d) $P(A) \cap P(B) = P(A \cap B)$.

PROOF.   Suggestion: First review proof strategies for inclusions and equalities; see especially 2.12–2.17. Also, as is always the case in proving theorems, it is essential that we recall the meanings of the expressions we are handling; that is, their **definitions**. All of the statements in the present theorem involve the power set of a set, so we remind ourselves: If X is a set, the *members* of $P(X)$ are the *subsets* of X. For example, statement (b) is equivalent to this: A is a subset of B if and only if every subset of A is a subset of B.

(a) We must show that $\emptyset \in P(A)$ and $A \in P(A)$; equivalently, $\emptyset \subseteq A$ and $A \subseteq A$. But we already know this by 2.14.

(b) We first prove "$\Rightarrow$." So assume $A \subseteq B$, and let $X \in P(A)$. (Here think, "And we want to show $X \in P(B)$, which is the same as showing

$X \subseteq B$." Then remember the hypothesis!) Then $X \subseteq A \subseteq B$, and so $X \subseteq B$; that is, $X \in P(B)$. We have therefore verified the implication

$$A \subseteq B \Rightarrow P(A) \subseteq P(B)$$

Conversely, assume $P(A) \subseteq P(B)$. We have the implication chain

$$x \in A \Rightarrow \{x\} \subseteq A \Rightarrow \{x\} \in P(A)$$
$$\Rightarrow \{x\} \in P(B) \Rightarrow \{x\} \subseteq B \Rightarrow x \in B$$

which gives the result.

(c) Since $A \subseteq A \cup B$ and $B \subseteq A \cup B$, by part (b) we know $P(A) \subseteq P(A \cup B)$ and $P(B) \subseteq P(A \cup B)$. Now apply Theorem 2.27(a).

(d) Since $A \cap B \subseteq A$, we have $P(A \cap B) \subseteq P(A)$ by part (b). Similarly, $P(A \cap B) \subseteq P(B)$, so Theorem 2.27(b) gives $P(A \cap B) \subseteq P(A) \cap P(B)$. Conversely, if $X \in P(A) \cap P(B)$ then $X \subseteq A$ and $X \subseteq B$, so $X \subseteq A \cap B$; that is, $X \in P(A \cap B)$. Therefore $P(A) \cap P(B) \subseteq P(A \cap B)$, and we have proved the desired equality. □

2.37 EXAMPLE. Let $A = \{1, 2\}$ and $B = \{2, 3\}$. Then $\{1, 2, 3\} \in P(A \cup B)$, while $\{1, 2, 3\} \notin P(A) \cup P(B)$. So the inclusion symbol in Theorem 2.36(c) cannot be replaced by equality.

Exercises

1. Let $A = \{1, 2, 3, 4\}$ and $B = \{4, 5, 6\}$. Determine the following sets.
   (a) $P(A \cap B)$
   (b) $P(B - A)$
   (c) $P(A) \cap P(B)$
   [Suggestion: Do part (c) in two ways as follows. First find $P(A)$ and $P(B)$ and determine their intersection; that's one way. Then find $A \cap B$ and obtain $P(A \cap B)$; that's the other way. By Theorem 2.36(d), these results are equal, but one approach involves considerably less work than the other.]

2. Determine each of the following sets.
   (a) $P(\{2\})$
   (b) $P(P(\{2\}))$
   (c) $P(P(P(\{2\})))$

3. Sam has one of each of the following: a penny, a nickel, a dime, a quarter, a half-dollar, a dollar bill, and a two-dollar bill. He will

definitely place a bet on his next poker hand. How many possibilities are there for the amount of his bet? Explain.

4. If each of the sets A and B contains an element not in the other, show that $P(A \cup B) \supset P(A) \cup P(B)$. (A Venn diagram may help here and in some other problems.)

5. Show that if $A \subset B$ then $P(A) \subset P(B)$.

6. (a) Show that if A and B are sets than $\emptyset \notin P(A) - P(B)$.
   (b) Deduce from part (a) that the difference of two power sets can never be a power set.
   (c) Prove that $P(A - B) \subseteq (P(A) - P(B)) \cup \{\emptyset\}$.

7. Under what conditions on sets A and B is it true that $P(A - B) = P(A)$? State and prove a condition that is necessary and sufficient.

8. Let A be a set, and suppose $x \notin A$. Describe $P(A \cup \{x\})$.

2.8 Ordered Pairs and Cartesian Products

There are many common procedures by which we pair, relate, or associate members of one or more sets with each other. (1) With a person's name we can associate his or her street address, or telephone number, or mother's maiden name, and so on. (2) To a positive real number w we assign a monetary amount p, the cost of postage required to send an item of weight w by first-class mail. (3) A traveling salesman planning to visit twenty cities makes a list that indicates the order in which he will visit the cities: the number n is paired with the nth city on his tour. (4) The formula $y = x^3 + e^x - \sin x$ describes a rule for pairing each real number x with a real number y. (5) Consider a line of people waiting to transact business with a bank teller. The line is more than a set of people: it has an *ordering*, which is an additional structure. For example, if one person in line cuts in front of another, then the order structure of the line has changed even though the same underlying set of people is involved. The ordering of the line can be determined by knowing who precedes whom for each two-person subset. For example, if we consider Smith's position relative to each other person's and determine that Smith is ahead of everyone except Jones, then we know that Jones is at the head of the line, followed immediately by Smith.

The notion of an "ordered pair" is central in all of the above examples. For instance, in example (4), if we start with $x = 0$ we get $y = 1$, but if we start with $x = 1$ we do not get $y = 0$. As is standard in analytic geometry, we say that the ordered pair $(0, 1)$ is associated with the given equation while the ordered pair $(1, 0)$ is not. Similarly, in example (5) we can associate an ordered pair (a, b) with the bank line if a is ahead of b in the line. Thus (Jones, Smith) is associated with the line, while (Smith, Jones) is not. But exactly what do we mean by *these* ordered pairs of names? How can we impose an order structure on an arbitrary two-element set? There is no difference in meaning between "shoe and sock" and "sock and shoe," while there *is* a distinction between "first sock, then shoe" and "first shoe, then sock." More generally, since $\{a, b\} = \{b, a\}$, something more is needed if we want to indicate that one element is to be viewed as preceding the other. Here is a start.

2.38 Quasi-definition. Let a and b be elements. The symbol (a, b) denotes an **ordered pair**, with the following understanding: if (c, d) is also an ordered pair, then

$(*)$ $\qquad\qquad (a, b) = (c, d) \Leftrightarrow a = c$ and $b = d$

What's "quasi" about 2.38? A close look shows that 2.38 does not really *define* an ordered pair. That is, *it doesn't really say what ordered pairs* ***are**; it just says what essential property ordered pairs should have, however we may choose to define them.*

2.39 Definition. Let a and b be elements. Then define

$$(a, b) = \{\{a\}, \{a, b\}\}$$

Here the elements a and b are called the **first** and **second coordinates**, respectively.

The following theorem and its corollary show that this definition of (a, b) achieves what we want: it attends to the order in which the elements are listed.

2.40 Theorem. $(a, b) = (c, d) \Leftrightarrow a = c$ and $b = d$.

PARTIAL PROOF. "$\Leftarrow$": if $a = c$ and $b = d$, then $\{a\} = \{c\}$ and $\{a, b\} = \{c, d\}$, and so $\{\{a\}, \{a, b\}\} = \{\{c\}, \{c, d\}\}$; that is, $(a, b) = (c, d)$.

We leave the converse ("$\Rightarrow$") as a tedious but worthwhile exercise in bracket shuffling. Suggestion: first consider the case $a = b$ (when $\{\{a\}, \{a, b\}\} = \{\{a\}\}$), and then consider the case $a \neq b$. $\qquad\square$

2.41 Corollary. $(a, b) = (b, a) \Leftrightarrow a = b$.

Of course, statements 2.40 and 2.41 are well known in the context of analytic geometry, where a point is described by an ordered pair of real numbers according to the point's position with respect to the axes. But the definition of ordered pair given in 2.39 frees the concept from geometrical constraints, so that we can apply it in other contexts. Later we will extend the notion of order to larger sets. This is important for a variety of purposes, including the practical problems of sorting and arranging large sets of data.

2.42 EXAMPLES.   (a) Suppose a group of numbered tennis players participate in a tournament. Losing a match eliminates an individual from contention. A record of the results can be given as a set S of ordered pairs: define

$$S = \{(m, n) \mid \text{ player } m \text{ defeated player } n\}$$

Thus, $(m, n) \in S$ is an abbreviation for the statement "player m defeated player n." If no one withdraws midtournament, the winner is the unique person whose number does not appear as the second coordinate of an element of S. The number of matches played by an individual is the number of elements of S in which his or her number appears as a first or second coordinate; and the total number of matches in the tournament is the number of elements of S. Question to ponder: Suppose N players enter the tournament. (Here N is a positive integer but not necessarily a power of 2.) How many matches will be played?

(b) Suppose a collection of numerical data is stored in a computer's memory. If the number m is stored in memory cell n, we make note of the ordered pair (m, n); then the set

$$T = \{(m, n) \mid m \text{ is stored at address } n\}$$

is a complete record of what numbers are where. The fact that the pairs are *ordered* is crucial if we are to avoid confusing a cell's contents with its address.

(Answer to the question in part (a): Each match has a loser, and each loser loses only once. So the number of matches is equal to the number of losers. But an N-player tournament has $N - 1$ losers, hence $N - 1$ matches.)

2.43 Definition.   The **Cartesian product** of sets A and B is the set of all ordered pairs with first coordinate in A and second coordinate in B.

Symbolically,

$$A \times B = \{(a, b)\mid a \in A \text{ and } b \in B\}$$

2.44 EXAMPLES. (a) Let $A = \{1, 2\}$ and $B = \{2, 3\}$. Then

$$A \times B = \{(1, 2), (1, 3), (2, 2), (2, 3)\}$$

and

$$B \times A = \{(2, 1), (2, 2), (3, 1), (3, 2)\}$$

So here $A \times B \neq B \times A$.

(b) The Cartesian product $\mathbb{R} \times \mathbb{R}$ is the set of all ordered pairs of real numbers. In analytic geometry, we view an ordered pair $(a, b) \in \mathbb{R} \times \mathbb{R}$ as the name of a point in the coordinatized xy-plane. Accordingly, in practice we speak of "the plane $\mathbb{R} \times \mathbb{R}$" and forget the formal definition of ordered pair. (This sort of thinking is familiar: we look at a family photograph album and exclaim "There's Shirley!" and not "There's a picture of the woman named Shirley!")

(c) A **closed interval** in $\mathbb{R}$ is a set of the form

$$[a, b] = \{x \in \mathbb{R}\mid a \leq x \leq b\}$$

In particular,

$$[0, 1] = \{x \in \mathbb{R}\mid 0 \leq x \leq 1\}$$

Then $[0, 1] \times [0, 1] = \{(x, y)\mid x, y \in [0, 1]\}$ is the **unit square** in $\mathbb{R} \times \mathbb{R}$, pictured as follows.

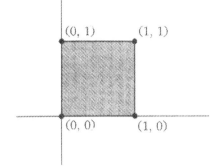

(d) In $\mathbb{R} \times \mathbb{R}$, consider the circle C_1 with radius 1 centered at the origin. (This is the **unit circle**.) Then

$$C_1 \times \mathbb{R} = \{((x, y), z) \mid x, y, z \in \mathbb{R} \text{ and } x^2 + y^2 = 1\}$$

We associate a typical element $((x, y), z)$ of $C_1 \times \mathbb{R}$ with the point (x, y, z) in coordinatized three-dimensional space. Once we do this we can interpret $C_1 \times \mathbb{R}$ as the circular cylinder of infinite length whose axis is the z-axis and whose radius is 1.

2.45 Theorem.   Let A, B, and C be sets. Then the following statements hold.

(a) $(A \cup B) \times C = (A \times C) \cup (B \times C)$
(b) $(A \cap B) \times C = (A \times C) \cap (B \times C)$
(c) $(A - B) \times C = (A \times C) - (B \times C)$
(d) If A and B are nonempty sets then

$$A \times B = B \times A \Leftrightarrow A = B$$

(e) If $A_1 \in P(A)$ and $B_1 \in P(B)$, then $A_1 \times B_1 \in P(A \times B)$.
(f) If A and B each have at least two elements, then not every element of $P(A \times B)$ has the form $A_1 \times B_1$ for some $A_1 \in P(A)$ and $B_1 \in P(B)$.
(g) $\emptyset \times A = \emptyset$

PROOF *(Partial Proof).*   First some general observations. To prove that a Cartesian product $R \times S$ is a subset of a given set T, the definition of set inclusion requires that the proof have the form

$$w \in R \times S \Rightarrow \cdots \Rightarrow w \in T$$

That is, the proof must start with "Let $w \in R \times S$" and conclude with "then $w \in T$." But we have the equivalence

$$w \in R \times S \Leftrightarrow w = (r, s) \quad \text{for some } r \in R \text{ and } s \in S$$

Accordingly, such proofs usually start with something like

$$\text{"}(r, s) \in R \times S \Rightarrow \text{"} \qquad \text{or} \qquad \text{"Let } (r, s) \in R \times S\text{"}$$

with the understanding that $r \in R$ and $s \in S$. Then "$(r, s) \in T$" will be the desired conclusion.

As we know from Theorem 2.17, to prove that sets X and Y are equal, we can first prove that $X \subseteq Y$ and then prove $Y \subseteq X$; that is, we prove the conditional statements $a \in X \Rightarrow a \in Y$ and $a \in Y \Rightarrow a \in X$. But we may be able to prove inclusion in both directions at once in the form $a \in X \Leftrightarrow a \in Y$. This bidirectional approach is always worth trying, because if it is successful (which will not always be the case) it may involve less writing. This will be our approach in the proof of part (a) here.

(a) $(x, y) \in (A \cup B) \times C \Leftrightarrow (x \in A \text{ or } x \in B) \text{ and } y \in C$

$\Leftrightarrow (x \in A \text{ and } y \in C) \text{ or}$
$(x \in B \text{ and } y \in C)$

$\Leftrightarrow (x, y) \in A \times C \text{ or } (x, y) \in B \times C$

$\Leftrightarrow (x, y) \in (A \times C) \cup (B \times C)$

The conclusion now follows from the definition of set equality. [Here the transition from the first line of the proof to the second line is via a *distributive law* from Chapter 1. See 1.34.]

(b) This part is left as an exercise.

(c) Exercise.

(d) First assume $A = B$. Then

$(x, y) \in A \times B \Leftrightarrow x \in A \text{ and } y \in B$

$\Leftrightarrow x \in B \text{ and } y \in A$ (here we use $A = B$)

$\Leftrightarrow (x, y) \in B \times A$

Therefore $A \times B = B \times A$, as desired. Conversely, suppose that $A \times B = B \times A$; let's give an indirect proof of the statement $A = B$. If $A \neq B$ then one of the sets A, B contains an element not in the other; say, $a \in A - B$. Pick any $b \in B$. (There *is* such an element b because B is nonempty by hypothesis.) Then $(a, b) \in A \times B$, and so $(a, b) \in B \times A$ (since we have assumed $A \times B = B \times A$). Hence $a \in B$, contradicting the way in which a was chosen. Thus the statement $A \neq B$ must be false.

(e) First note that the definition of the power set notation $P(\ )$ allows us to restate the proposition to be proved as follows:

$$A_1 \subseteq A \text{ and } B_1 \subseteq B \Rightarrow A_1 \times B_1 \subseteq A \times B$$

With this in mind, assume $A_1 \subseteq A$ and $B_1 \subseteq B$. Then

$$(x, y) \in A_1 \times B_1 \;\Rightarrow\; x \in A_1 \text{ and } y \in B_1$$
$$\Rightarrow\; x \in A \text{ and } y \in B \qquad \text{(from the hypothesis)}$$
$$\Rightarrow\; (x, y) \in A \times B$$

Therefore $A_1 \times B_1 \subseteq A \times B$, as claimed.

(f) Exercise.

(g) Exercise. □

Exercises

1. Let T be the collection of telephone lines for incoming calls at the Hotel Acme switchboard, and let R be the set of rooms in the hotel. Assume that each room has exactly one telephone.

   (a) Show that $T \times R$ can be interpreted as the set of all possible connections of incoming calls with room telephones.

   (b) Suppose four conversations are in progress. To what kind of subset of $T \times R$ does that correspond?

2. Show that if S is any set, then

$$\{1, 2\} \times S = (\{1\} \times S) \cup (\{2\} \times S)$$

3. Prove: $A \times B = \emptyset \Leftrightarrow A = \emptyset \text{ or } B = \emptyset$.

4. Describe the following subsets of $\mathbb{R} \times \mathbb{R}$ (viewed as the xy-plane) in words and pictures.

   (a) $[-2, 1] \times [3, 5]$

   (b) $\mathbb{Z} \times \mathbb{Z}$

   (c) $\mathbb{Z} \times \mathbb{R}$

   (d) $\mathbb{R} \times \mathbb{N}$

   (e) $[1, 2] \times \mathbb{R}$

   (f) $\mathbb{N} \times [1, 2]$

5. (a) Exhibit a subset S of $\{1, 2, 3\} \times \{1, 2, 3\}$ for which there are no sets $A, B \subseteq \{1, 2, 3\}$ such that $A \times B = S$.

   (b) Which of the following pictures represent(s) a set that has the form $A \times B$ for some $A, B \subseteq \mathbb{R}$?

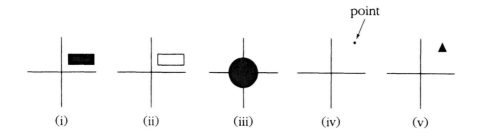

6. For elements a_1, a_2, a_3, define the *ordered triple* (a_1, a_2, a_3) by

$$(a_1, a_2, a_3) = ((a_1, a_2), a_3)$$

(a) Use the given definition to prove that if $(a_1, a_2, a_3) = (b_1, b_2, b_3)$ then $a_i = b_i$ for all i.

(b) Give a definition for the *ordered quadruple* (a_1, a_2, a_3, a_4) so that if $(a_1, a_2, a_3, a_4) = (b_1, b_2, b_3, b_4)$ then $a_i = b_i$ for all i. (Prove that your definition does the job.)

7. Prove assertions (b), (c), (f), and (g) of Theorem 2.45.

8. Prove the implication "$\Rightarrow$" in Theorem 2.40.

9. Prove the equality $(\bigcup_{i \in I} A_i) \times S = \bigcup_{i \in I} (A_i \times S)$.

2.9 Set Decomposition: Partitions and Relations

Zoologists study mammals, birds, reptiles, insects, and so on. Physiologists are concerned with body types: mesomorph, ectomorph, and endomorph. Mathematicians speak of even and odd integers; of rational and irrational numbers; of numbers that are positive, negative, or zero; and so on. People tend to classify and, indeed, *need* to classify: it helps us to sort out the universe. Our main goal in this section is to provide a mathematical framework for the notion of classification.

We begin with the concept of *partitioning* a set, which, according to standard English usage, means to break it into nonoverlapping pieces. (After World War II, Germany was partitioned into eastern and western regions. The office was partitioned in order to reduce the interaction among staff members.) Before giving a precise definition, here is a useful example.

2.46 EXAMPLE. Consider a three-piece jigsaw puzzle. How many different states of assembly are there? (Call two puzzle states different if one of them has two pieces interlocked that are not interlocked in the other.)

The answer is five, and here is a pictorial justification:

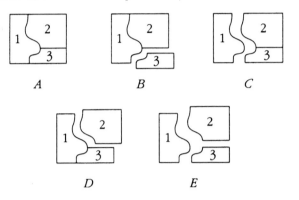

Now represent each cluster of interlocked pieces by the set containing the corresponding numbers. Then each of the pictures is represented by a family of such sets, as follows (here the Greek letter Π stands for *partition*):

$$\Pi_A = \{\{1, 2, 3\}\}$$

$$\Pi_B = \{\{1, 2\}, \{3\}\}$$

$$\Pi_C = \{\{2, 3\}, \{1\}\}$$

$$\Pi_D = \{\{1, 3\}, \{2\}\}$$

$$\Pi_E = \{\{1\}, \{2\}, \{3\}\}$$

Each of these is a family of nonempty sets whose union is the set $\{1, 2, 3\}$, and no two sets in the same family share any elements. We say that each of Π_A through Π_E is a *partition* of the set $\{1, 2, 3\}$.

The preceding example leads us to the following definition.

2.47 Definition.   Let S be a nonempty set. A **partition** Π of S is family $\Pi = \{A_i\}_{i \in I}$ of nonempty subsets of S satisfying these conditions:

$$\bigcup_{i \in I} A_i = S \qquad \text{(every member of } S \text{ belongs to some } A_i)$$

$$A_i \cap A_j = \emptyset \quad \text{if } i \neq j \qquad \text{(different pieces don't overlap)}$$

The A_i are called the **blocks** of the partition.

2.48 EXAMPLES.   (a) The set $S = \{1, 2, 3, 4\}$ has

$$\{\{1, 2, 3, 4\}\}$$

as its only one-block partition (that is, the only partition that has just one block.) It has 7 two-block partitions:

$$\{\{1\}, \{2, 3, 4\}\} \qquad \{\{2\}, \{1, 3, 4\}\} \qquad \{\{3, \}, \{1, 2, 4\}\}$$
$$\{\{4\}, \{1, 2, 3\}\} \qquad \{\{1, 2\}, \{3, 4\}\}$$
$$\{\{1, 3\}, \{2, 4\}\} \qquad \{\{1, 4\}, \{2, 3\}\}$$

It has 6 three-block partitions (Exercise: list them), and its only partition into four blocks is

$$\{\{1\}, \{2\}, \{3\}, \{4\}\}$$

(b) A jigsaw puzzle has two extreme states: full assembly and total disassembly. Similarly, a nonempty set S has two extreme partitions: the partition $\{S\}$ with only one block, and the partition into one-element blocks:

$$\{\{x\} \mid x \in S\}$$

(c) To work effectively with a large set S, we may need to partition S into smaller blocks that can be treated separately. For instance, if S is a set of real numbers, and our calculations require that we treat numbers differently according to sign, we use the partition $\Pi = \{A_1, A_2, A_3\}$, where

$$A_1 = \{x \in S \mid x > 0\} \qquad A_2 = \{x \in S \mid x < 0\} \qquad A_3 = \{0\}$$

Caution: This is a bona fide partition only if S contains positive numbers, negative numbers, and zero, because a partition's blocks are required to be nonempty.

(d) Let E be the standard xy-plane, and consider the families $\{L_i\}_{i \in \mathbb{R}}$, $\{H_r\}_{r \in \mathbb{R}}$, $\{C_r\}_{r \geq 0}$, and $\{D_r\}_{r \geq 0}$ discussed in Examples 2.28 and 2.29; call them F_1, F_2, F_3, and F_4, respectively. The family F_1 is a partition of E; for, the fact that every point is on some vertical line yields $\cup L_i = E$, and two different vertical lines are parallel and therefore don't intersect. But F_2 is not a partition of E, because distinct half-planes intersect. (Indeed, $H_r \cap H_s = H_s$ if $s \geq r$.) It is left to the reader to verify that F_3 is a partition of E and F_4 is not.

We usually decide to partition a set during the course of a procedure when there seems to be no unified method for handling all its elements simultaneously. A useful strategy is to construct a partition such that all the elements in a given block share a common feature that allows a unified treatment.

2.49 EXAMPLES. (a) The oddness or evenness of an integer is called its **parity**. The relation of "having the same parity" leads to a partition of $\mathbb{Z}$ into two blocks: the set of odd integers and the set of even integers.

(b) Let S be the set of points in the xy-plane that lie on neither axis. That is,

$$S = \{(x, y) \in \mathbb{R} \times \mathbb{R} \mid xy \neq 0\}$$

For points $P = (p_1, p_2)$ and $Q = (q_1, q_2)$ in S, we say that P and Q "are in the same quadrant" if $p_1 q_1 > 0$ and $p_2 q_2 > 0$. This partitions S into the usual four quadrants of analytic geometry. If we take as a fifth set the union of the x-axis and y-axis, we achieve a partition of $\mathbb{R} \times \mathbb{R}$ into five blocks:

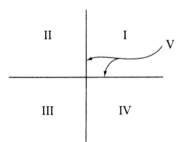

From these examples we see that the consideration of partitions leads us to study relations among elements in a set. But what exactly do we mean by a "relation"? Our objective now is to make this notion precise, to build a vocabulary for discussing the properties of relations, and to examine the interaction between relations and partitions.

Imagine that you are trying to teach the meaning of the words "larger" and "redder" to a child who has not yet learned "large" and "red." You have two apples, A_1 and A_2, to use as teaching materials. You notice that A_1 is larger than A_2, and you point this out to illustrate "larger." Then, when the child seems to understand, you move on to explain "redder" by pointing out that A_1 is redder than A_2. The result: the child comes to believe that "larger" and "redder" are synonyms. In fact, as long as the child works only with the set $S = \{A_1, A_2\}$ there is no harm in this belief, since the relations "is larger than" and "is redder than" on S both apply only to the ordered pair (A_1, A_2). Of course, to do a more effective teaching job you need a third apple, A_3. For instance, if A_3 is larger than A_1 but between A_1 and A_2 in redness, then you can distinguish between "larger" and "redder" by pointing out that on the set $\{A_1, A_2, A_3\}$, the relation "is larger than" is associated with the set of ordered pairs

$$\{(A_1, A_2), (A_3, A_1), (A_3, A_2)\}$$

while "is redder than" corresponds to the set of ordered pairs

$$\{(A_1, A_2), (A_1, A_3), (A_3, A_2)\}$$

(Of course, if you are working with a standard child you will need to use less formal terminology.) After this the child may still not have a clear understanding of the relations being defined (for that, he will need to work with sets with many more elements), but at least he will know that they are not synonyms. To sum up: the only way to distinguish between two relations on a given set is to know an ordered pair that belongs to one of the relations but not to the other. Now we can give a precise definition.

2.50 Definition. A **relation** R on a set S is a collection of ordered pairs of elements of S; that is, a subset $R \subseteq S \times S$. The assertion $(x, y) \in R$ is usually abbreviated xRy, and we say x **is related to** y **by** R. (If $(x, y) \notin R$ we write $x\not\!Ry$.)

2.51 EXAMPLES. (a) Let S be the set of all people and all dogs. Define a relation R on S by

$$pRd \Leftrightarrow (p \text{ is a person. } d \text{ is a dog, and } p \text{ owns } d)$$

Thus the relation of dog ownership is realized as a set of ordered pairs.

(b) For any set S, the relation $S \times S$ is called the **universal relation** on S, and the empty set $\emptyset$ is called the **empty relation** in this context. Neither is of serious interest. On the one hand, if everything is related to everything, then being related is no mark of distinction; on the other hand, if no two elements are related, why waste our time?

(c) The symbol "$<$" denotes a well-known relation on the set $\mathbb{R}$ of real numbers. In the formal sense of Definition 2.50, $<$ is a set of ordered pairs of real numbers, and the statement $a < b$ abbreviates the more cumbersome expression $(a, b) \in <$. Since it is our custom to picture $\mathbb{R} \times \mathbb{R}$ as the coordinatized xy-plane, we have the following formal portrait of the relation $<$ as a set of ordered pairs, where the dashed diagonal line is not included:

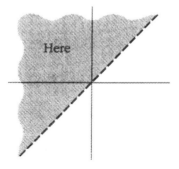

Similar considerations hold for the relation "$>$" on $\mathbb{R}$.

(d) Let L be the set of all living people. Define relations P and C on L as follows:

$$P = \{(x, y) \mid x \text{ is a parent of } y\}$$
$$C = \{(y, x) \mid y \text{ is a child of } x\}$$

Here $xPy \Leftrightarrow yCx$, and we say that each of P and C is the **inverse** of the other, written $P = C^{-1}$ and $C = P^{-1}$. Similarly, on the set $\mathbb{R}$ of real numbers, the relation $<$ is the inverse of the relation $>$.

Sometimes if we know that certain elements are paired in a given relation, that tells us something about other pairings. For example in $\mathbb{R}$, if $x \leq y$ and $y \leq z$ then $x \leq z$. The following definition gives names for three especially important properties of some relations.

2.52 Definition.   Let R be a relation on the set S. Then R is **reflexive** if xRx for all $x \in S$. The relation R is **symmetric** if for all $x, y \in S$, the implication $xRy \Rightarrow yRx$ is true. Finally, R is **transitive** if for all $x, y, z \in S$, the implication $(xRy \text{ and } yRz) \Rightarrow xRz$ is true.

2.53 EXAMPLES.   (a) Let P be the set of all people who have ever lived. Let A be the relation "is an ancestor of" (that is, $xAy \Leftrightarrow x$ is an ancestor of y) and let F be the relation "is a first cousin of." Then A is transitive but not reflexive or symmetric; and F is symmetric but not reflexive or transitive.

(b) (From a familiar children's game) Let

$$S = \{\text{rock, scissors, paper}\}$$

Define a relation B (read "beats") on S by

$$B = \{(\text{rock, scissors}), (\text{scissors, paper}), (\text{paper, rock})\}$$

In words: rock beats scissors, scissors beats paper, etc. The relation B is neither reflexive, symmetric, nor transitive. Incidentally, a similar phenomenon occurs in the ranking of professional tennis players. For instance, from the facts that Jones usually defeats Smith and Smith usually defeats Doe, we cannot conclude that Jones usually defeats Doe.

(c) Let $S = \{1, 2, 3\}$ and consider the following relations on S:

$$R_1 = \{(1, 1), (2, 2), (3, 3), (1, 2), (2, 3)\}$$
$$R_2 = \{(1, 2), (2, 3), (1, 3)\}$$
$$R_3 = \{(1, 2), (2, 1)\}$$

Then R_1 is reflexive, not symmetric (since $1R_1 2$ and $2\not R_1 1$), and not transitive (since $1R_1 2$ and $2R_1 3$, but $1\not R_1 3$). We claim that R_2 is transitive, but neither reflexive ($1\not R_2 1$) nor symmetric ($1R_2 2$ but $2\not R_2 1$). To verify transitivity of R_2, we must show that for every x, y, $z \in S$, the following implication is true:

$$(xR_2 y \text{ and } yR_2 z) \Rightarrow xR_2 z$$

Recall from Chapter 1 that an implication is true unless its hypothesis is true and its conclusion is false. But the implication's hypothesis is true only when $x = 1$, $y = 2$, $z = 3$, and in that case $xR_2 z$ is also true. Thus R_2 is transitive, as claimed. Finally, R_3 is symmetric but neither reflexive ($1\not R_3 1$) nor transitive [the implication ($1R_3 2$ and $2R_3 1$) $\Rightarrow 1R_3 1$ is false].

2.54 Exercise. Let $S = \{1, 2, 3\}$. For each pair of properties from the set

$$\{\text{reflexive, symmetric, transitive}\}$$

write down a nonempty relation on S that satisfies both properties in that pair but not the other property.

2.55 Definition.   A relation is an **equivalence relation** if it is reflexive, symmetric, and transitive. If ∼ is an equivalence relation and $x \sim y$, we say x and y are **equivalent** with respect to ∼. (The symbol "∼" is often used to denote relations, probably because it is quick to write. We will avoid using it in contexts where it might be mistaken for a negation symbol.)

2.56 EXAMPLES.   (a) Let Z be the set of all animals in a particular zoo, and define $x \sim y$ to mean that x and y are of the same species. The relation ∼ is reflexive because each animal is of the same species as itself. It is symmetric because if x and y are of the same species (thus $x \sim y$) then so are y and x (thus $y \sim x$). Finally, if x and y are of the same species, and y and z are, too, then so are x and z, and this verifies transitivity.

(b) On the set $S = \{1, 2, 3, 4\}$, the relation

$$R = \{(1, 2), (2, 1), (1, 1), (2, 2)\}$$

is symmetric and transitive (check this); but it is not reflexive since, for example, $3 \not{R} 3$. We can fortify this relation with reflexivity by adjoining more pairs: the larger relation

$$R_1 = R \cup \{(3, 3), (4, 4)\}$$

is reflexive. The relation R_1 inherits the symmetric and transitive properties of R, and R_1 is therefore an equivalence relation. Observe that R_1 was obtained by supplementing R with exactly what was essential (no more, no less) in order to get a reflexive relation containing R. We call R_1 the **reflexive closure** of R.

(c) Let S be the set of partially exposed stones in a stream that you wish to cross. For $x, y \in S$, define $x \sim y$ to mean that you can step directly from x to y without getting wet. Then ∼ is reflexive (once you're on a stone, you can hop on it) and symmetric, but *not* generally transitive: if you can step directly from x to y and from y to z, it does *not* generally follow that you can step directly from x to z. (Under what rock-and-stream conditions will ∼ be transitive?)

(d) Let S and ∼ be as in part (c). For $x, y \in S$, define $x \approx y$ to mean that you can step from x to y by a sequence of dry steps on members of S. Formally, $x \approx y$ means that there is a collection $x_1, x_2, \ldots, x_n$ of elements of S, with $x = x_1$ and $y = x_n$, such that $x_i \sim x_{i+1}$ for each

i satisfying $1 \leq i \leq n - 1$. The new relation $\approx$ is transitive, since if you get from x to y by stepping on members of S and then from y to z likewise, you have traveled from x to z by stepping on members of S. Like $\sim$, the relation $\approx$ is reflexive and symmetric; therefore $\approx$ is an equivalence relation. Notice that the relation $\approx$ has been obtained by supplementing $\sim$ with precisely those pairs needed to acquire transitivity. Accordingly, $\approx$ is called the **transitive closure** of $\sim$.

(e) On the set T of all triangles in a given plane, the relations of congruence and similarity are both equivalence relations.

2.57 Definition. If $\sim$ is an equivalence relation on a set S, the set of all elements of S that are equivalent (with respect to $\sim$) to a given element x constitute the **equivalence class** of x, denoted $[x]$. Thus

$$[x] = \{s \in S \mid s \sim x\}$$

For instance, in Example 2.56(a), if the zoo contains an elephant e, then the equivalence class $[e]$ is the set of all elephants in Z. In 2.56(b), the equivalence relation R_1 has the following equivalence classes:

$$[1] = [2] = \{1, 2\} \qquad [3] = \{3\} \qquad [4] = \{4\}$$

In part (e), if $\triangle$ is a triangle in the given plane, then, with respect to similarity, the equivalence class $[\triangle]$ consists of all the triangles in the plane that are similar to $\triangle$.

In each equivalence relation that we have discussed, notice that equivalence classes that are not equal have empty intersection. For instance, in Example 2.56(a) there is an equivalence class $[e]$ consisting of elephants and (probably) an equivalence class $[t]$ of tigers, and clearly $[e] \cap [t] = \emptyset$. In part (b), for relation R we have

$$[1] \cap [3] = \{1, 2\} \cap \{3\} = \emptyset$$

The following result generalizes the preceding observation.

2.58 Lemma. If $\sim$ is an equivalence relation and $[x] \neq [y]$, then

$$[x] \cap [y] = \emptyset$$

PROOF. We will prove the contrapositive. That is, assume $[x] \cap [y] \neq \emptyset$, and we will show that $[x] = [y]$. First we prove the inclusion $[x] \subseteq [y]$.

Let $s \in [x]$. Because $[x] \cap [y] \neq \emptyset$, there is an element $z \in [x] \cap [y]$. Thus $z \sim x$ and $z \sim y$ and so

$$z \in [x]$$
$$\downarrow$$
$$s \sim x \sim z \sim y$$
$$s \in [x] \quad z \in [y]$$

By the transitive property of $\sim$, it follows that $s \sim y$. (In greater detail: the statements $s \sim x$ and $x \sim z$ gives $s \sim z$, by transitivity; this, combined with $z \sim y$, gives $s \sim y$, again by transitivity.) Therefore $s \in [y]$, and we have shown the inclusion $[x] \subseteq [y]$. The converse inclusion $[x] \supseteq [y]$ is shown similarly, and it follows that $[x] = [y]$, as desired. $\square$

The equivalence relation "is of the same species" defined on a zoo Z [recall Example 2.56(a)] leads us to picture Z something like this:

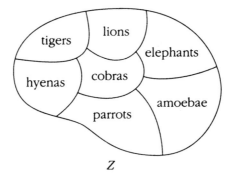

Z

Here we no longer think of Z as an unstructured assortment of animals; instead, the equivalence relation has enabled us to classify the members of Z and to cluster together all the animals of the same species. The resulting family of one-species sets (that is, the collection of "pieces" in the picture) constitutes a partition of Z. Similarly, the relation R_1 in Example 2.56(b) yields the decomposed set

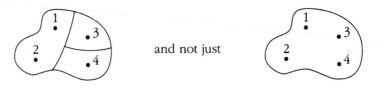

and not just

The procedure for partitioning sets via equivalence relations is made explicit in the following theorem.

2.59 Theorem. Let $\sim$ be an equivalence relation on a nonempty set S, and let Π be the family of equivalence classes determined by $\sim$. Then Π is a partition of S. (We call Π the partition **induced** by $\sim$.)

PROOF SKETCH. Begin by writing Π as an indexed set: $\Pi = \{C_i\}_{i \in I}$. By Lemma 2.58 we know that $C_i \cap C_j = \emptyset$ whenever $i \neq j$. To prove that Π is a partition it remains to check $\cup C_i = S$. Since each C_i is a subset of S, so is $\cup C_i$. (Verify this.) Conversely, if $s \in S$ then s belongs to some C_i, namely, to $[s]$ (since $s \sim s$ by reflexivity). Hence $s \in \cup C_i$, so $S \subseteq \cup C_i$, and therefore $S = \cup C_i$. □

Here is another way to design a visual representation for an equivalence relation $\sim$ on a set S of n elements. Draw a point (or **vertex**) corresponding to each member of S, and connect two vertices with an arc or line segment (or **edge**) if the corresponding members of S are related by $\sim$. For the sake of visual economy, it is customary not to draw an arc from each vertex to itself, since reflexivity is understood. The resulting collection of vertices and edges is called the **graph** of the equivalence relation $\sim$.

2.60 EXAMPLE. The equivalence relation

$$\sim = \{(1, 1), (2, 2), (3, 3), (4, 4), (5, 5), (6, 6), (1, 5), (5, 1), (2, 4),$$
$$(4, 2), (2, 6), (6, 2), (4, 6), (6, 4)\}$$

on the set $S = \{1, 2, 3, 4, 5, 6\}$ is represented by the graph

Each cluster of connected vertices represents an equivalence class, so the associated partition of S into equivalence classes is

$$\{\{1, 5\}, \{3\}, \{2, 4, 6\}\}$$

Notice how the graph and the partition display the essence of $\sim$ with an immediacy lacking in the original list of ordered pairs.

We have seen how an equivalence relation on a nonempty set S induces a partition of S into equivalence classes. Conversely, a partition of S can be used to *define* an equivalence relation. The next example is a model for this procedure, which is formalized in the subsequent theorem.

2.61 EXAMPLE. The principal of Portsmouth Junior High School assigns entering seventh-grade students to one of five homerooms by putting each student's name on a card, shuffling the deck, and dealing the deck into five piles. Once the assignments have been made, an equivalence relation emerges: students x and y are said to be related if they have the same homeroom.

2.62 Theorem. Let Π be a partition of the set S. For $x, y \in S$, define $x \sim y$ to mean that x and y belong to the same block of the partition Π. Then $\sim$ is an equivalence relation on S. (This is called the equivalence relation **induced** by the given partition.)

PROOF. Let $\Pi = \{A_i\}_{i \in I}$. Since Π is a partition, we know (by Definition 2.47) that $A_i \cap A_j = \emptyset$ when $i \neq j$, and also that $\cup A_i = S$. We must prove that the relation $\sim$ is reflexive, symmetric, and transitive.

If $x \in S$ then $x \in A_i$ for some i (since $S = \cup A_i$), and so by definition of $\sim$ we have $x \sim x$, proving reflexivity. For symmetry, if $x \sim y$ then

$$\{y, x\} = \{x, y\} \subseteq A_i \quad \text{for some } i \in I$$

and so $y \sim x$. Finally, transitivity: if $x \sim y$ and $y \sim z$ then $\{x, y\} \subseteq A_i$ and $\{y, z\} \subseteq A_j$ for some $i, j \in I$. But then $y \in A_i \cap A_j$, and therefore $i = j$ (from the definition of partition). Thus $\{x, z\} \subseteq A_i$; that is, $x \sim z$. $\square$

2.63 EXAMPLES. Let's review Examples 2.49 from the perspective of Theorem 2.62.

(a) The set $\mathbb{Z}$ of integers has a familiar partition into two blocks: $\mathbb{Z} = A \cup B$, with A the set of even integers and B the set of odd integers. The induced equivalence relation $x \sim y$ means that x and y are both even or both odd. (Another way to say it: $x \sim y$ if and only if $x - y$ is even.)

(b) Let S be the set of all points in the xy-plane that lie on neither axis. If $p_1, p_2 \in S$, define $p_1 \sim p_2$ to mean that p_1 and p_2 lie in the same quadrant. Then $\sim$ is an equivalence relation, since the four quadrants clearly partition S.

Exercises

1. Give three different partitions of each of the following sets. Do not use the trivial partition that has only one block. (Caution: Do not confuse the words "partition" and "block.")

   (a) The set $\mathbb{R}$ of real numbers

   (b) The set of all people

   (c) The set $\mathbb{Z}$ of integers

2. List all the partitions of the set $\{1, 2, 3, 4, 5\}$ that have no one-element blocks.

3. Label each of the following statements *true* or *false*.

   (a) $\{\{1, 2\}, \{3, 5\}\}$ is a partition of $\{1, 2, 3, 4, 5\}$.

   (b) $\{\{1, 2\}, \emptyset\}$ is a partition of $\{1, 2\}$.

   (c) $\{\{1, 2, 3, 4\}, \{-1\}\}$ is a partition of $\{-1, 1, 2, 3, 4\}$.

   (d) $\{\{1, 2\}, \{4, 1\}, \{3\}\}$ is a partition of $\{1, 2, 3, 4\}$.

4. Prove that if S is a set and A is a nonempty proper subset of S, then $\Pi = \{A, S - A\}$ is a partition of S.

5. If $\Pi_1 = \{A_i\}_{i \in I}$ and $\Pi_2 = \{B_j\}_{j \in J}$ are both partitions of S, we say Π_1 is **finer** than Π_2 if every A_i is contained in some B_j. [Formally, $(\forall i)(\exists j)(A_i \subseteq B_j)$. Intuitively, the blocks in Π_1 are pieces of the blocks in Π_2. Think of a finer grind of coffee bean.] For example, if $S = \{1, 2, 3, 4, 5\}$, the partition $\Pi_1 = \{\{1, 2\}, \{5\}, \{3, 4\}\}$ is finer than $\Pi_2 = \{\{1, 2, 5\}, \{3, 4\}\}$.

   (a) Give four different partitions Π_1, Π_2, Π_3, Π_4 of the set $\{1, 2, 3, 4, 5, 6\}$, with Π_i finer than Π_{i+1} for $i = 1, 2, 3$.

   (b) Do the same for the set $\mathbb{N}$ of natural numbers.

   (c) Prove that every set S has a *finest* partition Π. That is, Π has the property that if Π' is any partition of S, then Π is finer than Π'. (Suggestion: First do part (c) when $S = \{1, 2, 3\}$. Think of the smallest "pieces" into which S can be decomposed. Then do the exercise without restricting S.)

6. Let $S = \{1, 2, 3\}$. In each case give an example of a relation R on S that has the stated properties.

   (a) R is not symmetric, not reflexive, and not transitive.

   (b) R is transitive and reflexive, but not symmetric.

7. Let R be a relation on a set S. It can be shown that a unique relation R_1 exists on S with these properties:

   (a) $R_1 \supseteq R$

   (b) R_1 is reflexive

   (c) No proper subset of R_1 that contains R is reflexive.

The relation R_1 is called the **reflexive closure** of R. Now let $S = \{1, 2, 3, 4\}$, and define

$$R = \{(1, 2), (1, 3), (2, 3), (1, 4), (4, 1)\}$$

Determine the reflexive closure of R.

8. Repeat Exercise 7 with the word "reflexive" replaced by the word "symmetric" throughout.

9. Repeat Exercise 7 with the word "reflexive" replaced by the word "transitive" throughout.

10. Let C be a set of n cities. For cities, x, $y \in C$, define xRy to mean that there is a direct road from x to y that passes through no other cities along the way.

    (a) Must R be symmetric? Illustrate any negative answer with a diagram, representing cities by vertices and roads by directed (with arrowheads) arcs or line segments between the cities.

    (b) What road construction would have to be undertaken so that the resulting network of roads corresponds to the transitive closure of R? Otherwise put, what's the smallest amount of road construction that must be undertaken in order for the associated road-connection relation to be transitive?

11. We have seen (Example 2.60) how to represent an equivalence relation graphically. More generally, if R is *any* relation on an n-element set S, then R can be represented as follows. Start with a collection of n points in a plane, and label each point with the name of a different element of S; these points are the vertices of the graph. Consider each ordered pair of vertices, and connect vertices p and q with a directed edge from p to q if the ordered pair (p, q) belongs to R.

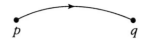

$p \qquad\qquad q$

After all such edges have been drawn, the resulting configuration is called a **directed graph** associated with R, and we will denote such a graph by $G(R)$.

    (a) Draw a directed graph for each relation in Example 2.53(c) and Example 2.56(b).

For each of the following, describe a property of $G(R)$ associated with the given condition on R.

    (b) R is symmetric.

(c) R is reflexive.

(d) R is transitive.

12. Let R and $G(R)$ be as in Exercise 11. Describe how to use $G(R)$ to obtain a directed graph for each of the following:

(a) the symmetric closure of R;

(b) the reflexive closure of R;

(c) the transitive closure of R;

(d) the inverse relation of R^{-1}.

13. Suppose R is a relation on the set $S = \{s_1, s_2, \ldots, s_n\}$. Denote the transitive closure of R by $\hat{R}$. Describe an algorithm (that is, an organized procedure) for determining all the elements $y \in S$ that satisfy the condition $s_1 \hat{R} y$. Your algorithm should involve repeated scanning of S to collect more elements that qualify. [Suggestion: For a start, notice that every element y that satisfies $s_1 R y$ also satisfies $s_1 \hat{R} y$. This gives an initial batch of elements. Then work with each of these elements in the same way that you worked with s_1, and repeat as often as necessary. Clarifying "in the same way" and "as often as necessary" is the essence of the problem. (Incidentally, the algorithm suggested here is called *breadth-first search*.)]

14. Let R be a relation on the set S. Show that if R is an equivalence relation then so is the inverse relation R^{-1}.

15. A relation R is **antisymmetric** if xRy and yRx together imply that $x = y$. A relation R on S is a **partial ordering** (or simply an **ordering**) if R is reflexive, antisymmetric, and transitive. For example, the relation "≤" on $\mathbb{R}$ is an ordering. Show that each of the following is an ordering.

(a) The inclusion relation "⊆" on the power set of a given set A.

(b) The *divisibility* relation on $\mathbb{N}$, defined as follows: if $a, b \in \mathbb{N}$, define $a \mid b$ (pronounced "a divides b") to mean that $b = ac$ for some $c \in \mathbb{N}$.

16. An ordering R on a set S (see Exercise 15) is a **linear ordering** (or **total ordering**) if every two elements of S are comparable; that is, for each $a, b \in S$ either aRb or bRa.

(a) Show that neither ordering in Exercise 15 is a total ordering. (Here assume that A has at least two elements.)

(b) Let W be the set of English words. To use a dictionary one must know the *alphabetical* (or *lexicographic*) ordering of W, which we will denote here by L. Define L precisely. (That is, carefully state the conditions under which one word precedes another in the dictionary.)

17. Let $\sim$ be an equivalence relation on the set $\{1, 2, 3\}$.

 (a) Suppose $\sim$ has exactly three ordered pairs. List them explicitly.

 (b) Is it possible that $\sim$ has exactly *four* ordered pairs? Explain.

 (c) What is the maximum possible number of ordered pairs in $\sim$? When $\sim$ is chosen with this maximum number of ordered pairs, what is the corresponding partition into equivalence classes?

18. Let S be a nonempty set. Verify that the empty relation $\emptyset$ is a symmetric and transitive relation on S, but not a reflexive relation.

19. Let A and B be sets. Many books define a *relation R from A to B* to be a subset $R \subseteq A \times B$. Show that such an R is a relation on $A \cup B$ according to Definition 2.50.

20. For each of the following, determine whether the given relation is or is not an equivalence relation. Then, if it *is* an equivalence relation, describe the partition it induces.

 (a) On the set H of human beings, define $x \sim y \Leftrightarrow x$ and y weigh within one pound of each other.

 (b) On the set C of all solid-color cars, define $x \sim y \Leftrightarrow x$ and y have the same color.

 (c) On the set $\mathbb{N}$ of positive integers, consider the *divisibility* relation defined in Exercise 15(b).

 (d) On the set $\mathbb{R}$ of real numbers, define $x \sim y \Leftrightarrow x^2 = y^2$.

 (e) On the set $\mathbb{R}$ of real numbers, define $x \sim y \Leftrightarrow xy < 0$.

 (f) On the plane $\mathbb{R} \times \mathbb{R}$, define $P \sim Q$ to mean that P and Q have the same y-coordinate.

21. Do Exercise 2.54.

22. Write out the definitions of the equivalence relations induced by the partitions $\{L_i\}_{i \in \mathbb{R}}$ and $\{C_r\}_{r \geq 0}$ discussed in Examples 2.28 and 2.29.

2.10 Mathematical Induction and Recursion

Mathematical induction is a powerful technique for proving statements about large sets, such as the set $\mathbb{N}$ of natural numbers. If we can prove that every natural number n has a certain property P, then we have in effect proved infinitely many theorems: $P(1), P(2), P(3), \ldots$. (Here we use $P(n)$ to denote the statement, "The integer n has property P.") The miracle of mathematical induction is that it enables us to carry out such a task in only a finite number of steps. Induction is closely linked to the notion of *recursion*, which is a structural framework for the definitions of many complex mathematical structures. (Recursion is also at the heart of many procedures in computer programming.) We begin with two intuitive examples that give the flavor of the inductive process.

2.64 EXAMPLES. (a) Imagine that you are swimming across a crocodile-infested lake, and your strength is fading. Suddenly a rescue helicopter arrives and drops down one end of a rope ladder. To be rescued, here is what you must do: (1) You must somehow grab the bottom step of the ladder; and (2) you must be able to get from each step to the next. The second statement needs amplification. Some steps may be slippery or otherwise special, and for your plan to be complete it must accommodate all of these difficulties. For example, getting from the first step to the second may require different strategy from the problem of getting from the eighth step for the ninth. Your plan must either handle individual differences separately or (better) be general enough to treat all cases with one set of instructions. However you do it, once you are assured that you can grab the bottom step and, having done that, that you can always get from where you are to the next level, then you know you will be rescued.

(2.65)

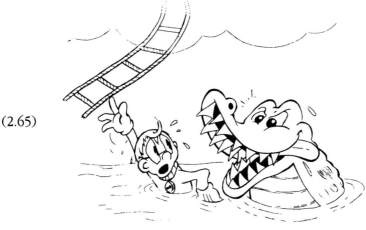

Mathematical Induction

(b) Imagine a massive line of people, beginning in front of you and extending out over the horizon, with everyone's feet embedded in cement. You believe that everyone in the line will soon catch a particular disease, and here is the outline of your proof to government officials. (1) You conduct a test showing that the first person in line has the disease. (2) You prove that the disease is *contagious*, which means that when one person catches the disease the next person will also catch it. In the manner of part (a), your proof of contagion must accommodate any special characteristics of the individuals in the line.

Our main goal in this section is to state and apply several versions of the principle of mathematical induction, which is just a formalization of the preceding examples. Though we state the principle without proof, we note that it can be deduced (in all its versions) from the following intuitively reasonable statement, called the *well-ordering principle* for $\mathbb{N}$:

Every nonempty set of natural numbers has a least element.

This principle was probably well known during the Stone Age in this form:

If everyone has a rock collection,
then someone has a smallest collection.

In what follows, we continue the convention of using $P(n)$ for the statement, "The number n has property P."

2.66 Principle of Mathematical Induction   (First Version).
Let $S \subseteq \mathbb{N}$, and suppose the following:

(a) $1 \in S$.

(b) For each $k \in \mathbb{N}$, the following implication is true:

$$k \in S \Rightarrow k + 1 \in S$$

Then $S = \mathbb{N}$.

If for some property P we have $S = \{x \in \mathbb{N} \mid P(x)\}$, then 2.66 can be reformulated as follows.

2.67 Principle of Mathematical Induction   (Second Version).
Suppose P is a property for which the following statements hold:

(a) $P(1)$.

(b) For each $k \in \mathbb{N}$, the following implication is true:

$$P(k) \Rightarrow P(k + 1)$$

Then $P(n)$ holds for every $n \in \mathbb{N}$.

Let's restate this version of the induction principle in words: To prove that every positive integer has a certain property, it's enough to show that the number 1 has the property, and then to show that whenever some number k has the property then $k + 1$ also has the property.

The act of verifying $P(1)$ is the **basis step** of the induction proof, and verifying statement (b) is the **induction step**. The statement $P(k)$ in part (b) is called the **induction hypothesis**. In the imagery of Figure 2.65, the basis step fastens our grip onto the bottom step of the ladder, and the induction step guarantees that once we reach any step, we can get to the next step. The result is that we can reach every step of the ladder. (In 2.66 and 2.67, the "ladder" has a step corresponding to each natural number.)

A technique we often use in proving the induction step is to express one or more parts of statement $P(k + 1)$ in terms of expressions involved in $P(k)$; then we can use the information supplied by $P(k)$. Incidentally, a proof by induction of a statement of the form "$P(n)$ is true for every $n \in \mathbb{N}$" is called a proof "by induction on n."

2.68 EXAMPLE. We claim that for every $n \in \mathbb{N}$,

$$1 + 2 + \cdots + n = \frac{n(n + 1)}{2}$$

This proposition is suggested by the following observation:

$$1 + 2 + 3 + \cdots + 100 = \underbrace{(1 + 100)}_{101} + \underbrace{(2 + 99)}_{101} + \underbrace{(3 + 98)}_{101}$$

$$+ \cdots + \underbrace{(50 + 51)}_{101}$$

$$= 50 \cdot 101 = \frac{100}{2} \cdot 101$$

More generally, if n is any even natural number, it is easy to believe the equation

$$(*) \qquad 1 + 2 + \cdots + n = \underbrace{1 + n}_{n+1} + \underbrace{2 + (n-1)}_{n+1} + \underbrace{3 + (n-2)}_{n+1} + \cdots$$

a sum of $n/2$ terms each equal to $n + 1$; hence the claim. A similar argument can be made if n is odd. (Try this.) Geometrically inclined individuals may be more convinced by a picture:

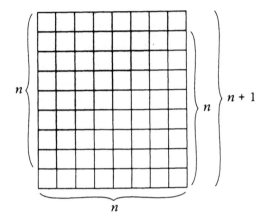

The sum $1 + 2 + \cdots + n$ is half of the rectangle's area. (Just count the white squares.)

Each of these arguments provides some insight, but each has a weak moment. The dots at the right end of $(*)$ are unsatisfying. Also, the picture actually shows an 8×9 rectangle, and perhaps we have been seduced by a special property of 8×9 rectangles that doesn't carry over to $n \times (n + 1)$ rectangles for all n. Now let's actually prove the result using mathematical induction.

DETAILED PROOF WITH SUBCONSCIOUS REMARKS. We will verify statements (a) and (b) in 2.67. Here the basis $P(1)$ is the statement $1 = 1 \cdot (1 + 1)/2$, which is clearly true. Now assume the induction hypothesis $P(k)$; that is, assume the statement is true in the case $n = k$: $1 + 2 + \cdots + k = k(k + 1)/2$. (We have already shown that $k = 1$ is such a number, but now we're assuming that k is an *unspecified* positive integer that has property P. Perhaps $k = 1$, perhaps $k = 3592$; we make no assumption about its exact value. All we assume is that k is *some* positive integer with property P.)

We must deduce that $P(k + 1)$ holds; that $1 + 2 + \cdots + (k + 1) = (k + 1)[(k + 1) + 1]/2$. We now have

$$1 + 2 + \cdots + (k + 1) = (1 + 2 + \cdots + k) + (k + 1) \quad \text{(this sets us up to apply } P(k)\text{)}$$

$$= \frac{k(k + 1)}{2} + (k + 1) \quad \text{(by induction hypothesis } P(k)\text{)}$$

$$= \frac{k(k + 1) + 2(k + 1)}{2}$$

$$= \frac{k^2 + 3k + 2}{2}$$

$$= \frac{(k + 1)(k + 2)}{2}$$

$$= \frac{(k + 1)[(k + 1) + 1]}{2} \quad \text{(by arithmetic)}$$

So $P(k + 1)$ holds, and we're done. $\quad \square$

More Standard, Concentrated Proof (Without the Mumbling)

$$P(1): \quad 1 = \frac{1 + 1}{2}$$

Assume $P(k)$: $1 + \cdots + k = k(k + 1)/2$. Then

$$1 + 2 + \cdots + (k + 1) = (1 + 2 + \cdots + k) + (k + 1)$$

$$= \frac{k(k + 1)}{2} + (k + 1) \quad \text{(by } P(k)\text{)}$$

$$= \frac{(k + 1)(k + 2)}{2}$$

which proves $P(k + 1)$. $\quad \square$

Remember, proving that we can get from one step of a ladder to the next does not prove that we can get *on* the ladder! In a proof by induction, the induction step of the proof tells us how to move up the ladder; but the basis step is needed to get us *onto* the ladder in the first place. Similarly, a proof of the conditional statement "$P(k) \Rightarrow P(k + 1)$" is not a proof of $P(k)$. In fact, for values of k for which $P(k)$ is false, the statement "$P(k) \Rightarrow P(k + 1)$" is *automatically* true; that is why we focus on thoses cases in which $P(k)$ is true. Thus the line "assume $P(k)$" is legitimate and does not represent a gap in the logic.

2.69 EXAMPLE.   Look for a pattern in the following data.

Arithmetic   *Geometry*

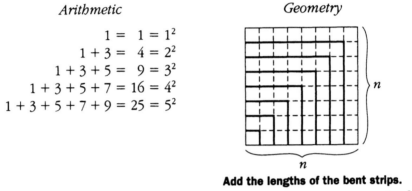

$$
\begin{aligned}
1 &= 1 = 1^2 \\
1 + 3 &= 4 = 2^2 \\
1 + 3 + 5 &= 9 = 3^2 \\
1 + 3 + 5 + 7 &= 16 = 4^2 \\
1 + 3 + 5 + 7 + 9 &= 25 = 5^2
\end{aligned}
$$

Add the lengths of the bent strips.
(There are *n* of them, and the sum is n^2.)

Based on this data, it is natural to make the following conjecture:

The sum of the first n odd natural numbers is n^2.

Notice the equalities

$$1 = 2(1) - 1; \qquad 3 = 2(2) - 1; \qquad 5 = 2(3) - 1; \qquad 7 = 2(4) - 1$$

Thus the ith odd natural number is the number $2(i) - 1$. The conjecture can now be restated like this:

$$\text{For all } n \in \mathbb{N}, \quad 1 + 3 + 5 + \cdots + (2n - 1) = n^2$$

Now for the proof by induction. Let $P(n)$ denote the equation to be proved for each n. Then, as desired,

$$P(1): \quad 2(1) - 1 = 1 = 1^2$$

Now assume $P(k)$: $1 + \cdots + (2k - 1) = k^2$. [We must prove $P(k + 1)$, that is, we must prove this equation: $1 + \cdots + (2(k + 1) - 1) = (k + 1)^2$.]

We have

$$1 + \cdots + \left(2(k+1) - 1\right) = \underbrace{1 + \cdots + (2k-1)}_{k^2} + \underbrace{\left(2(k+1) - 1\right)}_{2k+1}$$

$$= k^2 + 2k + 1 = (k+1)^2$$

The proof of the implication $P(k) \Rightarrow P(k+1)$ is now complete. $\quad\square$

Sometimes we want to prove a property to be true for every integer greater than or equal to some integer N, and for this purpose the following variant of the induction principle is needed. Notice that 2.67 is the special case of 2.70 in which $N = 1$.

2.70 Principle of Mathematical Induction (Third Version). Let N be a fixed integer. Suppose P is a property for which the following two statements hold:

(a) $P(N)$

(b) For all integers $k \geq N$, the implication

$$P(k) \Rightarrow P(k+1)$$

is true.

Then $P(n)$ is true for all integers $n \geq N$.

2.71 Theorem. If S is a set with n elements then the power set $P(S)$ has 2^n elements.

PROOF. We will use induction in the format of 2.70 with $N = 0$. Here a set with m elements will be called an m-set; and in order to avoid confusion about the meaning of $P(\ )$, in this proof we use $P(\ )$ only for the power set notation, and not for "property P holds for ...".

First consider the case $n = 0$. The only 0-set is $\emptyset$, and $P(\emptyset) = \{\emptyset\}$ is a 1-set ($1 = 2^0$). Now assume the result is true for $n = k$: the power set of a k-set is a 2^k-set. Let S be a $(k+1)$-set. Fix an element $s_0 \in S$. Then $S = \{s_0\} \cup T$, where T is a k-set. With each subset $A \subseteq T$ we associate two subsets of S, namely, A and $A \cup \{s_0\}$. This accounts for every subset of S. (Why?) Thus S has twice as many subsets as T. But by the induction hypothesis for k-sets, T has 2^k subsets, and therefore S has $2 \cdot 2^k = 2^{k+1}$ subsets. $\quad\square$

We will extend this result on the comparative sizes of a set and its power set in Chapter 4 (see Cantor's theorem).

In constructing an induction proof, it is not always an easy matter to recognize how to use the induction hypothesis $P(k)$ in proving $P(k + 1)$. The following example is a result in elementary number theory; here the key to the arithmetic juggling is the addition of zero to an expression in such a way as to force the quantity in $P(k)$ to appear. Recall that an integer x is a **multiple** of an integer y if $x = yt$ for some integer t.

2.72 EXAMPLE.   Prove that for every integer $n \geq 0$, the number $4^{2n+1} + 3^{n+2}$ is a multiple of 13.

PROOF.   We use induction on n, starting with $n = 0$.

$$P(0): \quad 4^{2(0)+1} + 3^{0+2} = 4 + 9 = 13 = 13 \cdot 1$$

Assume $P(k)$: $4^{2k+1} + 3^{k+2} = 13t$ for some integer t. We must prove

$$P(k + 1): \quad 4^{2(k+1)+1} + 3^{(k+1)+2} \text{ is a multiple of 13.}$$

We have

$$4^{2(k+1)+1} + 3^{(k+1)+2} = 4^{(2k+1)+2} + 3^{(k+2)+1}$$

$$= 4^2(4^{2k+1}) + 4^2 \underbrace{(3^{k+2} - 3^{k+2})}_{0} + 3 \cdot 3^{k+2}$$

$$= 4^2(4^{2k+1} + 3^{k+2}) + 3^{k+2}(-4^2 + 3)$$

$$= 16 \cdot 13t + 3^{k+2} \cdot (-13) \qquad \text{(by } P(k)\text{)}$$

$$= 13(16t - 3^{k+2}), \quad \text{a multiple of 13} \qquad \square$$

Sometimes we want to carry out an induction argument, but we need more than $P(k)$ to deduce $P(k + 1)$. For this purpose the following formulation of the induction principle is useful.

2.73 Principle of Mathematical Induction   (Fourth Version). Let N be a fixed integer. Suppose P is a property for which the following two statements are true:

(a) $P(N)$

(b) For every integer $k \geq N$, if $P(t)$ is true for all integers t satisfying $N \leq t \leq k$, then also $P(k + 1)$ is true.

Then $P(n)$ is true for every integer $n \geq N$.

Once again we illustrate with a result from number theory. Recall that a **prime number** is an integer $p > 1$ that has no integer factorization $p = ab$ in which $a > 1$ and $b > 1$.

2.74 Theorem. Every integer $n \geq 2$ is a product of prime numbers. (Here a prime number is itself to be viewed as a one-factor product of prime numbers.)

PROOF. We argue by induction on n, using 2.73. The number 2 is clearly prime, so the result holds when $n = 2$.

Now suppose for some $k \geq 2$ that every integer t satisfying $2 \leq t \leq k$ is a product of primes; we must now show $k + 1$ to be a product of primes. If $k + 1$ is prime we are done. Otherwise write $k + 1 = ab$, with $a > 1$ and $b > 1$. Then in fact $2 \leq a \leq k$ and $2 \leq b \leq k$, so by the induction hypothesis, a and b are both products of primes, say, $a = p_1 \ldots p_r$ and $b = p_{r+1} \cdots p_s$, where the p's are primes. Then $k + 1 = ab = p_1 \cdots p_r \cdot p_{r+1} \cdots p_s$, and the proof is complete. $\square$

Notice in the proof of Theorem 2.74 that $P(k)$ by itself would not have enabled us to prove $P(k + 1)$, since there is no obvious link between the factorizations of k and $k+1$. Accordingly, we used mathematical induction in the form given by 2.73; a direct application of 2.67 could not have done the job. Having said that, we also note (without proof) that all forms of the induction principle stated here are equivalent, in the sense that any one of the four can be used to prove any of the others.

We conclude this section with a brief discussion of recursion, an induction-like format for certain mathematical definitions. Suppose for each positive integer n we want to calculate the sum $s_n = 1 + 2 + 3 \cdots + n$. Having cranked out $s_{10} = 55$, how should we then compute s_{11}? Rather than start from scratch ("1 plus 2 plus 3 plus 4" and so on), surely the most efficient thing to do would be simply to add 11 to 55. More generally, having computed s_k for some k, then $s_{k+1} = (k + 1) + s_k$. In other words, the procedure for computing the required value associated with a given number > 1 consists of first carrying out the procedure for the predecessor of the number and then adding the given number to this result. We say that the numbers s_n are defined *recursively* by the following equations:

$$s_1 = 1$$

$$s_{k+1} = (k + 1) + s_k$$

This definition gives us a procedure for computing s_n for each $n \in \mathbb{N}$.

More generally, suppose a nu ber a_i is given for each $i \in \mathbb{N}$. The intuitive expression $a_1 + a_2 + \cdots + a_n$ is usually abbreviated

$$\textbf{summation symbol:} \quad \sum_{i=1}^{n} a_i$$

The following recursive scheme formally defines this symbol for each $n \in \mathbb{N}$. In effect, the definition is a "program" for evaluating the symbol.

$$\sum_{i=1}^{1} a_i = a_1$$

$$\sum_{i=1}^{k+1} a_i = \left(\sum_{i=1}^{k} a_i \right) + a_{k+1}$$

Like induction, recursion deals with a sequence of instances by first "initializing" and then considering subsequent instances in terms of what has come before. We finish this section with a few more examples of recursive definitions.

We recursively define the

$$\textbf{product symbol:} \quad \prod_{i=1}^{n} a_i \qquad \text{and} \qquad \textbf{factorial symbol:} \quad n!$$

respectively, by

$$\left. \begin{array}{l} \prod_{i=1}^{1} a_i = a_1 \\[2ex] \prod_{i=1}^{k+1} a_i = \left(\prod_{i=1}^{k} a_i \right) \cdot a_{k+1} \end{array} \right\} \quad \text{and} \quad \left\{ \begin{array}{l} 0! = 1 \\[1ex] (k + 1)! = k!(k + 1) \end{array} \right.$$

In a line of text, the sum and product symbols will usually appear as $\sum_{i=1}^{n} a_i$ and $\prod_{i=1}^{n} a_i$, respectively.

Similariy, we can define families of sets recursively. For example,

$$A_1 = \{1, 5\}$$

$$A_{k+1} = P(A_k) \qquad (P(\ ) \text{ is the power set notation})$$

defines a set A_n for each $n \in \mathbb{N}$.

We will return to recursion when we discuss *sequences* in Chapter 3.

Exercises

1. Use mathematical induction to prove the following statement for every $n \in \mathbb{N}$:

$$1^2 + 2^2 + \cdots + n^2 = \frac{n(n+1)(2n+1)}{6}$$

2. Prove for every integer $n \geq 1$:

$$1^3 + 2^3 + \cdots + n^3 = \left(\frac{n(n+1)}{2}\right)^2$$

3. Prove that the inequality $n^2 \geq n$ holds *for every integer.*

4. Prove that for every integer $n \geq 0$ the number $n^4 - 4n^2$ is divisible by 3.

5. Assume that $S \subseteq \mathbb{N}$ and $3 \in S$, and assume further that the implication

$$x \in S \implies x + 3 \in S$$

is true. Deduce that

$$\{3n \mid n \in \mathbb{N}\} \subseteq S$$

6. Prove for every integer $n \geq 2$:

$$\frac{1}{1 \cdot 2} + \frac{1}{2 \cdot 3} + \cdots + \frac{1}{(n-1)n} = 1 - \frac{1}{n}$$

7. Prove that $2^n > n^3$ for every integer $n \geq 10$.

8. What is wrong (if anything) with the following induction argument?
   Proposition. All horses are the same color.
   "Proof" outline. It suffices to show for every $n \in \mathbb{N}$ that in any collection of n horses, all n of them are the same color. If $n = 1$

the result is trivial. Now assume that in any collection of k horses, all k horses are the same color. Consider a set of $k + 1$ horses. By the induction hypothesis, the first k horses are the same color and the last k horses are the same color. But the first and last are the same color as the middle horses.

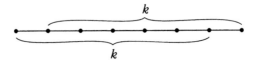

Therefore all the horses are the same color.

9. It is claimed that every positive real number α has the property $\alpha^{n-1} = 1$ for all $n \in \mathbb{N}$, and here is a "proof" using the principle of mathematical induction (fourth version). If $n = 1$ we have $\alpha^{n-1} = \alpha^{1-1} = \alpha^0 = 1$, as desired. Now suppose the result has been checked for all values of n satisfying $1 \le n \le k$. Then

$$\alpha^{(k+1)-1} = \alpha^k = \frac{\alpha^{k-1} \cdot \alpha^{k-1}}{\alpha^{k-2}}$$

$$= \frac{1 \cdot 1}{1} \qquad \text{(by the induction hypothesis)}$$

$$= 1 \quad \square$$

Is the claim now proved? Explain.

10. For each $i \in \mathbb{N}$, assume a_i is a positive real number. There is ambiguity to the exponential expression

(*) $$a_n^{a_{n-1}^{\cdot^{\cdot^{\cdot^{a_2^{a_1}}}}}}$$

(For example, does 2^{3^4} mean $2^{(3^4)} = 2^{81}$ or $(2^3)^4 = 2^{12}$?) Write a recursive procedure for computing (*), with the interpretation that the exponent of each a_i is everything above it.

11. Use the well-ordering principle to prove the principle of mathematical induction as stated in 2.67. (Suggestion: Suppose there is a nonempty set A of natural numbers n for which $P(n)$ is *false*. Apply the well-ordering principle to A to get a contradiction of the hypothesis of 2.67.)

12. For each $i \in N$, let $a_i = 3^{i-2}$. Evaluate

$$\sum_{i=1}^{5} a_i \qquad \text{and} \qquad \prod_{i=1}^{5} a_i$$

13. Assume that $a > 0$ and $n \in \mathbb{N}$; and for each $i \in \mathbb{N}$ let $b_i \in \mathbb{R}$. Use mathematical induction and the laws of exponents to prove that

$$\prod_{i=1}^{n} a^{b_i} = a^{\left(\sum_{i=1}^{n} b_i\right)} \qquad \text{for all } n \in \mathbb{N}$$

(Here the left-hand expression means $\prod_{i=1}^{n} c_i$, where $c_i = a^{b_i}$.)

14. If we were to compute the gigantic integer $N = 100!$, how many zeroes would appear on the right-hand side of N? That is, N would have the form $m \cdot 10^k$, where m is not a multiple of 10; your job is to determine k.

FUNCTIONS

A group of Hungarian aristocrats lost their way hiking in the Alps. One of them, it is said, took out a map, and after studying it for a long time, exclaimed: "Now I know where we are!" "Where?" asked the others. "See that big mountain over there? We are right on top of it."

GEORGE GAMOW
One Two Three . . . Infinity

3.1 Definitions and Examples

In Chapter 2 we introduced sets: what they are, how to build new ones from old ones, and how to decompose them into subsets. In this chapter we will begin to consider more dynamic set interactions, called *functions*, which link the elements of one set to elements of another in a rather special way.

The theory of functions provides the foundation for what is called *mathematical modelling*, whereby one mathematical object represents certain features of another or of some nonmathematical object, perhaps with the elimination of some distracting complexities. Moreover, functions give a mathematically precise framework for the intuitive idea of *transformation*. Ordered pairs are fundamental for everything that we will be discussing here.

117

3.1 EXAMPLES.   (a) Each member of a television studio audience takes a numbered raffle ticket from a well-mixed bowl; this associates a unique number with each member of the audience. A complete record of this data is a list of ordered pairs of the form {(John Doe, 467). (Molly Brown, 93)...}, with one pair for each audience member.

(b) Pair each real number with its square; this process produces the set of all ordered pairs of the form (x, x^2) for $x \in \mathbb{R}$.

Notice that in Example 3.1(a), no two people are paired with the same number, while in 3.1(b) a nonzero number x and its negative are both paired with x^2. Both examples in 3.1 are functions, according to the definition about to be given, but we will find it useful to remain aware of this distinction between them.

Now we are ready for a precise definition of function. First recall that the *Cartesian product* $A \times B$ of sets A and B is the set of all ordered pairs of the form (a, b), with $a \in A$ and $b \in B$.

3.2 Definition.   Let A and B be sets. A **function** f **from** A **to** B is a set of ordered pairs

$$f \subseteq A \times B$$

with the property that for each element x in A there is exactly one element y in B such that $(x, y) \in f$. The statement "f is a function from A to B" is usually represented symbolically by

$$f : A \to B \qquad \text{or} \qquad A \xrightarrow{f} B$$

In Example 3.1(a), the given set of ordered pairs is a function from the audience to the set of ticket numbers; and in 3.1(b) the given set of pairs is a function from $\mathbb{R}$ to $\mathbb{R}$.

Suppose f is a function from A to B. Then A is called the **domain** of f, denoted **dom** f; its members are the first coordinates of the ordered pairs belonging to f. If $(x, y) \in f$ we usually write $y = f(x)$ and call y the **image** of x; and x is a **pre-image** of y. In Example 3.1(a) the domain is the audience, and $f(\text{Molly Brown}) = 93$. In Example 3.1(b) the domain is the set $\mathbb{R}$ of real numbers, and $f(-.2) = f(.2) = .04$; so $-.2$ and $.2$ are both preimages of $.04$.

Notice that in 3.1(a) there is no abbreviated way to present the function: all the pairs must be listed if we are to know what the number assignments are. On the other hand, in 3.1(b) an explicit listing of all the pairs is impossible, but we can .completely describe the function by giving the rule

$$f(x) = x^2 \quad \text{for all } x \in \mathbb{R}$$

Thus it is sometimes convenient to view a function as a set of ordered pairs, as in the definition; and at other times we will view a function f from A to B as *a rule or formula for pairing each member of A with a unique element of B.* Also, we may think of f as a kind of programmed machine that emits a unique element of B whenever an element of A is fed in: input x always yields output $f(x)$.

If $y = f(x)$, we sometimes say that f **transforms** or **takes** x to y denoted by $x \overset{f}{\longmapsto} y$ or $x \longmapsto y$. We also say that f **acts** or **operates** on the members of its domain. An unnamed function from A to B is often indicated by $A \to B$. Functions are also called **mappings, maps,** or **transformations**.

3.3 EXAMPLES. (a) Suppose $S \subseteq T$. Define a function i from S to T by

$$i(x) = x \quad \text{for all } x \in S$$

This is called the **inclusion mapping**. If, in this setting, $S = T$, we write $i = i_s$ and call it the **identity mapping** on S.

(b) Given nonempty sets A and B, fix an element $b_0 \in B$ and define a function f from A to B by

$$f(a) = b_0 \quad \text{for all } a \in A$$

As a set of ordered pairs, $f = \{(a, b_0) \mid a \in A\}$. This is called the **constant function** with value b_0.

(c) Let F be the set of all the living fathers of living daughters, and let D be the set of all the living daughters of living fathers. Define

$$g = \{(x, y) \mid x \in F \text{ and } y \text{ is the daughter of } x\}$$

Is g a function from F to D? (Pause and think, *then* read on.) We have $g \subseteq F \times D$, and for each $x \in F$ there is a $y \in D$ such that $(x, y) \in g$. So far so good. But if a father x has two living daughters, say with the delightful names y_1 and y_2, then $(x, y_1) \in g$ *and* $(x, y_2) \in g$, contradicting the "exactly one" condition in the definition of function.

Therefore g is *not* a function. On the other hand, if

$$h = \{(y, x) \mid y \in D \text{ and } x \text{ is the father of } y\}$$

then h is a function from D to F, since every daughter has exactly one father.

(d) What happens when we depress a key on a computer keyboard? Clearly the answer depends on two things: the state of the machine (for example, the model, the data that has already been fed in) and our choice of key. That is, the new state is determined by the ordered pair (q, σ), where q is the former state and σ is the input symbol. Thus if S denotes the set of all possible states of the machine, and Σ denotes the set of keyboard symbols, there is a function

$$\delta : S \times \Sigma \longrightarrow S$$

defined as follows: $\delta((q, \sigma)) = q'$ means that if the symbol σ is received as input when the machine is in state q, then the machine will go to state q'. The function δ is called the **transition function** for the machine. Notice a new wrinkle in this example: the members of the domain of δ are themselves ordered pairs. In this situation it is customary to suppress one pair of parentheses and write $\delta(q, \sigma)$ instead of $\delta((q, \sigma))$. We will follow this practice from now on.

(e) Let S be the set of all propositions, that is, the set of all truth-valued statements. Define the **truth-value function**

$$v : S \longrightarrow \{T, F\}$$

by

$$v(P) = \begin{cases} T & \text{if } P \text{ is a true proposition} \\ F & \text{if } P \text{ is a false proposition} \end{cases}$$

As we saw in Chapter 1, if we know the values taken by v on some propositions, we can deduce its values on others. For instance, if $v(P) = T$ and $v(Q) = F$, then $v(P \wedge Q) = F$ and $v(P \vee Q) = T$.

(f) A function $f : \mathbb{R} \to \mathbb{R}$ is said to be a **polynomial function of degree** n if there are real numbers $a_0, a_1, \ldots, a_n$, with $a_n \neq 0$, such that

$$(*) \qquad f(x) = a_n x^n + a_{n-1} x^{n-1} + \cdots + a_1 x + a_0$$

for all $x \in \mathbb{R}$. The numbers $a_0, a_1, \ldots, a_n$ are called the **coefficients** of f. (It is a fact, but not an *obvious* one, that the coefficients of f are uniquely determined by f. That is, the formula for f cannot be rewritten using other coefficients in place of the given ones without producing a different function. We will omit the proof here.)

A function $f : A \to B$ can be informally represented by a picture, as follows:

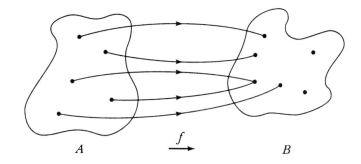

with the understanding that each point in A is taken by f to the point in B to which it is connected in the picture. If A and B are sets of real numbers, then $f \subseteq A \times B \subseteq \mathbb{R} \times \mathbb{R}$, and the pairs $(x, y) \in f$ can be represented as points in the usual coordinatized plane. The resulting diagram is the **graph** of f. For example, the graph of the function $f(x) = x^2$ is following familiar parabola.

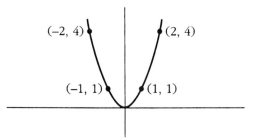

So the graph of a function $\mathbb{R} \to \mathbb{R}$ is just a pictorial representation of the ordered pairs belonging to it.

3.4 EXAMPLE. A function whose domain or image is not a set of numbers may not be representable by a graph in any obvious way. For instance, if A is the set of all college sophomores (as you read this sentence), B is the set of all photographs ever taken, and $f : A \to B$ pairs each sophomore with the picture he or she has seen most recently, there is no evident "*x*-axis" on which to locate the sophomores, nor is there a "*y*-axis" that holds the photographs. There are many interesting and important functions that don't involve numbers (and hence don't involve graphs), and we will therefore need to develop a language for describing functions in a way that is not "graph-dependent."

We have defined a function as a set of ordered pairs satisfying certain conditions; accordingly, functions f and g are **equal** if they are the same sets of ordered pairs. Let's reformulate this statement. Notice that dom f consists of all the first-coordinate elements x in the pairs (x, y) belonging to f and g. The equation $f = g$ also implies that each element $x \in$ dom f is taken to (that is, paired with) the same element by f as it is by g. It follows that

$$(3.5) \qquad f = g \quad \Leftrightarrow \quad \begin{cases} \text{dom } f = \text{dom } g \\ \qquad \text{and} \\ f(x) = g(x) \quad \forall x \in \text{dom } f \end{cases}$$

In computer jargon: functions f and g are equal if they have the same sets of acceptable input and produce the same output for each piece of input.

3.6 EXAMPLE.   Consider functions f, g, h defined by

$$f(x) = x^2 - 1 \quad \forall x \in \mathbb{Z}$$

$$g(x) = x^2 - 1 \quad \forall x \in \mathbb{R}$$

$$h(x) = (x + 1)(x - 1) \quad \forall x \in \mathbb{R}$$

Here $g = h$: both functions have domain $\mathbb{R}$, and $g(x) = h(x)$ for all $x \in \mathbb{R}$. Thus the truth of "$g = h$" follows from 3.5, but *not* from the less precise view of a function as a "rule or formula." (Indeed, the given formulas for g and h dictate different computational procedures.) But $f \neq g$ since dom $f = \mathbb{Z} \neq \mathbb{R} = $ dom g. (That is, f and g have different sets of acceptable input.)

The functions f and g in Example 3.6 operate via the same formula, but f applies that formula to a more restricted domain; accordingly, f is called the **restriction** of g to $\mathbb{Z}$, denoted $f = g|_{\mathbb{Z}}$. More generally:

3.7 Definition.   Let f and g be functions. Suppose that dom $f = A \subseteq$ dom $g = B$, and $f(x) = g(x)$ for all $x \in A$. Then f is called the

restriction of g to A, written $f = g|_A$; and g is called an **extension of f to B**.

3.8 EXAMPLES. (a) Let $f = \{(1, 3), (3, 2)\}$ and $g = \{(1, 3), (2, 2), (3, 2)\}$. Then f and g are functions, with dom $f = \{1, 3\}$ and dom $g = \{1, 2, 3\}$. Moreover, $f(1) = g(1) = 3$ and $f(3) = g(3) = 2$. Therefore $f = g|_{\{1,3\}}$.

(b) For any real number x, let $[x]$ denote the greatest integer less than or equal to x. Thus $[\pi] = 3$, $[\sqrt{2}] = 1$, $[-2.4] = -3$, and $[-5] = -5$. The function $f: \mathbb{R} \to \mathbb{R}$ given by $x \mapsto [x]$ is called the **greatest integer function**. Notice that $[x] = x$ for all $x \in \mathbb{Z}$; thus $f|_{\mathbb{Z}} = i_{\mathbb{Z}}$, the identity function on $\mathbb{Z}$. (See Example 3.3(a).) It follows that the greatest integer function and the identity function $i_{\mathbb{R}}$ are both extensions of $i_{\mathbb{Z}}$ to $\mathbb{R}$.

Exercises

1. Let $A = \{1, 2, 3, 4\}$ and $B = \{2, \pi, e\}$. Which of the following sets of ordered pairs are functions from A to B? Explain each case in which your answer is negative.
   (a) $f = \{(1, \pi), (3, \pi), (4, \pi), (2, e)\}$
   (b) $g = \{(1, e), (2, e), (3, \pi), (2, e), (4, 2)\}$
   (c) $h = \{(1, 2), (2, 2), (3, \pi), (4, 2), (1, \pi)\}$
   (d) $j = \{(2, \pi), (3, e)\}$.
2. (a) Give sets A and B such that the following set f is a function from A to B: $f = \{(3, 2), (1, 1), (8, 5), (9, -4), (\pi, 1)\}$.
   (b) With f as in part (a), $f(8) = $ _____ and the pre-image(s) of 2 is (are) _____.
3. Let X and Y be nonempty sets. Show that the Cartesian product $X \times Y$ is a function if and only if Y has exactly one element.
4. For functions whose domains are sets of real numbers, it is common practice to use a formula to describe a function's pairing rule, with the understanding that the domain of the function is the set of all real numbers for which the formula gives a unique real number, unless further restrictions are imposed. For example, the function f given by $f(x) = \sqrt{x - 3}$ has domain $\{x \in \mathbb{R} \mid x \geq 3\}$, for if $x \geq 3$ the formula gives a unique real number, while if $x < 3$ then $x - 3 < 0$ and no square root exists. (Recall that $\sqrt{w}$ is the nonnegative real number whose square is w.) In each of the following, determine the domains of f and g, and then use statement 3.5 in the text to determine whether f and g are equal.

(a) $f(x) = 1, \quad g(x) = \dfrac{x - 5}{x - 5}$

(b) $f(x) = \sqrt{x}, \quad g(x) = \sqrt{|x|}$

(c) $f(x) = |x|, \quad g(x) = \sqrt{x^2}$

(d) $f(x) = x^2 - x - 6, \quad g(x) = (x - 4)(x + 3) + 6$

(e) $f(x) = x^2, \quad g(x) = \begin{cases} x^2 & \text{if } x \text{ is rational} \\ 0 & \text{if } x \text{ is irrational} \end{cases}$

5. Let S and T be sets of three elements. How many functions are there from S to T? Justify briefly.

6. Suppose a function $f : A \to B$ is given. Define a relation $\sim$ on A as follows:

$$a_1 \sim a_2 \quad \Leftrightarrow \quad f(a_1) = f(a_2)$$

(a) Prove that $\sim$ is an *equivalence relation* on A.

Since $\sim$ is an equivalence relation, it induces a *partition* of A into equivalence classes. Describe these equivalence classes in each of the following cases.

(b) A is the set of all solid-color cars, B is the set of all colors, $f(x)$ is the color of x.

(c) $A = B = \mathbb{R}, \ f(x) = x^2$

(d) $A = B = \mathbb{R}, \ f(x) = |x|$

(e) $A = \mathbb{R} \times \mathbb{R}, \ B = P(\mathbb{R})$ (the *power set* of $\mathbb{R}$), $f(x, y) = \{x, y\}$

(f) $A = \mathbb{R} \times \mathbb{R}, \ B = \mathbb{R}, \ f(x, y) = x + y$

(g) $A = \mathbb{R} \times \mathbb{R}, \ B = \mathbb{R}, \ f(x, y) = x^2 + y^2$

7. Let S be a set. For each subset $A \subseteq S$ define a function $\chi_A : S \to \{0, 1\}$, called the **characteristic function** of A, as follows:

$$\chi_A(x) = \begin{cases} 1 & \text{if } x \in A \\ 0 & \text{if } x \notin A \end{cases}$$

For example, if $S = \{1, 2, 3, 4\}$ and $A = \{1, 2, 4\}$, then $\chi_a(1) = \chi_A(2) = \chi_A(4) = 1$ and $\chi_A(3) = 0$.

(a) Give the formulas for the characteristic functions $\chi_\emptyset$ and χ_S.

(b) Let A' denote the complement of A in S. Compare the formulas for χ_A and $\chi_{A'}$.

(c) Show that if A and B are subsets of S then

$$A = B \quad \Leftrightarrow \quad \chi_A = \chi_B$$

(The proof will involve the careful consideration of *set equality*, which appears in the left-hand statement, and *function equality*, which appears in the right-hand statement.)

(d) Show that if A and B are subsets of S then

$$\chi_{A \cap B}(x) = \chi_A(x) \cdot \chi_B(x) \quad \forall x \in S$$

$$\chi_{A \cup B}(x) = \chi_A(x) + \chi_B(x) - \chi_A(x)\chi_B(x) \quad \forall x \in S$$

(Suggestion: Draw a Venn diagram that represents A and B sitting inside S. Then compare the values obtained on both sides of the alleged equations as x is considered in different sections of the diagram.)

8. This exercise uses the notation of Example 3.3(d).

   (a) Fix $q_0 \in S$. What is the intuitive meaning of the following set?

   $$\{\delta(q_0, \sigma) \mid \sigma \in \Sigma\}$$

   (b) Fix $\sigma_0 \in \Sigma$. What is the intuitive meaning of the following set?

   $$\{\delta(q, \sigma_0) \mid q \in S\}$$

   (c) Suppose that with the machine initially in state q_0, the symbol σ_1 is typed on the keyboard, and then the symbol σ_2 is typed. (That is, the two-letter "word" $\sigma_1 \sigma_2$ is typed.) Write an expression that represents the resulting state of the machine.

   (d) Generalize part (c) by writing an expression that represents the resulting state when the n-letter word $\sigma_1 \sigma_2 \cdots \sigma_n$ is input. Assume that the initial state is q_0.

9. This exercise deals with properties of the **greatest integer function**, $f(x) = [x]$. (See Example 3.8(b).)

   (a) Write a simple formula for $[\alpha] + [-\alpha]$, where $\alpha \in \mathbb{R}$.

   (b) Show that if n is an integer then

   $$n + [\alpha] = [n + \alpha] \quad \text{for all } \alpha \in \mathbb{R}$$

   (c) Suppose α is a real number that is not an integer, and suppose further that $\alpha > 2$. Show that there is a real number β in the interval $(1, 2)$ such that

   $$[\alpha][\beta] < [[\alpha]\beta]$$

   (d) Let n and m be positive integers. Show (without proving all the details) that there are exactly $[n/m]$ integers x that are multiples of m and satisfy the inequality $1 \leq x \leq n$.

(e) Part (d) can be used to show that the highest power of 7 that is a divisor of 1000! is

$$\left[\frac{1000}{7}\right] + \left[\frac{1000}{49}\right] + \left[\frac{1000}{343}\right] = 142 + 20 + 2 = 164$$

(That is, 7^{164} is a divisor of 1000!, but 7^{165} is not.) Give a convincing explanation of why this is so.

10. This exercise concerns two functions that, like the greatest integer function, assign a nearby integer to each real number. Give a formula for each of them in terms of the greatest integer function.

   (a) The **nearest integer function**: $f(x)$ is the nearest integer to x; if x is midway between two integers, $f(x)$ is the larger of the two.

   (b) The **ceiling function**: $f(x)$ is the smallest integer that is greater than or equal to x.

   [The greatest integer function is also called the **floor function**. The notations $\lfloor x \rfloor$ and $\lceil x \rceil$ are sometimes used for the floor and ceiling of x, respectively. (The zealous reader may wish to call $\lfloor x \rfloor - 1$ and $\lceil x \rceil + 1$ the "basement" and "attic" of x, respectively, but this is not standard terminology.)]

11. If A and B are sets, let B^A denote the set of all functions from A to B.

   (a) Determine the set $\{1, 2\}^{\{1,2\}}$. That is, list its members explicitly.

   (b) Show that if A, B, C are sets, and $A \subseteq B$, then $A^C \subseteq B^C$.

   (c) Show that the sets $\{1, 2\}^{\{1,2\}}$ and $\{1, 2\}^{\{1,2,3\}}$ are disjoint.

   (d) Generalize part (c) by showing that if $B \neq C$ then $A^B \cap A^C = \emptyset$.

   (e) Show that if A is a nonempty set then $\emptyset^A = \emptyset$.

   (f) Show that if B is any set then $B^{\emptyset} = \{\emptyset\}$.

3.2 Surjections, Injections, Bijections, Sequences

A function $f : A \to B$ might not use every element of B as an image of some element of A. The subset of B consisting of all those elements of B that *are* images is called the **range** or **image** of f, usually denoted $f(A)$ or **im** f. Thus

$$f(A) = \text{im } f = \{f(a) \mid a \in A\}$$

If we view f as a set of ordered pairs (as in Definition 3.2) then we have

$$\text{im } f = \{b \in B \mid (a, b) \in f \text{ for some } a \in A\}$$
$$= \{b \in B \mid f(a) = b \text{ for some } a \in A\}$$

More generally, if $S \subseteq A$ we write

(3.9) $$f(S) = \{f(x) \mid x \in S\}$$

In a picture:

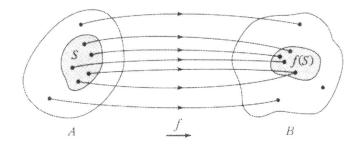

For example, for the trigonometric function sin: $\mathbb{R} \to \mathbb{R}$, we have dom(sin) = $\mathbb{R}$, with sin($\mathbb{R}$) = $[-1, 1]$, and sin($[0, \pi/2]$) = $[0, 1]$.

A function $f: A \to B$ is said to be **surjective with respect to** B or **onto** B if $f(A) = B$; equivalently, for each $b \in B$ there exists an element $a \in A$ such that $f(a) = b$. If the set B is understood from the context, we usually say more briefly that such a function f is **surjective** or **onto**, and f is said to be a **surjection**. Notice that the definition dictates a method for *proving* that a function f is surjective: we pick an element $b \in B$, and then we show that its being in B guarantees the existence of an element $a \in A$ such that $f(a) = b$. (In fact *every* function takes its domain onto its range. Therefore a statement to the effect that a given function $f: A \to B$ is "onto" actually gives us information only because B has been specified, so that we know the answer to the question "'Onto *what?*")

3.10 EXAMPLES. (a) The function $f: \mathbb{R} \to \mathbb{R}$ given by the formula $f(x) = x^2$ is not surjective, because if $y < 0$ no element $x \in \mathbb{R}$ can be found such that $f(x) = y$.

(b) The function $g: \mathbb{R} \to \mathbb{R}$ given by $g(x) = x + 1$ is surjective, because for each $y \in \mathbb{R}$ we have $g(y - 1) = (y - 1) + 1 = y$. On the other hand, the function $h: \mathbb{N} \to \mathbb{N}$ defined by $h(x) = x + 1$ is *not* surjective, since there is no $x \in \mathbb{N}$ such that $h(x) = 1$.

(c) Let A be an n-element set, with $n \in \mathbb{N}$, and let B be a two-element set. How many nonsurjective functions are there from A to B?

SOLUTION.   Suppose $B = \{b_1, b_2\}$. If a function $f : A \to B$ is not surjective, then either $f(a) = b_1$ for all $a \in A$ or $f(a) = b_2$ for all $a \in A$. (Otherwise, there would exist elements a_1 and a_2 such that $f(a_1) = b_1$ and $f(a_2) = b_2$, and this would imply that f is surjective, contrary to the hypothesis.) Thus there are exactly *two* nonsurjective functions from A to B, namely the two constant functions. (See Example 3.3(b).)

(d) In Chapter 2 we discussed indexed sets without giving the notion a precise definition. Now that we have functions available for use, we can remedy the situation. If S and I are sets and $f : I \to S$ is a surjective function, we say that f has **indexed** the set S by I. Once such an f has been given, we usually write s_i instead of $f(i)$. Return to Examples 2.28 and 2.29 for an abundant supply of indexed sets. For instance, in 2.29(b) we used C_r for the circle with radius r and center $(0, 0)$ in the xy-plane. In our present notation, S is the set of circles centered at $(0, 0)$ and I is the set of nonnegative real numbers; for each $r \in I$, we have $f(r) = C_r$.

3.11 Definition.   A function $f : A \to B$ is said to be **one-to-one** (abbreviated **1-1**), **injective**, or an **injection** if the following implication is true for every $a_1, a_2 \in A$:

$$f(a_1) = f(a_2) \quad \Rightarrow \quad a_1 = a_2$$

In words: elements of A with the same image must be equal. The contrapositive is equally useful:

$$a_1 \neq a_2 \quad \Rightarrow \quad f(a_1) \neq f(a_2)$$

That is, different elements in the domain yield different images.

3.12 EXAMPLES.   (a) The function $f : \mathbb{R} \to \mathbb{R}$ given by $f(x) = x^3$ is injective.

PROOF.   We will verify the first implication in Definition 3.11 for $f(x) = x^3$. We have

$$
\begin{aligned}
f(x_1) = f(x_2) \quad &\Rightarrow \quad x_1^3 = x_2^3 \\
&\Rightarrow \quad x_1^3 - x_2^3 = 0 \\
&\Rightarrow \quad (x_1 - x_2)(x_1^2 + x_1 x_2 + x_2^2) = 0 \\
&\Rightarrow \quad x_1 - x_2 = 0 \quad \text{or} \quad x_1^2 + x_1 x_2 + x_2^2 = 0
\end{aligned}
$$

To conclude that $x_1 = x_2$, it remains to prove the implication

(∗) $$x_1^2 + x_1 x_2 + x_2^2 = 0 \quad \Rightarrow \quad x_1 = x_2$$

The hypothesis of (∗) yields

(∗∗) $$\begin{aligned} 0 &= x_1^2 + x_1 x_2 + x_2^2 \\ &= (x_1^2 + x_1 x_2) + x_2^2 \\ &= (x_1^2 + x_1 x_2 + \tfrac{1}{4} x_2^2) + (x_2^2 - \tfrac{1}{4} x_2^2) \\ &= (x_1 + \tfrac{1}{2} x_2)^2 + \tfrac{3}{4} x_2^2 \end{aligned}$$

Because squares of nonzero real numbers are positive, we conclude that $x_2 = 0$, and then that $x_1 = 0$. □

Argument (∗∗) is an instance of a useful algebraic trick called *completing the square*. Readers who find the method unappealing have other options. For instance, the proof of (∗) can be broken into separate cases as follows. If exactly one of x_1, x_2 is nonzero the hypothesis of (∗) is false, so (∗) is automatically true. If neither x_1 nor x_2 is zero and $|x_1| \le |x_2|$, then $x_2^2 + x_1 x_2 \ge 0$, hence $x_1^2 + x_1 x_2 + x_2^2 > 0$, a contradiction. The case $|x_2| \le |x_1|$ is similar. Alternatively, readers who have studied calculus can use the derivative $f'(x)$ to show that $f(x) = x^3$ is strictly increasing and then observe that a strictly increasing function is injective (why?).

(b) Let Σ stand for the usual English alphabet. A *four-letter word over* Σ is a function $w: \{1, 2, 3, 4\} \to \Sigma$. If $w(i) = a_i$ for $1 \le i \le 4$, we write

$$w = a_1 a_2 a_3 a_4$$

For example, the word w given by $1 \mapsto$ s, $2 \mapsto$ p, $3 \mapsto$ a, $4 \mapsto$ r is written

$$\text{spar}$$

Now we let W_4 denote the set of four-letter words over Σ, and we let $P(\Sigma)$ denote the power set of Σ (that is, the set of all subsets of Σ). We define a function $f: W_4 \to P(\Sigma)$ by

$$f(a_1 a_2 a_3 a_4) = \{a_1, a_2, a_3, a_4\}$$

That is, the image of a word is its set of letters. Then f is not injective, because two different words can have the same letters. [For instance,

$f(\text{bozo}) = f(\text{zoob}) = \{b, z, o\}$.] And f is not surjective, because no set of five or more letters is in the image of f.

(c) Return for a moment to the discussion of indexing in Example 3.10(d). Notice that there is no requirement that an indexing function be injective. For example, let S be the set of all lines through the origin in the xy-plane and suppose, for each $\alpha \in \mathbb{R}$ that $f(\alpha)$ is the line through $(0, 0)$ at angle α (radians) with the positive x-axis. Then S is indexed by $\mathbb{R}$ by means of f, and $s_\alpha = s_{\alpha + n\pi}$ for all integers n.

Many practical problems amount to asking whether a function exists that satisfies certain constraints, and we will now briefly consider the *marriage problem* as an example. Let $X = \{x_1, \ldots, x_n\}$ and Y be the sets of unmarried women and men, respectively, in a given region. Suppose that each woman x_i determines the set $M_i \subseteq Y$ of all men she considers acceptable for marriage. The problem is this: Is every woman able to marry an acceptable man, assuming that bigamy is illegal? [Readers whose present concerns are more with jobs than with marriage can rephrase the preceding problem as follows. Let $X = \{x_i\}_{1 \le i \le n}$ be the set of applicants for jobs, let Y be the set of available jobs, and let M_i denote the set of available jobs for which x_i is qualified. Can everyone be hired?]

We can mathematically model the marriage problem with sets and functions as follows: Let $I = \{1, \ldots, n\}$, and suppose we are given a family $\{M_i\}_{i \in I}$ of nonempty sets; find an injective function $f : I \to \cup_{i \in I} M_i$ such that $f(i) \in M_i$ for $i = 1, \ldots, n$. (Here injectivity corresponds to the requirement that no two women marry the same man; and the condition $f(i) \in M_i$ assures that each woman marries a man acceptable to her.) The set $\{f(1), \ldots, f(n)\}$ is called a **system of distinct representatives** for the family $\{M_i\}_{i \in I}$.

There are some conditions that must be avoided in order to achieve a happy solution to the marriage problem. For instance, if $M_1 = M_2 = M_3 = \{y_1, y_2\}$ then no solution is possible, for x_1, x_2, and x_3 cannot all find husbands from the two-element set $\{y_1, y_2\}$. So it is clearly necessary that the set $M_1 \cup M_2 \cup M_3$ contain at least three elements. More generally, for each k satisfying $1 \le k \le n$, each union of k of the M_i's must contain at least k elements. In 1935, the mathematician Philip Hall showed that this condition on unions is in fact sufficient to guarantee the existence of a solution to the marriage problem. The proof is beyond the scope of our present treatment; but for the curious, we will now illustrate a method for solving problems of this kind. (Our method is an example of what is called a **greedy algorithm**; such algorithms are characterized by proceeding at each step in a way that seems optimal in some sense at that moment without concern about future difficulties, then revising the initial choices later on if necessary.)

3.13 EXAMPLE. Find a system of distinct representatives for the following family of sets: $\{1\}, \{1, 2, 3\}, \{3, 4\}, \{2, 4, 5\}, \{3, 6\}, \{1, 4, 7\}, \{6\}$.

SOLUTION. We start by moving through the sets in the order in which they are listed, and in each case we choose as representative the smallest number compatible with the choices already made. This results in the respective choices

$$1, 2, 3, 4, 6, 7$$

for the first six sets. But now we are stuck: we can't make the required choice of 6 for the representative of the final set, since 6 was already chosen. Therefore we must amend our selection to

$$1, 2, 3, 4, \cancel{6}, 7$$
$$3$$

which requires the change

$$1, 2, \cancel{3}, 4, \cancel{6}, 7$$
$$4 \qquad 3$$

which in turn demands

$$1, 2, \cancel{3}, \cancel{4}, \cancel{6}, 7$$
$$4 \; 5 \; 3$$

Now we are free to select 6 as the representative of the final set, giving us the list

$$1, 2, 4, 5, 3, 7, 6$$

as our system of distinct representatives of the respective sets.

3.14 Definition. A function $f : A \to B$ is said to be **bijective**, a **bijection**, or a **one-to-one correspondence** if it is both injective and surjective.

It is a useful exercise to check that when the definitions of injection and surjection are stated in terms of ordered pairs, the following characterization of bijections emerges:

(3.14) A set $f \subseteq A \times B$ is a bijection from A to B if and only if each $a \in A$ is the first coordinate of exactly one pair belonging to f and each $b \in B$ is the second coordinate of exactly one pair belonging to f.

3.16 EXAMPLE. Let $A = \{1, 2, 3\}$ and $B = \{r, s, t, u\}$. Consider

$$f = \{(1, r), (2, u), (3, s)\} \qquad g = \{(1, r), (2, r), (3, u)\}$$
$$h = \{(1, r), (1, s), (2, u), (3, t)\} \qquad j = \{(1, r), (2, s)\}$$

Here f and g are functions from A to B, and f is injective but g is not, since $g(1) = g(2) = r$. Neither f nor g is surjective, since $t \notin f(A) \cup g(A)$. The set h is not a function, since 1 is paired by h with two different elements of B. Finally, j is not a function from A to B (since dom $j \neq A$), but j *is* an injective function from $\{1, 2\}$ to B.

None of the given sets of pairs is a bijection from A to B, but f is a bijection from A to $\{r, u, s\}$. More generally, *any* injective function is a bijection from its domain onto its range. (Check this.)

At the end of Chapter 2 we discussed the use of recursion to define certain families of mathematical objects; we will now employ recursion in the definition of functions.

Notation. If n is a natural number, we write

$$\mathbb{N}_n = \{x \in \mathbb{N} \mid 1 \leq x \leq n\} = \{1, 2, \ldots, n\}$$

3.17 Definition. Let A be a set. A **finite sequence** in A is a function $f: \mathbb{N}_n \to A$ for some $n \in \mathbb{N}$. (This is also called a **sequence of length n**.) An **infinite sequence** in A is a function $f: \mathbb{N} \to A$. We will follow the standard practice of using the word **sequence** for both varieties.

If f is a sequence in A, we usually write $f(1) = a_1$, $f(2) = a_2$, and so on. If f is an infinite sequence we visualize it as a never-ending list:

$$a_1, a_2, a_3, \ldots$$

If f is a sequence of length n, we usually denote f by the symbol

$$(a_1, a_2, \ldots, a_n)$$

and call it an **n-tuple**, with a_i its ith **coordinate**. By our criteria for function equality (see 3.5), it follows that

$$(a_1, \ldots, a_n) = (b_1, \ldots, b_n) \quad \Leftrightarrow \quad a_i = b_i \text{ for each } i, \ 1 \le i \le n$$

We sometimes denote a sequence of length n by $\{a_i\}_{1 \le i \le n}$ and an infinite sequence by $\{a_n\}_{n \in \mathbb{N}}$ or $\{a_n\}_{n \ge 1}$. (The letters i and n are the world's most popular subscripts.) More informally and less precisely, both kinds of sequences are often denoted $\{a_n\}$. The element a_n is also called the **nth term** of the sequence.

A recursive definition of a sequence $\{a_n\}$ begins by specifying one or more initial terms $a_1, \ldots, a_N$ explicitly; it then gives a formula that defines each succeeding term $a_{N+1}, a_{N+2}, \ldots$ in terms of its predecessors.

3.18 EXAMPLE. We will now consider a recursive procedure for computing the square root of a positive number m. We start by guessing a number r satisfying $0 < r \le m$. If the guess is correct (that is, $r = \sqrt{m}$) then $m/r = r$. If the guess is wrong, then either m/r is too small and r is too large, or vice versa. (Why?) The correct answer must therefore lie between r and m/r, so we use the average, $\frac{1}{2}\left(r + \frac{m}{r}\right)$, as the next guess, and continue in this fashion. This is called the **divide-and-average** method for computing $\sqrt{m}$. More compactly, we define a sequence $\{a_n\}$ recursively as follows:

$$a_1 = 1 \qquad \text{(a thought-free initial guess)}$$

$$a_{k+1} = \frac{1}{2}\left(a_k + \frac{m}{a_k}\right)$$

For instance, if $m = 3$ the first few terms of the sequence $\{a_n\}$ are

$$a_1 = 1$$

$$a_2 = \frac{1}{2}\left(1 + \frac{3}{1}\right) = 2$$

$$a_3 = \frac{1}{2}\left(2 + \frac{3}{2}\right) = \frac{7}{4}$$

$$a_4 = \frac{1}{2}\left(\frac{7}{4} + \frac{3}{\frac{7}{4}}\right) = \frac{97}{56}$$

$$a_5 = \frac{1}{2}\left(\frac{97}{56} + \frac{3}{\frac{97}{56}}\right) = \frac{18{,}817}{10{,}864}$$

Compare the last number with the value of $\sqrt{3}$ on a calculator.

3.19 EXAMPLE.   Consider the set $\mathbb{N} \times \mathbb{N}$, which we picture as the collection of all points with integer coordinates in the first quadrant.

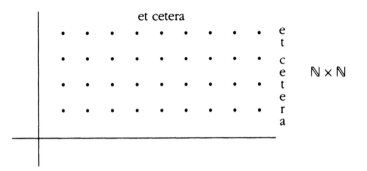

Can we list these points in some sort of order so that they are the terms in an infinite sequence? That is, is there a surjective function $f : \mathbb{N} \to \mathbb{N} \times \mathbb{N}$? As a first attempt, we might start by listing the points in the first column: $(1,1), (1,2), (1,3), \ldots$. But this is doomed to failure: we never escape from the first column! Similarly, a horizontal excursion through the bottom row, $(1,1), (2,1), (3,1), \ldots$, doesn't do the job. Success comes by moving along diagonals as pictured here:

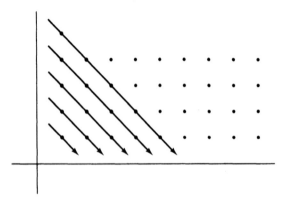

We start on the little diagonal at the lower left and then move down the next higher diagonal, then down the next, and so on. Notice that points (a, b) and (c, d) are on the same diagonal if and only if $a + b = c + d$; in that event, (a, b) precedes (c, d) as we move down their common diagonal if and only if $a < c$. The point (a, b) is on an *earlier* diagonal than (c, d) if and only if $a + b < c + d$. So the list we are constructing satisfies this rule: (a, b) precedes (c, d) on the list if and only if

$$a + b < c + d \quad \text{or} \quad a + b = c + d \quad \text{and} \quad a < c$$

Now we will give a recursive definition of the desired function $f : \mathbb{N} \to \mathbb{N} \times \mathbb{N}$ to generate the list we just described. Define $f(1) = (1, 1)$; and if $f(k) = (a, b)$ define

$$(*) \qquad f(k + 1) = \begin{cases} (a + 1, b - 1) & \text{if } b > 1 \\ (1, a + 1) & \text{if } b = 1 \end{cases}$$

Thus $f(2) = (1, 2)$, $f(3) = (2, 1)$, $f(4) = (1, 3)$, and so on. Formula $(*)$ tells us that $f(k + 1)$ follows $f(k)$ as we move down $f(k)$'s diagonal, unless $f(k)$ is already at the bottom, in which case $f(k + 1)$ is at the top of the next diagonal. We assert that f is surjective, and we will prove this by contradiction. If f is *not* surjective, move along the diagonals in succession until the first (a, b) is reached that is not in $f(\mathbb{N})$.[*] If $a \neq 1$ then $(a-1, b+1)$ precedes (a, b) on the same diagonal, so $(a-1, b+1) = f(k)$ for some $k \in \mathbb{N}$. But then an application of $(*)$ gives $f(k + 1) = (a, b)$, contradicting the assumption that $(a, b) \notin f(\mathbb{N})$. If $a = 1$ then $(b-1, 1)$ is at the bottom of the preceding diagonal, so $(b - 1, 1) = f(k)$ for some k, and then $(*)$ yields $f(k + 1) = (1, b) = (a, b)$, again a contradiction. Thus our assumption that f is not surjective is false, and we are done. It can also be shown that f is injective, but the details are technical and we omit them. (The argument uses $(*)$ to show that if $k_1 < k_2$ then either $f(k_2)$ is below $f(k_1)$ on the same diagonal or $f(k_2)$ is on some subsequent diagonal.)

Many problems in mathematics and computer science boil down to determining a procedure for listing a given set of objects as the terms in a sequence. It is therefore important to know that certain sets *cannot* be so listed; the following example provides an illustration.

---

[*]That is, among all those points (x, y) not in $f(\mathbb{N})$, consider those whose coordinate sum $x + y$ is minimal, and among those choose the point (a, b) with smallest first coordinate.

3.20 EXAMPLE. Let F denote the set of all functions from $\mathbb{N}$ to $\mathbb{N}$. Can the members of F be listed as a sequence? More precisely, is there a surjective function $g\colon \mathbb{N} \to F$? *Suppose there is such a function g*; then for each $n \in \mathbb{N}$ let's write g_n instead of $g(n)$. So we can list the functions from $\mathbb{N}$ to $\mathbb{N}$: $g_1, g_2, g_3, \ldots$. Now define a function $h\colon \mathbb{N} \to \mathbb{N}$ by the formula

$$h(n) = g_n(n) + 1 \quad \text{for all } n \in \mathbb{N}$$

Then $h \in F$, and therefore $h = g_k$ for some $k \in \mathbb{N}$. But

$$h(k) = g_k(k) + 1 \neq g_k(k)$$

and therefore $h \neq g_k$, a contradiction! Conclusion: no surjection $g\colon \mathbb{N} \to F$ exists, and therefore *no* procedure exists for listing the functions from $\mathbb{N}$ to $\mathbb{N}$.

The main idea underlying Example 3.19 is called **diagonalization**, a method first used by Georg Cantor in the nineteenth century. Cantor's idea is an adaptation of this fact: every row of a checkerboard contains a square on the main diagonal.

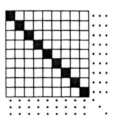

Cantor's gameboard

Each of the functions $g_n\colon \mathbb{N} \to \mathbb{N}$ in Example 3.19 is represented by a row of numbers:

$$g_n(1) \quad g_n(2) \quad g_n(3) \quad g_n(4) \quad \cdots$$

That is, g_n is represented by the nth row of the following array:

$$
\begin{array}{cccccc}
g_1(1) & g_1(2) & g_1(3) & g_1(4) & g_1(5) & \cdots \\
g_2(1) & g_2(2) & g_2(3) & g_2(4) & g_2(5) & \cdots \\
g_3(1) & g_3(2) & g_3(3) & g_3(4) & g_3(5) & \cdots \\
\vdots & \vdots & \vdots & \ddots & \vdots &
\end{array}
$$

An important slant on sequences

The function $h: \mathbb{N} \to \mathbb{N}$ in Example 3.19 is represented by the sequence

$$h(1) \quad h(2) \quad h(3) \quad h(4) \quad h(5) \quad \ldots$$

Then if h were one of the g_n, one of the terms $h(1), h(2), h(3), \ldots$ would be on the diagonal of the array; but that possibility has been eliminated by the manner in which we defined h.

We will hear more from Cantor in Chapter 4.

Exercises

1. Determine the image of each function in Exercise 4 of Section 3.1. (No proofs required.)

2. Let N be the set of all living nephews of living aunts, and let A be the set of all living aunts of living nephews.
   (a) Define a function from N to A.
   (b) Is your function injective?
   (c) Is your function surjective?
   (d) What condition on the numbers of elements in N and A would guarantee the existence of an injection $N \to A$? Explain briefly.
   (e) Repeat part (d), but replace "injection" with *surjection*.

3. In each case, state without proof whether the given function is injective, surjective, bijective.
   (a) $f: \mathbb{N} \to \mathbb{N}$ given by $f(x) = x^3$.
   (b) $g: \{1, 2, 3\} \to \{-2, 5, 6\}$ given by $g = \{(1, 5), (2, -2), (3, 6)\}$.
   (c) $h: \{1, 2, 3\} \to \{-2, 5, 6\}$ given by $h = \{(3, 5), (2, -2), (1, 5)\}$.

4. Let S and T be sets with three elements and two elements, respectively. In each case state the answer and justify briefly.
   (a) How many functions are there from S to T?
   (b) How many injections are there from S to T?
   (c) How many injections are there from T to S?
   (d) How many surjections are there from S to T?
   (e) How many surjections are there from T to S?
   (f) Guess the answers to (a) and (b) if S has m elements and T has n elements.

5. A function $f: A \to B$ is a subset of $A \times B$, hence a subset of $(A \cup B) \times (A \cup B)$. In the terminology of Chapter 2, f is a **relation** on $A \cup B$. Therefore f has an **inverse relation** (see Example 2.51(d)):

$$f^{-1} = \{(b, a) \mid (a, b) \in f\}.$$

(a) Write down the inverses g^{-1} and h^{-1} of the functions g and h in Exercise 3.

(b) Show that if f is not injective then f^{-1} is not a function.

(c) Show that if f is injective but not surjective then f^{-1} is a function whose domain is a proper subset of B.

6. For each part of this exercise, exhibit sets A, B, and C, with $C \subset A$, and a function $f : A \to B$ satisfying the given conditions. Or, if no such function exists, *show* that none exists. (There is no need to get fancy here. In each case where such an f exists, an example can be constructed in which each of the sets A, B, C has at most two elements.)

(a) f is surjective and the restriction $f|_C$ is surjective.

(b) f is surjective but $f|_C$ is not surjective.

(c) f is injective and $f|_C$ is injective.

(d) f is injective but $f|_C$ is not injective.

7. Show that the system of distinct representatives produced by the solution to the problem in 3.13 is the only acceptable answer.

8. For each family of sets, either find a system of distinct representatives or show that none exists.

(a) $\{2,5\}, \{2,3,4,5,6\}, \{1,3,5\}, \{1,4,5\}, \{2\}$

(b) $\{1,4\}, \{2,3,4,5,6\}, \{2,4,5,6\}, \{4,6\}, \{1,4,6\}, \{1,4,6\}$

9. Let a and b be real numbers. Consider a function $f : \mathbb{R} \to \mathbb{R}$ given by the formula $f(x) = ax + b$.

(a) Under what conditions on a and b is f a bijection from $\mathbb{R}$ to $\mathbb{R}$? (For instance, what if $a = 0$?)

(b) Under what conditions on a and b is the restriction $f|_\mathbb{Z}$ a bijection from $\mathbb{Z}$ to $\mathbb{Z}$?

(c) Under what conditions on a and b is the restriction $f|_\mathbb{N}$ a bijection from $\mathbb{N}$ to $\mathbb{N}$?

10. Let Π denote the xy-plane, let O denote the origin, let $\Pi^* = \Pi - \{O\}$ (the "punctured plane"), and let L denote the set of all lines through O. For each point $P \in \Pi^*$, let $f(P)$ be the line containing the segment OP. Show that the function $f : \Pi^* \to L$ is not a bijection, and then find a set $S \subset \Pi^*$ such that the restriction $f|_S$ *is* a bijection from S to L.

11. (This exercise requires the definition of an *ordering* on a set S. This was given in Exercise 15 of Section 2.9.) First an example: Suppose that each of five parachute jumpers is assigned a different number from 1 to 5. Jumper number 1 will jump first, then jumper number 2,

and so on. The standard ordering on the set $\{1, 2, 3, 4, 5\}$ has *induced* an ordering on the set of jumpers. This is the idea underlying this exercise.

Show that if $\leq$ is an ordering on S and $f: S \rightarrow T$ is a bijection, then f can be used to define an ordering $<$ on T satisfying this property:

$$s_1 \leq s_2 \Leftrightarrow f(s_1) < f(s_2) \quad \forall s_1, s_2 \in S.$$

(Your answer should start with something like this: "If $t_1, t_2 \in T$, define $t_1 < t_2$ as follows:....")

12. The definition of n-tuple given in this section may produce confusion when $n = 2$, because our definition of the 2-tuple (a_1, a_2) differs from our definition of the ordered pair (a_1, a_2) in Chapter 2. This can be remedied with a different definition of n-tuple as follows: Define the 1-tuple $(a_1) = \{a_1\}$. Define the 2-tuple (a_1, a_2) to be the ordered pair (a_1, a_2). In general, if the k-tuple $(a_1, a_2, \ldots, a_k)$ has been defined, define the $(k + 1)$-tuple $(a_1, \ldots, a_k, a_{k+1})$ to be the ordered pair

$$((a_1, \ldots, a_k), a_{k+1})$$

Prove by induction on n that this recursive definition of n-tuple retains the following essential property:

$$(a_1, \ldots, a_n) = (b_1, \ldots, b_n) \quad \Leftrightarrow \quad a_i = b_i \text{ for each } i, \ 1 \leq i \leq n$$

13. Information transmitted electronically is usually encoded in the form of n-tuples of 0s and 1s, often called **n-bit strings**. For brevity, commas and parentheses are omitted; thus 01101011 is an 8-bit string. A **code of length n** is a set of such strings, and the members of a code are called **codewords**. To aid in the detection and correction of errors, it is useful to have different codewords differ in more than one coordinate. (The same is true in ordinary English: a one-letter typing error in "house" can yield "horse" or "mouse" and lead to confusion, whereas a one-letter error in "Mississippi" will probably be detected and corrected.) Define the **distance** between two n-bit strings to be the number of coordinates in which they differ. More formally, let $\mathbb{Z}_2^n$ denote the set of n-bit strings, and define a function $d: \mathbb{Z}_2^n \times \mathbb{Z}_2^n \rightarrow \mathbb{Z}$ by

$$d(a_1 a_2 \ldots a_n, b_1 b_2 \ldots b_n) = \sum_{i=1}^{n} |a_i - b_i|$$

where $a_i, b_i \in \{0, 1\}$ for each i. [Example: $d(1101, 1001) = 2$.] Prove that the function d has the following properties:

(a) $d(s_1, s_2) \geq 0$ (here the s's are strings)

(b) $d(s_1, s_2) = 0 \Leftrightarrow s_1 = s_2$

(c) $d(s_1, s_2) = d(s_2, s_1)$

(d) For all $s_1, s_2, s_3 \in \mathbb{Z}_2^n$

$$d(s_1, s_3) \leq d(s_1, s_2) + d(s_2, s_3)$$ (the **triangle inequality**)

(Suggestion: Use induction on n, starting with $n = 1$.)

14. Use the divide-and-average method to compute $\sqrt{5}$, correct to five decimal places. (No calculators allowed!)

15. Suppose you are using the divide-and-average method to compute a square root, and you want your answer to be correct to n decimal places. (That is, you want all the digits through the first n digits to the right of the decimal point to be correct.) How can you test your current estimate to see whether it is good enough? Explain.

16. Give a recursive definition of each of the following sequences.

    (a) $1, 3, 5, 7, 9, 11, 13, 15, 17, \ldots$

    (b) $1, 1, 3, 3, 5, 5, 7, 7, 9, 9, \ldots$

    (c) $2, 3, 5, 8, 12, 17, 23, 30, 38, \ldots$

    (d) $1, 1, 2, 3, 5, 8, 13, 21, 34, 55, \ldots$ (the *Fibonacci numbers*)

17. Suppose $f: \mathbb{N} \rightarrow A$ and $g: \mathbb{N} \rightarrow B$ are surjections. Prove that there is a surjection $h: \mathbb{N} \rightarrow A \cup B$. [Suggestion: Consider the list $f(1), g(1), f(2), g(2), \ldots$]

18. Show that there is a one-to-one correspondence between $\mathbb{N}$ and the following set of integers, written here in decimal form:

$$\{2, 11, 101, 1001, 10001, 100001, \ldots\}$$

19. In the first quadrant, draw a connected path starting at $(1, 1)$ that, if continued, would pass through all of $\mathbb{N} \times \mathbb{N}$. (That is, any prechosen point in $\mathbb{N} \times \mathbb{N}$ will eventually be reached.) Your path should have *only horizontal and vertical segments*, and no point should be covered more than once. No proof is required; but be sure to draw enough so that the method for continuing the path is clear to the reader.

20. Write a recursive definition of a sequence whose range is the set of points in the fourth quadrant with integer coordinates. Your formula should correspond to moving along diagonals as pictured here. (Suggestion: review formula ($*$) in Example 3.18.)

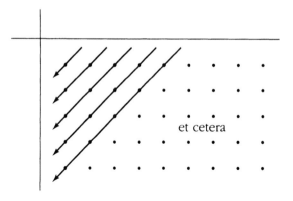

21. Draw a connected path starting at $(0, 0)$ that, if continued, would pass through all of $\mathbb{Z} \times \mathbb{Z}$.

3.3 Composition of Functions

Suppose we are given functions $f: A \rightarrow B$ and $g: B \rightarrow C$; then each element $x \in A$ is paired by f with a unique element $y \in B$, and y is in turn paired by g with a unique element $z \in C$. It is natural to view x as paired with z by this two-stage process, and the result is a new function called the **composition** of f and g, denoted $g \circ f$. More formally, we define $g \circ f: A \rightarrow C$ by the rule

(3.21) $$(g \circ f)(x) = g(f(x)), \quad \forall x \in A$$

The intuitive picture:

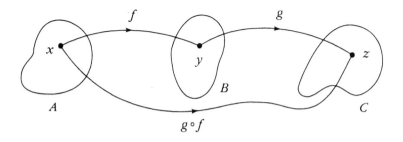

A consequence of our definition is that $\mathrm{dom}(g \circ f) = \mathrm{dom}\, f$. A function expressed as a composition is said to be *composite*.

3.22 EXAMPLES. (a) Suppose $f: \mathbb{R} \to \mathbb{R}$ and $g: \mathbb{R} \to \mathbb{R}$ are defined by the formulas

$$f(x) = x + 3 \quad \forall x \in \mathbb{R} \qquad \text{and} \qquad g(x) = x^2 \quad \forall x \in \mathbb{R}$$

Then for each $x \in \mathbb{R}$ we have

$$(f \circ g)(x) = f(g(x)) = f(x^2) = x^2 + 3$$

and

$$(g \circ f)(x) = g(f(x)) = g(x + 3) = (x + 3)^2 = x^2 + 6x + 9$$

Note that here $g \circ f \neq f \circ g$ since, for example, $(f \circ g)(1) = 4$, while $(g \circ f)(1) = 16$. (We remark that $(f \circ g)(-1) = (g \circ f)(-1) = 4$; so unequal functions with a common domain need not disagree at every point of that domain.)

(b) Consider functions f and g from $\mathbb{R} \times \mathbb{R}$ to $\mathbb{R} \times \mathbb{R}$ defined by $f(x, y) = (x, 0)$ and $g(x, y) = (0, y)$ for all $(x, y) \in \mathbb{R} \times \mathbb{R}$. (The functions f and g are called the **projections** onto the horizontal and vertical axes, respectively.) Here we have

$$(f \circ g)(x, y) = f(g(x, y)) = f(0, y) = (0, 0)$$

and similarly $(g \circ f)(x, y) = (0, 0)$ for all $(x, y) \in \mathbb{R} \times \mathbb{R}$. Therefore in this example we have $f \circ g = g \circ f$.

In elementary arithmetic we have the dual notions of multiplication and factorization: We can multiply two integers and produce a single product, and we can factor some integers into products of smaller integers. Similarly, we can compose certain functions to get one function, and we can express some functions as compositions of simpler ones. A complicated procedure is sometimes more manageable if it is decomposed into simpler steps.

3.23 EXAMPLE. Consider the function $f: \mathbb{R} \to \mathbb{R}$ given by $f(x) = (x^2 + 1)^3$. Then we can express f in a variety of ways as a composition of functions from $\mathbb{R}$ to $\mathbb{R}$, and here are some samples:

$$f = h \circ u = s \circ r = (s \circ h) \circ g = s \circ (h \circ g)$$

where $g(x) = x^2, h(x) = x + 1, r(x) = x^2 + 1, s(x) = x^3$, and $u(x) = x^6 + 3x^4 + 3x^2$. Let's check in detail that $f = (s \circ h) \circ g$ to illustrate the method; the other equalities are left for the reader. For each $x \in \mathbb{R}$ we have

$$
\left.
\begin{aligned}
((s \circ h) \circ g)(x) &= (s \circ h)(g(x)) \\
&= s(h(g(x)))
\end{aligned}
\right\} \quad \text{(from the definition of function composition)}
$$

$$
\begin{aligned}
&= s(h(x^2)) && \text{(since } g \text{ acts by squaring)} \\
&= s(x^2 + 1) && \text{(since } h \text{ acts by adding 1)} \\
&= (x^2 + 1)^3 && \text{(since } s \text{ acts by cubing)} \\
&= f(x) && \text{(by definition of } f)
\end{aligned}
$$

This shows that $(s \circ h) \circ g$ and f have the same action on each element of their common domain $\mathbb{R}$. Therefore $(s \circ h) \circ g = f$ by 3.5.

We verbalize the existence of functions f and g such that $f \circ g \neq g \circ f$ by saying that composition of functions is not **commutative**. Mathematicians use this word in a variety of settings, with varying degrees of precision. In general, objects or procedures are said to **commute** with one another if the order in which they appear in a statement makes no crucial difference. For example, 3 and 5 commute with each other additively but not with respect to division: $3 + 5 = 5 + 3$, but $5 \div 3 \neq 3 \div 5$. The procedures of putting on socks and shoes do not commute with each other. We will give a more precise definition of commutative operations in Chapter 6.

The computation displayed in Example 3.22 is an exercise in parenthesis juggling (a favorite sport (of (some) mathematicians)), and the key part comes in the first two lines, in which $((s \circ h) \circ g)(x)$ is transformed into $s(h(g(x)))$. A similar computation will show that $(s \circ (h \circ g))(x)$ is also equal to $s(h(g(x)))$, from which it follows that $(s \circ h) \circ g = s \circ (h \circ g)$. Because the formulas that define s, h, and g are nowhere involved in this deduction, we sense that our example is an instance of a more general law, and the following theorem makes that law explicit.

3.24 Theorem (Associative Law of Function Composition). Given functions $f : A \rightarrow B$, $g : B \rightarrow C$, and $h : C \rightarrow D$; then

$$
h \circ (g \circ f) = (h \circ g) \circ f
$$

PROOF.   We have

$$\mathrm{dom}(h \circ (g \circ f)) = \mathrm{dom}((h \circ g) \circ f) = A$$

(Why?) So to complete the proof we must verify that $(h \circ (g \circ f))(x) = ((h \circ g) \circ f)(x)$ for all $x \in A$. But the definition of composition gives

$$(h \circ (g \circ f))(x) = h((g \circ f)(x)) = h(g(f(x)))$$
$$= (h \circ g)(f(x)) = ((h \circ g) \circ f)(x),$$

and this storm of parentheses completes the proof.   □

Thanks to Theorem 3.23, the composite functions $h \circ (g \circ f)$ and $(h \circ g) \circ f$ can now be written $h \circ g \circ f$ without fear of confusion.

The following theorem shows what happens when one injection or surjection is composed with another. We will apply these results again and again in the subsequent chapters.

3.25 Theorem.   Let $f : A \to B$ and $g : B \to C$ be functions.

(a) If f and g are injections then $g \circ f : A \to C$ is an injection.

(b) If f and g are surjections then so is $g \circ f$.

(c) If f and g are bijections then so is $g \circ f$.

PROOF.   (a) Let $a_1, a_2 \in A$. We have the following series of implications:

$$(g \circ f)(a_1) = (g \circ f)(a_2) \Rightarrow g(f(a_1)) = g(f(a_2)) \quad \text{(by definition of composition)}$$
$$\Rightarrow f(a_1) = f(a_2) \quad \text{(since g is injective)}$$
$$\Rightarrow a_1 = a_2 \quad \text{(since f is injective)}$$

Therefore $g \circ f$ is injective.

(b) Let $c \in C$. We must find an $a \in A$ such that $(g \circ f)(a) = c$. Since g is onto C, there is an element $b \in B$ such that $g(b) = c$. Then, since f is onto B, there exists $a \in A$ such that $f(a) = b$. Thus

$$(g \circ f)(a) = g(f(a)) = g(b) = c$$

(c) This part follows immediately from the preceding parts.   □

3.26 EXAMPLE. Let $\mathbb{Q}^+$ denote the set of positive rational numbers. In Example 3.18 we exhibited a surjection $f: \mathbb{N} \twoheadrightarrow \mathbb{N} \times \mathbb{N}$. Now define a function $g: \mathbb{N} \times \mathbb{N} \to \mathbb{Q}^+$ by the rule $(a, b) \mapsto a/b$. Check that g is surjective. (But g is not injective since, for example, $g(2, 3) = g(4, 6) = 2/3$.) By Theorem 3.24(b), it follows that the function $g \circ f: \mathbb{N} \to \mathbb{Q}^+$ is surjective. Imagine that each point representing a natural number n on the real line is physically uprooted and replanted on top of the point representing the image $(g \circ f)(n)$. Then surjectivity of $g \circ f$ shows the remarkable fact that there are enough integer points on the positive real axis to completely cover all the rational points. Let's say it pictorially:

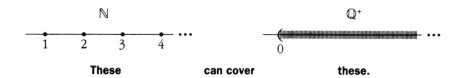

These   **can cover**   **these.**

Suppose A and B are sets and $f: A \to B$ is a bijection. We now define a new function, the **inverse** of f, denoted f^{-1}, that transforms each element of B back to the element of A from which it came. There *is* such an element of A since f is surjective; and it is unique because f is injective. More formally, define $f^{-1}: B \to A$ by

(3.27) $$f^{-1} = \{(b, a) \in B \times A \mid (a, b) \in f\}$$

Now we can see that f^{-1} has the desired action:

$$f^{-1}(b) = a \Leftrightarrow (b, a) \in f^{-1} \Leftrightarrow (a, b) \in f \Leftrightarrow f(a) = b$$

It follows from 3.14 that f^{-1}, like f, is a bijection.*

The next theorem shows that the actions of f and f^{-1} cancel each other, and that f^{-1} is the *only* function having that behavior with respect to f. Recall that i_A denotes the identity function on A.

3.28 Theorem. Let $f: A \to B$ and $g: B \to A$. then the following two statements are equivalent:

(a) f is a bijection and $g = f^{-1}$.
(b) $g \circ f = i_A$ and $f \circ g = i_B$.

PROOF. Assume statement (a) is true. We will prove the equation $g \circ f = i_A$. (The proof of $f \circ g = i_B$ is similar, and it is left to the reader.) Pick any

---

*Injectivity of f is essential in order for f^{-1} to be a function; surjectivity of f is required in order to have dom $f^{-1} = B$. See Exercise 5 in Section 3.2 for further discussion.

element $a \in A$; say, $f(a) = b \in B$. Then

$$(g \circ f)(a) = (f^{-1} \circ f)(a) = f^{-1}(f(a)) = f^{-1}(b) = a = i_A(a)$$

therefore $g \circ f$ and i_A agree on all elements of their common domain A, and so $g \circ f = i_A$, as desired.

Now suppose statement (b) is true. Then for all $a_1, a_2 \in A$ we have the implications

$$f(a_1) = f(a_2) \Rightarrow g(f(a_1)) = g(f(a_2))$$
$$\Rightarrow a_1 = a_2 \quad (\text{since } g \circ f = i_A)$$

hence f is injective. Moreover, if $b \in B$ then $g(b) \in A$ and $f(g(b)) = b$ (since $f \circ g = i_B$), so f is surjective. Thus f is a bijection, so we know that the function f^{-1} exists; it remains to prove that $g = f^{-1}$.

Observe that both $g \circ i_B$ and g have domain B; and for each $b \in B$ we have $(g \circ i_B)(b) = g(i_B(b)) = g(b)$. Therefore $g \circ i_B = g$; similarly, check that $i_A \circ f^{-1} = f^{-1}$. The conclusion now follows from a chain of equalities:

$$g = g \circ i_B = g \circ (f \circ f^{-1}) = (g \circ f) \circ f^{-1} = i_A \circ f^{-1} = f^{-1} \quad \square$$

3.29 Corollary (Corollary (Cancellation Laws)).   Let f be a bijection. Then

$$f \circ g = f \circ h \Rightarrow g = h \quad \text{(left cancellation)}$$
$$r \circ f = s \circ f \Rightarrow r = s \quad \text{(right cancellation)}$$

PROOF.   Exercise. (Major hint: Compose appropriately with f^{-1}.) $\square$

If a bijection f is given by a formula of the form $f(x) = y$, then computing f^{-1} amounts to determining a formula that tells us how to transform y back to x. For this we reverse the steps leading from x to y, starting with the last step and backing up from there. A mnemonic: to invert "put on socks, put on shoes, walk from A to B," we walk from B to A, take off shoes, take off socks." For example, consider

$$\mathbb{R}^+ = \{x \in \mathbb{R} \mid x \geq 0\} \quad \text{and} \quad B = \{x \in \mathbb{R} \mid x \geq 5\}$$

and define $f : \mathbb{R}^+ \to B$ by $y = f(x) = x^2 + 5$. This formula says "square, add 5" so f^{-1} tells us "subtract 5, take square root." That is,

$$y = x^2 + 5 \quad \Rightarrow \quad y - 5 = x^2 \quad \Rightarrow \quad \sqrt{y - 5} = x$$

(The assumption $x \geq 0$ is crucial in the last step.) thus $x = f^{-1}(y) = \sqrt{y-5}$. Although the letters we use to represent points in the domain and range of a function are arbitrary, it is a common (but not universal) custom to use x and y, respectively, for these. With this convention our formula becomes $y = f^{-1}(x) = \sqrt{x-5}$.

In summary, the procedure for determining inverses can be stated briefly like this: *If a bijection f is given by $y = f(x)$, then the formula for f^{-1} is obtained by solving for x in terms of y. If so desired, the variables can then be relabeled by using the letter y in place of x, and x in place of y.*

The following theorem reinforces our understanding that we undo the results of "put on sock, then put on shoe" with "take off shoe, *then* take off sock."

3.30 Theorem. Let $f : A \rightarrow B$ and $g : B \rightarrow C$ be bijections. Then $(g \circ f)^{-1} = f^{-1} \circ g^{-1}$.

PROOF. We make repeated use of the associative law for composition of functions:

$$(f^{-1} \circ g^{-1}) \circ (g \circ f) = f^{-1} \circ (g^{-1} \circ (g \circ f)) = f^{-1} \circ ((g^{-1} \circ g) \circ f)$$

$$= f^{-1} \circ (i_B \circ f) = f^{-1} \circ f = i_A$$

Similarly, check that $(g \circ f) \circ (f^{-1} \circ g^{-1}) = i_C$. Now use Theorem 3.27. $\square$

Exercises

1. Because $(g \circ f)(x) = g(f(x))$ for all $x \in \operatorname{dom} f$, the strict definition of composition requires that $f(x) \in \operatorname{dom} g$ for all $x \in \operatorname{dom} f$. It is common practice to be sloppy and *not* require this, with the understanding that the domain of $g \circ f$ is the set of all $x \in \operatorname{dom} f$ for which $g(f(x))$ makes sense. For example, if f and g act on real numbers by the formulas $f(x) = x - 5$ and $g(x) = \sqrt{x-4}$, then

$$(g \circ f)(x) = g(f(x)) = \sqrt{(x-5)-4} = \sqrt{x-9}$$

hence $\operatorname{dom} g \circ f = \{x \mid x \geq 9\}$. In each of the following cases, write the formula for $g \circ f$ and compute its domain. (The domain of each given function is understood to be the set of all real numbers for which the formula produces a value.)

(a) $f(x) = x^2, \qquad g(x) = \sqrt{x}$

(b) $f(x) = \sqrt{x}, \qquad g(x) = x^2$

(c) $f(x) = \sin x, \qquad g(x) = 1/x^2$

(d) $f(x) = \begin{cases} \pi/2 & \text{if } x \in \mathbb{Q} \\ \pi/4 & \text{if } x \notin \mathbb{Q} \end{cases} \qquad g(x) = \tan x$

2. Express each of the following functions as a composition of two functions, neither of which is the identity function.

   (a) $f(x) = (x^2 + \cos x)^3$

   (b) $f(x) = x^5 - 7x + 1$

   (c) $f(x) = x^2(10)^{2x}$

   (d) $f(x) = 5/x\sqrt{x-1}$

3. (a) Give examples of functions f and g from $\mathbb{R}$ to $\mathbb{R}$ that do not commute with respect to composition (not the example in the text, please).

   (b) Give examples of functions f and g from $\mathbb{R}$ to $\mathbb{R}$ (with $f \neq g$) that *do* commute with respect to composition.

4. Suppose that f and g are different constant functions from S to S, where S is a nonempty set. Show that $f \circ g \neq g \circ f$.

5. If $a, b \in \mathbb{R}$, define $a * b$ to be the result of rounding the product ab to the nearest tenth. For example, $3.7 * 12.9 = 47.7$. Verify that

$$(8.2 * 9.2) * 10.2 \neq 8.2 * (9.2 * 10.2)$$

   (This exercise is here as a moral lesson: it warns us that this section's associative law actually requires proof. There are instances in which we might wish for such a law but not have our wish granted.).

6. Just for fun, forget for a moment that you know the associative law for composition of functions, and verify that $f \circ (g \circ h) = (f \circ g) \circ h$ when

$$f(x) = \sin x^3, \qquad g(x) = \frac{x^2 - 5}{x + 1}, \qquad h(x) = \sqrt[4]{3x}$$

7. Suppose $f: A \to B$ and $g: B \to C$ are functions.

   (a) Show that if $g \circ f$ is injective then f is injective.

   (b) Show that if $g \circ f$ is surjective then g is surjective.

8. In each part of this exercise, give examples of sets A, B, C and functions $f: A \to B$ and $g: B \to C$ satisfying the indicated properties.

   (a) g is not injective but $g \circ f$ *is* injective.

   (b) f is not surjective but $g \circ f$ *is* surjective.

   (Suggestions: Work with sets having at most three elements; draw pictures.)

9. Define functions f and g from $\mathbb{Z}$ to $\mathbb{Z}$ such that f is not surjective and yet $g \circ f$ is surjective.

10. In our statement of the cancellation laws (3.28), the function f was taken to be a bijection. Now we ask whether this condition is essential.

    (a) Are the cancellation laws valid when f is surjective but not injective? Consider both laws, and in each case either prove that the law holds for such a function f or give a counterexample.

    (b) Repeat part (a) with f injective but not surjective.

11. Let $A = B = \{1, 2, 3, 4\}$, and let $f : A \to B$ be the function

    $$f = \{(1, 3), (2, 4), (3, 2), (4, 1)\}$$

    If f is a bijection, determine f^{-1}. If f is not a bijection, *show* that it isn't.

12. The function f acts on real numbers according to the formula

    $$f(x) = x^{1/4} + 3$$

    Determine the domain and range of this function, and give a formula for f^{-1}.

13. Refer to Theorem 3.29. Instead of the rule given there, a natural dream would be to have the rule $(g \circ f)^{-1} = g^{-1} \circ f^{-1}$.

    (a) Show that this statement can be made to fail solely on account of incompatibility of domains and ranges.

    (b) Give an example of a set S and bijections f and g from S to S, with $f \neq g$, such that the dream comes true:

    $$(f \circ g)^{-1} = f^{-1} \circ g^{-1}$$

    (c) Regain your senses by giving bijections from S to S such that

    $$(f \circ g)^{-1} \neq f^{-1} \circ g^{-1}$$

14. A function is a set of ordered pairs (satisfying certain conditions), so the **union** of two functions f and g is also a set of ordered pairs. It is therefore reasonable to ask whether $f \cup g$ is also a function and, if it is, to consider how its properties relate to the properties of f and g. This exercise considers these issues.

    Assume $f : A \to B$ and $g : C \to D$. All the examples requested in this exercise can be produced using sets A, B, C, D that have at most two elements each.

(a) Show that if $A \cap C = \emptyset$, then $(f \cup g): A \cup C \to B \cup D$.

(b) Give an example in which $A \cap C \ne \emptyset$ and $f \cup g$ is not a function.

(c) Give an example in which $A \cap C \ne \emptyset$ and $(f \cup g): A \cup C \to B \cup D$.

For the remaining parts, assume that $f \cup g$ *is* a function from $A \cup C$ to $B \cup D$.

(d) Show that if f and g are surjective then $f \cup g$ is surjective.

(e) Show that if $f \cup g$ is injective then f and g are injective.

(f) Show that if $f \cup g$ is a bijection then $(f \cup g)^{-1} = f^{-1} \cup g^{-1}$.

(g) Give an example in which $f \cup g$ is injective.

(h) Give an example in which f and g are injective but $f \cup g$ is not injective.

15. Prove the left and right cancellation laws (Corollary 3.28).

FINITE AND INFINITE SETS

"No room! No room!" they cried out when they saw Alice coming. "There's *plenty* of room!" said Alice indignantly, and she sat down in a large armchair at one end of the table.

LEWIS CARROLL
Alices Adventures in Wonderland

4.1 Cardinality; Fundamental Counting Principles

Learning to count is one of our first great intellectual triumphs. But what exactly are we doing when we count? Can the process be generalized in a way that lets us compare sets that are larger than numbers can describe? What is meant by an infinite set? Are all infinite sets essentially the same size? Exploring these mysteries (the topic of *cardinality*) is our central goal in this chapter. As we proceed we will examine many of the fundamental principles of counting that we have viewed as intuitively obvious since childhood. (Example: You have n objects, and you give some of them to a friend; then you have given your friend at most n objects.) This will lay the foundation for the many practical counting procedures that we will develop here and in Chapter 5. In Section 4.5 we will use our work on functions and cardinality to initiate the study of languages and automata, fundamental topics in the theory of computation.

Two primitive shepherds want to determine whose flock is larger, but counting is unknown to them. How can they proceed? Here is a way. They could guide the flocks (call them A and B) into adjoining pens, then select one sheep from A and one from B and link them with a cord. They would repeat this pairing procedure until one of the flocks has been used up. If one of the flocks has remaining unpaired sheep, that flock is larger; if no unpaired sheep remain in either flock, then A and B are the same size.

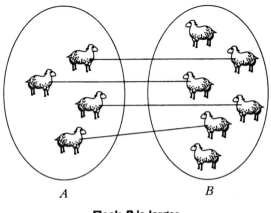

Flock *B* is larger.

While we're on this subject we can all agree on one more assertion: If flocks A and B are the same size and someone adds a sheep to A but not to B, then A will have more sheep than B.

Now imagine that there is a hotel with infinitely many rooms along an unending corridor: a first room, a second room, and so on. Imagine further that there is a person occupying each room; so we can reasonably say that there are exactly as many guests as there are rooms. You arrive at the hotel seeking a room, and the manager tells you, "At the moment the rooms are all occupied, but we always have room for one more." Whereupon she speaks into an intercom connected to all the rooms, saying, "At the sound of the bell, each guest should step out into the corridor and move into the next room in line." This clears out the first room, and you have a place to stay. Notice that although you thought you had enlarged the collection of guests by your presence, there are still as many hotel rooms as there are guests. (Contrast this remark with the closing assertion on the flocks of sheep example.)

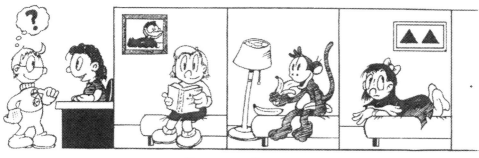

Always room for one more . . .

The two examples just discussed (particularly the second one) show that the matter of set comparison—saying that one set has more, fewer, or the same number of elements as another—involves some subtleties, and we will now give a careful treatment of these ideas.

4.1 Definition. Sets A and B are said to have the same **cardinality** or **cardinal number** if there is a bijection $f : A \rightarrow B$. In this situation we also say that A and B are **equipotent** sets, abbreviated $A \approx B$, or that they are **in one-to-one correspondence**. The negation of this statement is written $A \not\approx B$.

The following theorem provides three useful properties of equipotence.

4.2 Theorem. Let A, B, C be sets. Then

(a) $A \approx A$,

(b) $A \approx B \Rightarrow B \approx A$,

(c) $A \approx B$ and $B \approx C \Rightarrow A \approx C$.

Consequently, if S is any collection of sets, then equipotence is an equivalence relation on S.

PROOF. (a) The mapping $i_A : A \rightarrow A$ is a bijection.

(b) If $f : A \rightarrow B$ is a bijection, then so is $f^{-1} : B \rightarrow A$.

(c) If $f : A \rightarrow B$ and $g : B \rightarrow C$ are bijections, then so is $g \circ f : A \rightarrow C$.

Statements (a), (b), and (c) say (respectively) that the relation $\approx$ on S is reflexive, symmetric, and transitive; hence an equivalence relation. $\square$

4.3 EXAMPLE. Let S be the set of seats at the Acme Theater, and let P be the set of people waiting to be seated for the next show. The assertion $P \approx S$ means that there is a seat for everyone, with no seats to spare. If $P \not\approx S$ then either there are too many people (no function $P \to S$ is injective) or, no matter how the people distribute themselves in the seats, there will be empty seats remaining (no function $P \to S$ is surjective).

4.4 EXAMPLE. Let X be a set with ten elements, let S be the set of all seven-element subsets of X, and let T be the set of all three-element subsets of X. Then $S \approx T$.

PROOF OUTLINE. For each $A \in S$, let A' denote the complement of A in X. Then $A' \in T$, and the function $S \to T$ given by $A \mapsto A'$ is a bijection from S to T. $\square$

Intuitively, we usually view two equipotent sets as having the same size or the same number of elements. But there are weaknesses in this idea, as the next examples show.

4.5 EXAMPLES.   (a) Let E denote the set of even integers, and define $f: \mathbb{Z} \to E$ by $f(n) = 2n$. Then f is a bijection (check this), and therefore $\mathbb{Z} \approx E$. Notice the miracle here: We have taken $\mathbb{Z}$, thrown out half of it (namely all the odd integers), and we are left with a subset E that is still in one-to-one correspondence with $\mathbb{Z}$. Therefore $\mathbb{Z}$ is an example of a set that, in a sense, is no larger than half of itself!

(b) If $a, b \in \mathbb{R}$, with $a < b$, consider the **open interval**

$$I_a^b = \{x \in \mathbb{R} \mid a < x < b\}$$

Define $f: I_a^b \to I_0^1$ by

$$x \overset{f}{\longmapsto} \frac{x - a}{b - a}$$

If $x_1 < x_2$ then clearly $f(x_1) < f(x_2)$, and so f is injective. Also f is surjective. For suppose $t \in I_0^1$; then define $x = a + t(b - a)$ and check that $x \in I_a^b$ and $f(x) = t$. Therefore $I_a^b \approx I_0^1$. (Intuitively, f stretches or contracts I_a^b to cover I_0^1 precisely.)

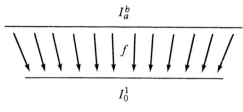

A visit to the shrink

In particular, this result gives $I_{-\pi/2}^{\pi/2} \approx I_0^1$; so by Theorem 4.2 we obtain the equipotence $I_a^b \approx I_{-\pi/2}^{\pi/2}$. But we know from trigonometry that the mapping $I_{-\pi/2}^{\pi/2} \to \mathbb{R}$ given by $x \mapsto \tan x$ is a bijection, and hence $I_{-\pi/2}^{\pi/2} \approx \mathbb{R}$. Therefore, again by Theorem 4.2, we have $I_a^b \approx \mathbb{R}$. Our conclusion:

(4.6) Every open interval, no matter how short, is in one-to-one correspondence with the set $\mathbb{R}$ of real numbers. Therefore any two open intervals have the same cardinality (even if one interval is properly contained in the other).

For each integer $n \geq 0$, define

$$\mathbb{N}_n = \{x \in \mathbb{N} \mid 1 \leq x \leq n\}$$

Then $\mathbb{N}_0 = \emptyset$, and clearly $\mathbb{N}_m \subseteq \mathbb{N}_n$ if $m \leq n$.

4.7 Definition. A set S is said to be **finite** if $S \approx \mathbb{N}_n$ for some $n \geq 0$, and in this case we write $\#S = n$. (The expression $\#S$ is verbalized "the number of elements in S.") A set is **infinite** if it is not finite. To **count** a finite set S is to establish a bijection $f : \mathbb{N}_n \to S$ for some $n \in \mathbb{N}$ or to recognize that S is empty. (This is a precise mathematical formulation of the counting process used by every elementary school child.)

The next few theorems on counting provide a useful exercise in humility. In each case the intuitive formulation of the result is a statement that seems obvious, yet the proof is challenging.

4.8 Theorem. Let n and m be nonnegative integers, with $n > m$.

(a) There is no injection from $\mathbb{N}_n$ to $\mathbb{N}_m$, and hence $\mathbb{N}_n \not\approx \mathbb{N}_m$.

(b) If A is a set and $\#A = n$, then $\#A \neq m$. (Intuitively: *If a finite set is correctly counted twice, the results will be the same.*)

PROOF.   (a) We use induction on n, starting with $n = 1$. If $n = 1$ then $m = 0$, and there is no injection (indeed, no *function*) from $\mathbb{N}_1$ to $\mathbb{N}_0$, for such a function would have to pair the element 1 in $\mathbb{N}_1$ with an element of $\mathbb{N}_0$; but since $\mathbb{N}_0 = \emptyset$, this is impossible.

Assume the result to be true when $n = k$; that is, if $0 \le m < k$ there is no injection from $\mathbb{N}_k$ to $\mathbb{N}_m$. Suppose there *is* an injection $f : \mathbb{N}_{k+1} \to \mathbb{N}_m$ for some $m < k + 1$; we seek a contradiction. First note that we must have $m \ge 1$, since (as in the case $n = 1$) no function exists from $\mathbb{N}_{k+1}$ to $\mathbb{N}_0 = \emptyset$. Now let $g : \mathbb{N}_m \to \mathbb{N}_m$ be the bijection that interchanges m with $f(k + 1)$ and fixes everything else; that is, define g by

$$g(x) = \begin{cases} f(k + 1) & \text{if } x = m \\ m & \text{if } x = f(k + 1) \\ x & \text{otherwise} \end{cases}$$

(So g is just the identity mapping on $\mathbb{N}_m$ if $f(k + 1) = m$.) Then $g \circ f : \mathbb{N}_{k+1} \to \mathbb{N}_m$ is an injection, since f and g are injections, and $(g \circ f)(k + 1) = m$. Therefore the restriction $(g \circ f)|_{\mathbb{N}_k}$ is an injection from $\mathbb{N}_k$ to $\mathbb{N}_{m-1}$. But $m - 1 < k$, so the existence of such a function contradicts the induction hypothesis. Thus an injection such as f cannot exist, and this completes the induction argument.

(b) If we had $\#A = n$ and $\#A = m$, then we would have $\mathbb{N}_n \approx A \approx \mathbb{N}_m$, an impossibility by part (a). $\square$

4.9 Corollary (The Pigeonhole Principle).   Let A and B be nonempty finite sets, with $\#A > \#B$. Then there is no injection from A to B. Thus for any function $A \to B$, some element in B has at least two preimages. (Intuitively: *If n pigeons fly into m pigeonholes and $n > m$, then some pigeonhole receives at least two pigeons.* Here the "pigeons" are the elements of A, the "pigeonholes" are the elements of B, and "flying" is the pairing action of the function.)

PROOF.   Suppose $\#A = n$ and $\#B = m$, with $n > m$. Then there are bijections $f : \mathbb{N}_n \to A$ and $g : B \to \mathbb{N}_m$. (Why?) If there were an injection $h : A \to B$, then the function

$$g \circ h \circ f : \mathbb{N}_n \to \mathbb{N}_m$$

would also be an injection, contradicting Theorem 4.8. Therefore no such h exists. $\square$

4.10 EXAMPLES. (a) The game of musical chairs is played with n people and $n-1$ chairs. Each chair can hold only one person. The players march around the chairs to music until the music is suddenly stopped, whereupon each player attempts to sit in a chair. By the pigeonhole principle, someone loses. (Let's go through the argument carefully. The pigeonhole principle says that there is no injection from the set P of n players to the set C of $n-1$ chairs, so at least one player must remain unseated in any attempt to seat everyone. On the other hand, if p_0 is an unseated player then $\#(P - \{p_0\}) = \#C = n-1$. Therefore there *is* an injection $P - \{p_0\} \to C$, so there is only one loser in a given round of the game.) The game now repeats with $n-1$ players and $n-2$ chairs, and the foolishness continues until only one player remains: the winner.

(b) In any set of eleven integers, there are two whose difference is divisible by 10. Proof idea: by the pigeonhole principle, two of the integers have the same right-hand digit, hence their difference is divisible by 10. (Here the set A of "pigeons" is the given set of eleven integers, the set of "pigeonholes" is the set $B = \{0, 1, \ldots, 9\}$ of possible right-hand digits, and the relevant function $A \to B$ takes each integer to its right-hand digit.)

(c) A cheese cube with 2-inch edges is finely chopped, and nine mice are each fed one of the resulting crumbs. We claim that two of those crumbs were at most $\sqrt{3}$ inches from each other in the original cube. To see this, imagine the original cube partitioned into eight cubes with 1-inch edges, as shown here:

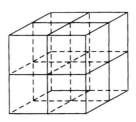

By the pigeonhole principle, two crumbs are from the same small cube, and those two crumbs are at most as far apart as the little cube's diagonally opposite corners. Invocation of Pythagoras's theorem completes the proof of the claim. (Check this.)

Recall that the symbol $\subset$ denotes *strict* set inclusion, so if $A \subset B$, then B contains at least one element not in A.

4.11 Theorem. Every subset of $\mathbb{N}_n$ is finite; and if $A \subset \mathbb{N}_n$ then $\#A = m$ for some $m < n$.

Before proving this theorem, we pause to note that our terminology and notation make this theorem seem more obvious than it is, and it is in part the *job* of terminology and notation to do this. (See the quotation from Alfred North Whitehead on page 54). But the assertion "$\#A = m$ for some $m < n$" has a precise meaning spelled out in 4.7, and there are details we must check before we can call the assertion "obvious" with at least a moderately clear conscience. A less suggestive notation would have made it more evident that there is work to be done in order to prove this theorem. Consider the following comment from Bertrand Russell (and compare it with the earlier statement by his pal Whitehead):

> Symbolism is useful because it makes things difficult. Now in the beginning everything is self-evident, and it is hard to see whether one self-evident proposition follows from another or not. Obviousness is always the enemy to correctness. Hence we must invent a new and difficult symbolism in which nothing is obvious.

PROOF OF THEOREM 4.11. It suffices to prove the second assertion. (The first is an immediate consequence of it.) We use mathematical induction, starting with $n = 0$.

If $n = 0$ the result is true because the set $\mathbb{N}_0 = \emptyset$ has no proper subsets. Now suppose the result is true when $n = k$, and consider a subset $A \subset \mathbb{N}_{k+1}$. We must show that $\#A = m$ for some $m \le k$.

Case (1). Suppose $k + 1 \notin A$. Then $A \subseteq \mathbb{N}_k$. If $A = \mathbb{N}_k$ then $\#A = k$; and if $A \subset \mathbb{N}_k$ the induction hypothesis yields $\#A = m$ for some $m < k$, and we are done.

Case (2). Suppose $k + 1 \in A$. Then $A = \{k + 1\} \cup (A \cap \mathbb{N}_k)$, and $A \cap \mathbb{N}_k \subset \mathbb{N}_k$ (since if $A \cap \mathbb{N}_k = \mathbb{N}_k$ we would have $A = \mathbb{N}_{k+1}$, contradicting the hypothesis that $A \subset \mathbb{N}_{k+1}$). From the induction hypothesis, we know that $\#(A \cap \mathbb{N}_k) = s$ for some $s \le k - 1$; thus there is a bijection $f : A \cap \mathbb{N}_k \to \mathbb{N}_s$. Now define a function $g : A \to \mathbb{N}_{s+1}$ by

$$g(x) = \begin{cases} f(x) & \text{if } x \in A \cap \mathbb{N}_k \\ s + 1 & \text{if } x = k + 1 \end{cases}$$

Then g is a bijection (why?), and therefore $\#A = s + 1 \le k$. □

The intuition underlying the last part of the proof of Theorem 4.11 (specifically, the definition of g in terms of f) is this: Suppose we have counted a given finite set and found that it has s elements. If someone now tosses a new element into our set, then instead of counting everything all over again we retain our record of the original count and call the new element the $(n + 1)$st element.

The following result is understood and believed by every first-grade child on the basis of experience: If you have a finite set of objects and you count some, but not all, of the objects, then your answer will be less than the total number. This is the intuitive meaning of assertion (c) of the following theorem.

4.12 Theorem. (a) Every subset of a finite set is finite.

(b) Every set containing an infinite set is infinite.

(c) If $A \subset B$ and B is finite then $\#A < \#B$.

PROOF. (a) Suppose $A \subseteq B$ and B is finite. Then from the definition of "finite" there is a bijection $f : B \rightarrow \mathbb{N}_n$ for some integer n. The restricted function $f|_A$ is injective, and it is a bijection from A to $f(A)$. By Theorem 4.11 we have $f(A) \approx \mathbb{N}_m$ for some integer $m \leq n$. Thus we have

$$A \approx f(A) \approx \mathbb{N}_m$$

Therefore $A \approx \mathbb{N}_m$, and so A is finite.

(b) Let $A \subseteq B$. In part (a) we proved the implication

$$B \text{ finite} \quad \Rightarrow \quad A \text{ finite}$$

The statement "A infinite $\Rightarrow B$ infinite" is just the contrapositive of this, so we are done.

(c) The proof is essentially the same as the proof of statement (a), except that now $f(A) \subset \mathbb{N}_n$. Check the details. □

Before proceeding further, let's display an infinite set for everyone to admire.

4.13 Theorem. The set $\mathbb{N}$ of natural numbers is infinite.

PROOF *(by Contradiction)*. If $\mathbb{N}$ is finite then there is a bijection $f : \mathbb{N} \rightarrow \mathbb{N}_m$ for some natural number m. Pick any natural number n such that $n > m$. Then $f|_{\mathbb{N}_n}$ is an injection from $\mathbb{N}_n$ into $\mathbb{N}_m$, and this is an impossibility by Theorem 4.8(a). □

4.14 Theorem. If A and B are disjoint finite sets, then $A \cup B$ is finite and

$$\#(A \cup B) = \#A + \#B$$

PROOF. Suppose $\#A = m$ and $\#B = n$. Then there exist bijections

$$f : \mathbb{N}_m \to A \qquad \text{and} \qquad g : \mathbb{N}_n \to B$$

Now define a function $h : \mathbb{N}_{m+n} \to A \cup B$ by

$$h(i) = \begin{cases} f(i) & \text{if } 1 \le i \le m \\ g(i - m) & \text{if } m + 1 \le i \le m + n \end{cases}$$

It is a short exercise to check that h is a bijection. Once this has been done, it follows that $\#(A \cup B) = m + n = \#A + \#B$. $\qquad \square$

Recall that sets $A_1, \ldots, A_m$ are said to be **pairwise disjoint** if $A_i \cap A_j = \emptyset$ whenever $i \ne j$.

4.15 Corollary. If $A_1, \ldots, A_m$ are pairwise disjoint finite sets, then $\bigcup_{i=1}^{m} A_i$ is finite and

$$\# \left(\bigcup_{i=1}^{m} A_i \right) = \#A_1 + \cdots + \#A_m$$

PROOF OUTLINE. When $m = 1$ we have $\bigcup_{i=1}^{1} A_i = A_1$, so here the theorem asserts that $\#A_1 = \#A_1$, which is true (since $A_1 \approx A_1$). The case $m = 2$ is covered by Theorem 4.14, and the general case follows by induction on m. $\qquad \square$

4.16 Corollary. If A and B are finite sets (not necessarily disjoint), then $A \cup B$ is finite and

$$\#(A \cup B) = \#A + \#B - \#(A \cap B)$$

PROOF. Express $A \cup B$ as the union of three pairwise disjoint sets:

$$A \cup B = \underbrace{(A - B) \cup \overbrace{(A \cap B)}^{B} \cup (B - A)}_{A}$$

(The Venn diagram for $A \cup B$ leads naturally to this decomposition.) Then

$$\#(A \cup B) = \#(A - B) + \#(A \cap B) + \#(B - A) \qquad \text{(by Corollary 4.15)}$$
$$= \underbrace{[\#(A - B) + \#(A \cap B)]}_{\#A} + \underbrace{[\#(B - A) + \#(A \cap B)]}_{\#B} - \#(A \cap B)$$

This gives the result. □

A more intuitive argument in support of 4.16 goes as follows. We start out computation of $\#(A \cup B)$ by first adding the number of elements in A to the number of elements in B; this assures that all elements of $A \cup B$ are included in our count. Then, upon noticing that the elements in $A \cap B$ have been counted twice, we subtract $\#(A \cap B)$ from the sum. Corollary 4.16 is an instance of the *inclusion–exclusion principle*, a general formula for the number of elements in the union of a finite number of finite sets. (We'll consider the case of three sets in Exercise 7 at the end of this section, and the general case in Chapter 6).

4.17 Theorem. If $\#A = m$ and $\#B = n$, then $\#(A \times B) = mn$

Proof Outline. If $A = \emptyset$ then also $A \times B = \emptyset$, and the result follows from the fact that $\#\emptyset = 0$. Otherwise we have $A = \{a_1, \dots, a_m\}$, say, and then $A \times B = \cup_{i=1}^{m}(\{a_i\} \times B)$, a union of m pairwise disjoint sets, each with the same cardinality as B. Apply Corollary 4.15. □

Theorem 4.17 provides the following fundamental counting principle:

A shop offering m ice cream flavors and n flavored sauces can serve mn kinds of ice cream sundaes.

Here is a rather technical-sounding extension of Theorem 4.17 that has an intuitive interpretation making it an extremely important tool in the solution of many practical problems.

4.18 Theorem. Let $A = \{a_1, \dots, a_m\}$; and for each i satisfying $1 \le i \le n$, let B_i be a set with $\#B_i = n$. Then

$$\#\left(\cup_{i=1}^{m}(\{a_i\} \times B_i)\right) = mn$$

Intuitive Interpretation. *Suppose two choices are to be made in succession. If there are m possibilities for the first choice and, once the first* *choice has been made, n possibilities for the second, then there are mn possibilities for the ordered pair of choices.*

PROOF. Put $S_i = \{a_i\} \times B_i$, for $1 \le i \le m$. Then the sets S_i are pairwise disjoint (why?), and for each i we have $\#S_i = n$. The conclusion now follows from Corollary 4.15. (As for the intuitive interpretation, view the a_i as the possible initial choices; and, having chosen some a_i, view the elements of B_i as the possible second choices. Then the elements of $\bigcup_{i=1}^{m}(\{a_i\} \times B_i)$ are the possible ordered pairs of choices.) □

4.19 EXAMPLES. To estimate the weight of a typical goldfish in a tank of 100 fish, it is decided to sweep a one-fish net through the tank until a fish is caught, record the weight of the captured fish, and then repeat the whole process once more. (The average of the two weights will be used as the estimate.)

(a) If the first fish is dropped back into the tank before the next selection is made, then by 4.18 there are $100 \times 100 = 10,000$ possibilities for the ordered pair of fish being chosen. (This is an example of **sampling with replacement**: there is the possibility that the same fish will be chosen twice.)

(b) If the first fish is kept out of the tank while the second fish is selected, then there are $100 \times 99 = 9,900$ possibilities for the ordered pair. (This is **sampling without replacement**.)

(c) Now suppose there are two tanks of fish, each with 100 fish, and *one* fish is to be chosen. How many possible choices are there? This situation is covered *not* by 4.18 but by Theorem 4.14, which tells us that there are 200 fish in all, and so 200 is our answer.

Now we can extend our discussion to decision procedures of arbitrary length. Recall from Chapter 3 that if n is a positive integer, an **n-tuple** $(a_1, \ldots, a_n)$ is a sequence of length n. (See Exercise 10 in Section 3.2 for an alternative definition.)

4.20 Definition. Let $A_1, \ldots, A_n$ be sets. The **Cartesian product**

$$A_1 \times \cdots \times A_n$$

is the set of all n-tuples $(a_1, \ldots, a_n)$ such that $a_i \in A_i$ for $1 \le i \le n$.

The following generalization of Theorem 4.17 can be proved by induction on n; we omit the details.

4.21 Theorem. Suppose $A_1, \ldots, A_n$ are finite sets, with $\#A_i = m_i$ for $1 \le i \le n$. Then the Cartesian product $A_1 \times \cdots \times A_n$ is also finite, and

$$\#(A_1 \times \cdots \times A_n) = m_1 m_2 \cdots m_n$$

There is also a natural extension of Theorem 4.18, as follows.

4.22 Product Rule. Suppose that n consecutive choices are to be made. Suppose further that there are m_1 possibilities for the first choice, and that for each k satisfying $2 \le k \le n$, there are m_k possibilities for the kth choice, no matter how the first $k - 1$ choices were made. Then there are exactly $m_1 m_2 \cdots m_n$ possibilities for the sequence of n choices.

4.23 EXAMPLE. A state motor vehicle bureau has decided that all automobile license plates must have exactly seven characters. The bureau directors agree that the characters will be chosen from the English alphabet or from the numerals $0, 1, \ldots, 9$, but the directors are still discussing whether the characters should satisfy some further conditions. In each of the following cases we will determine the number of licenses that satisfy the given condition.

(a) Each character can be any letter or numeral.
(b) The first three characters are letters and the last four are numerals.
(c) Three consecutive characters (not necessarily the first three) are letters and the others are numerals.
(d) Exactly three characters are letters and the others are numerals.
(e) Suppose the agreement that each license will have exactly seven characters is abandoned. Instead it is decided that a license must have *at most* seven characters, and each character can be any letter or numeral. (No car will get a blank license.)

SOLUTION. (a) Since there are 26 letters and 10 numerals, there are 36 possibilities for each character. (This is evident; but the underlying theorem is 4.14.) By 4.22 (with $n = 7$ and $m_i = 36$ for $1 \le i \le 7$), we see that there are 36^7 possible configurations.

(b) Here there are 26^3 possible letter configurations and 10^4 numeral configurations, so there are $(26^3)(10^4)$ possibilities in all.

(c) First it must be decided which character (counting from the left, say) will be the first one to be a letter; there are five such possibilities, and this choice dictates the locations of the other two letters. Once this decision has been made, there are $(26^3)(10^4)$ possibilities for the characters, by the same reasoning as in case (b). So altogether there are $5(26^3)(10^4)$ possibilities.

(d) Once it is decided which three places will hold the letters, as before there will be $(26^3)(10^4)$ possible choices. In how many ways can we choose the three positions out of seven in which to insert the letters? In Chapter 5, when we discuss *combinations*, we will see that there are 35 ways to do this. Accepting this for now, our present answer is $(35)(26^3)(10^4)$.

(e) Imagine the one-character plates in one pile, the two-character plates in a second pile, and so on. By the argument in case (a), we see that the kth pile will have 36^k plates. Altogether this gives a grand total of

$$36 + 36^2 + 36^3 + 36^4 + 36^5 + 36^6 + 36^7$$

possibilities.

4.24 EXAMPLE *(for Card Players).* A *straight* hand in poker consists of five cards in consecutive numerical order, for example,

$$3, 4, 5, 6, 7 \quad \text{and} \quad 10, J, Q, K, A$$

are straights. (Suits are irrelevant.) How many straights are there in all?

SOLUTION. There are ten possibilities for the lowest numerical value of a card in a straight. (An ace can have numerical value 1 or 14.) Once that lowest number has been determined, there are four cards in the deck corresponding to each of the five relevant numerical values. Therefore there are $(10)(4^5) = 10,240$ straights in a poker deck.

Exercises

Throughout this exercise set, the letters A, B, C, D will denote sets. Do not assume them to be finite unless that condition is given explicitly.

1. (a) Write a brief explanation of what it means to *count* a finite set. Your answer should be understandable to a fourth grade child who has never heard of functions.

    (b) Express the meaning of statement 4.2(c) in a form accessible to an elementary school child who has never heard of functions.

2. Let L and M be lines in the xy-plane. Prove that $L \approx M$. (Suggestion: First show that every line is equipotent to $\mathbb{R}$.)

3. (a) Exhibit a bijection from $\mathbb{Z}$ to the set of all integers that are 2 more than a multiple of 5.

   (b) Write a formula for the inverse of the bijection in part (a).

4. Prove the following statements.

   (a) $A \times B \approx B \times A$

   (b) If $A \approx C$ and $B \approx D$ then $A \times B \approx C \times D$.

   (c) $(A \times B) \times C \approx A \times (B \times C)$

   (d) If w is any element then $\{w\} \times A \approx A$.

5. Exhibit specific bijections that prove the following statements.

   (a) $[0, 1] \approx [2, 7]$

   (b) $\mathbb{Z} \approx$ the set of even natural numbers.

   (c) $[0, 2\pi) \approx \{(x, y) \mid x^2 + y^2 = 1\}$

6. Define a bijection from the interval $[-2, 8]$ onto the interval $[3, 5]$.

7. (For students who have had differential calculus) Outline the argument showing that the mapping $I_{-\pi/2}^{\pi/2} \to \mathbb{R}$ given by $x \mapsto \tan x$ is a bijection. (This fact is used in Example 4.5(b).)

8. Suppose that m and n are positive integers, with $m \le n$, and assume $\#A = n$. Prove that the number of m-element subsets of A is equal to the number of $(n - m)$-element subsets of A. (Example 4.4 and Theorem 4.14 may help you.)

9. If A, B, and C are finite sets, write a formula for the number of elements in $A \cup B \cup C$. Your formula may use addition, subtraction, and intersection, but not *union*. (Suggestion: A double application of 4.16 will do the job. Alternatively, draw a Venn diagram and think about it.)

10. A study of 115 breakfast eaters shows that 85 also eat lunch, 58 use dental floss regularly, and 27 subscribe to a morning newspaper. Among those who also eat lunch, 52 floss regularly and 15 get the morning paper, and 10 lunch eaters both floss and get the paper. Four flossers neither eat lunch nor get the paper.

    (a) How many of those in the study neither eat lunch, nor floss regularly, nor get the morning paper?

    (b) How many of those who use dental floss regularly also get the morning paper?

    (c) How many of those who get the morning paper neither use dental floss regularly nor eat lunch?

11. Prove that if $A_1, A_2, \ldots, A_n$ are finite sets, then $\bigcup_{i=1}^{n} A_i$ is finite and $\#(\bigcup_{i=1}^{n} A_i) \le \#A_1 + \cdots + \#A_n$. (Use induction on n.)

For Exercises 12, 13, and 14, imagine that you are familiar with the set of nonnegative integers, but that you have never heard of the operations of addition, subtraction, and multiplication.

12. Define the *sum* of nonnegative integers m and n as follows. Take disjoint sets A and B, with $\#A = m$ and $\#B = n$, and define

$$m + n = \#(A \cup B)$$

(a) Show that if a different pair of disjoint sets A_1 and B_1 are used, with $\#A_1 = m$ and $\#B_1 = n$, then the same value of $m + n$ will result.

(b) Show that the associative law of addition,

$$(m + n) + p = m + (n + p)$$

is a consequence of the definition of addition given in this exercise. (Here m, n, and p are understood to be nonnegative integers.)

13. Let m and n be integers with $n > m \ge 0$, and define the *difference* $n - m$ as follows. Take sets A and B such that $\#A = m$, $\#B = n$, and $A \subset B$; then define

$$n - m = \#(B - A)$$

(Here the "minus" sign on the left is the symbol being defined; the "minus" sign on the right denotes set difference.) Show that with "$-$" as defined here and "$+$" as in the previous problem, the following equation holds:

$$m + (n - m) = n$$

14. Let m and n be nonnegative integers, and define the *product* mn as follows. Suppose sets A and B are such that $\#A = m$ and $\#B = n$; then define

$$mn = \#(A \times B)$$

(a) Show that it follows from this definition that $mn = nm$.

(b) Show that from the definition of product given here and the definition of sum in Exercise 12, it follows that

$$m(n + k) = mn + mk$$

when m, n, and k are nonnegative integers.

15. (a) Show that in any group of eight people there are two (at least) who were born on the same day of the week.

    (b) How large a group of people must we consider in order to be sure that at least n of them were born on the same day of the week? (Here n is a positive integer.) Explain.

16. Define a **codeword** of length three to be a three-digit string of 0s and 1s. For instance, 011 and 101 are codewords.

    (a) Show that there are eight codewords of length three.

    (b) Define the **distance** between two codewords to be the number of digits in which they differ. For instance, the distance between 011 and 101 is 2. Show that there does not exist a set of five different codewords of length three, each of which has distance of at least 2 from each of the others. (Do *not* attempt to list all the five-element sets of codewords and eliminate them one by one. Instead, proceed by contradiction: suppose there *is* such a set, use the pigeonhole principle to show that at least three of these five codewords have the same first digit, and then go on to consider the second and third digits of these three codewords to deduce a contradiction.)

17. A camper's afternoon at Camp Sweatless begins with an hour of dabbling in one of seven art media, followed by attendance at one of the camp's nine films, and then consumption of a massive "snack." (The camper chooses one from a menu with seventeen possibilities.)

    (a) How many variations are possible in an afternoon's fun schedule?

    (b) Suppose that a new camp director is appointed who allows each camper the additional freedom to choose the order of his or her activities (for example, perhaps first a movie, then a snack, then art). How many variations are possible under this new arrangement?

18. The well-known mail order retailer M. M. Pease carries men's shirts in seven different sleeve lengths and five different collar sizes; and for women's shirts (these are shaped differently from the men's) there are eight different sizes and four different collar styles. (Don't be concerned with colors here.)

(a) How many variations in shirt construction are there altogether?

(b) Suppose the men's shirts can be purchased with two or three initials, or without initials. How many varieties of men's shirts are there in all, if you count two shirts as different if they are identically sized but have different initials? (And count differently sized shirts as different.)

(c) One quarter of all the varieties of women's shirts can be purchased with a pocket as an extra feature. Counting these as different from the shirts without pockets, how many different women's shirts are there?

19. Ten people are in a room, and each person shakes everyone else's hand. It is argued that altogether 90 handshakes have occurred, because each of ten people shakes nine hands, making 90 in all. Do you agree? Explain.

20. Suppose there are two 100-fish tanks, and one fish is to be chosen from each tank.

(a) How many ways are there to make the selection, assuming that the order in which the fish are chosen is irrelevant? (That is, all that matters is which two fish are chosen, not which is chosen first.)

(b) How many ways are there to make the selection if order *is* relevant?

21. Let A^B denote the set of all functions from B to A.

(a) Suppose $\#A = m$ and $\#B = n$. Then use the counting principles of this section to show that

$$\#(A^B) = m^n$$

(b) Determine the number of injections from B to A, assuming that $\#A = m$ and $\#B = n$. Here you will need to use the fact (to be proved in Chapter 5) that if $n \leq m$, the number of n-element subsets of an m-element set is

$$\frac{m!}{n!(m-n)!}$$

(c) (Challenging) Without any restrictions on the sets A, B, C, show that

$$(A \times B)^C \approx A^C \times B^C$$

22. (a) Suppose $\sim$ is an equivalence relation on an infinite set S, and suppose the relation partitions the set into a finite number of equivalence classes. Deduce that some equivalence class must contain an infinite number of elements.

    (b) Suppose $\sim$ is an equivalence relation on an infinite set S, with no further conditions. Must some equivalence class be infinite?

23. (a) Without writing anything down, convince yourself that in any set of 15 people there will be three people born on the same day of the week; and in a set of 22 people there will be four born on the same day of the week.

    (b) With part (a) in mind as a model, state (without proof) a generalized version of the Pigeonhole Principle involving functions from a set of $mn + 1$ elements to a set of m elements.

    (c) Show that if $f : A \rightarrow B$ and b_1, b_2 are distinct elements of B, then

$$f^{-1}(b_1) \cap f^{-1}(b_2) = \emptyset$$

    (d) Prove the generalized Pigeonhole Principle that you stated in part (b). (Suggestion: Consider a proof by contradiction. Part (c) may be useful.)

4.2 Comparing Sets, Finite or Infinite

Our focus in this chapter up to now has been the measurement and comparison of finite sets. The strategy has been to assign to each set a number that represents the set's size and then to compare sets by comparing their associated numbers. But the size of an *infinite* set is not represented by a number. So, while our intuition might lead us to declare that every infinite set is larger than every finite set, our methods thus far will yield only knitted brows when we contemplate comparing one infinite set with another. Our first goal in this section is therefore to reformulate our criteria for comparing set magnitudes so that we can compare *any* two sets, finite *or* infinite; and we want to do this in a way that is consistent with what we have achieved so far in the finite case. We will see that just as finite sets come in different sizes, so do infinite sets; and in fact there are infinitely many different levels of infinity! (Our brief taste of infinite sets in Example 4.5 might have led us to believe otherwise.) At the end of the chapter we will have a look at the impact of some of these remarkable concepts on theoretical computer science, when we briefly consider *languages* and the problem of *language specification*.

We begin with a slightly unnerving but useful lemma that shows the empty set to possess surprising vigor.

4.25 Lemma. If A is any set, then $\emptyset$ is an injective function from $\emptyset$ to A.

PROOF. First we show that $\emptyset$ is a function from $\emptyset$ to A by checking the conditions of Definition 3.2. We have $\emptyset \subseteq \emptyset \times A$ (in fact, $\emptyset = \emptyset \times A$). Moreover, for every element x, the conditional statement

$$x \in \emptyset \quad \Rightarrow \quad (x, y) \in \emptyset \quad \text{for exactly one } y \in A$$

has a false hypothesis and is therefore true. Thus $\emptyset$ satisfies Definition 3.2 and is a function from $\emptyset$ to A.
The proof of injectivity has a similar flavor: the statement

$$\left(x_1, x_2 \in \emptyset \quad \text{and} \quad \emptyset(x_1) = \emptyset(x_2) \right) \quad \Rightarrow \quad x_1 = x_2$$

is true because its hypothesis is false.   □

The following theorem provides the key to our broadening of the criteria for set comparison in order to accommodate infinite sets. The proof freely uses the basic properties of bijections and inverse functions. (See especially Theorem 3.24 and the material following 3.25.)

4.26 Theorem. Let A and B be finite sets. Then

(a) $\#A \leq \#B \;\Leftrightarrow\;$ There is an injection from A to B,
(b) $\#A = \#B \;\Leftrightarrow\; A \approx B$,
(c) $\#A < \#B \;\Leftrightarrow\;$ There is an injection but no bijection from A to B.

PROOF. Write $\#A = m$ and $\#B = n$. So there are bijections

$$\mathbb{N}_m \xrightarrow{f} A \quad \text{and} \quad \mathbb{N}_n \xrightarrow{g} B$$

(a) If $m \leq n$ there is an injection $j \colon \mathbb{N}_m \to \mathbb{N}_n$. (For instance, take j to be the inclusion mapping; see Example 3.3(a). Or use Lemma 4.25 if $m = 0$.) Then the mapping

$$A \xrightarrow{\;g \circ j \circ f^{-1}\;} B$$

is an injection, as desired. Conversely, if $h: A \rightarrow B$ is an injection, then so is

$$\mathbb{N}_m \xrightarrow{g^{-1} \circ h \circ f} \mathbb{N}_n$$

and therefore $m \leq n$ by Theorem 4.8.

Now to prove statement (b), repeat the proof of (a) using "$=$" in place of "$\leq$" and "bijection" in place of "injection."

Finally, we check (c). Assume $m < n$. If there were a bijection $h: A \rightarrow B$, then $g^{-1} \circ h \circ f: \mathbb{N}_m \rightarrow \mathbb{N}_n$ would also be bijective, and this is impossible by 4.8. The converse is an immediate consequence of statements (a) and (b).   □

Notice that the conditions in Theorem 4.26 on the right side of the "$\Leftrightarrow$" symbols make sense *whether or not the sets A and B are finite.* Accordingly, we can use these conditions to rewrite our criteria for set comparison, with full confidence that they will be consistent with the criteria we have been using for finite sets.

4.27 Definition. Let A and B be sets (finite or infinite). Define the expressions $\#A \leq \#B$, $\#A = \#B$, and $\#A < \#B$ by statements 4.26(a), (b), and (c), respectively.

The expressions defined in 4.27 are read as if they are relations between numbers (which they are, as we have seen, when the sets are finite). For example, the second expression is read, "the cardinality of A is less than or equal to the cardinality of B," or, more casually, "The number of elements in A is ...." Intuitively, the expression $\#A < \#B$ means that B is larger than A, because the existence of an injection $A \rightarrow B$ tells us that there are enough elements in B to pair each element of A with a different member of B, while the fact that no injection is surjective means that after any such pairing, there are elements of B left over.

We have given meaning to the statement $\#A < \#B$ (and the other statements in 4.27) without explicitly defining the symbol $\#A$ when A is infinite. (To do so would take us deeper into the foundations of mathematics than we intend to go here.) Is this really so strange? After all, it is possible to demonstrate that one object weighs less than another without knowing the weight of either. (See the following picture.) We have merely generalized the criterion of comparison used by the primitive shepherds discussed at the start of the chapter.

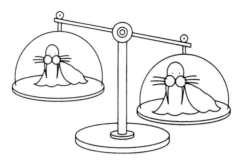

How to compare two walruses

It is natural to suppose that the standard laws of numerical inequalities extend to expressions such as those in 4.27. Indeed, it is easy to see that for every set A we have $\#A \leq \#A$, since the identity mapping is an injection from A to A. We also have

$$\#A \leq \#B \text{ and } \#B \leq \#C \quad \Rightarrow \quad \#A \leq \#C,$$

for the hypothesis provides injections $A \to B$ and $B \to C$, whose composition is injective by 3.24(a). But to handle the *strict* inequalities we need the following theorem, proved independently by E. Schröder and F. Bernstein in the 1890s. We omit the proof,[*] but we remark that if the sets involved are finite, the theorem is an immediate consequence of the pigeonhole principle. Incidentally, we will continue to write $A \approx B$ instead of the slightly longer $\#A = \#B$; there is no harm in this since the expressions are equivalent.

4.28 Schröder–Bernstein Theorem. Let A and B be sets. Then

$$\#A \leq \#B \quad \text{and} \quad \#B \leq \#A \quad \Rightarrow \quad A \approx B$$

4.29 EXAMPLE. Consider the open interval $(0, 1)$ and the closed interval $[0, 1]$. We claim that

$$[0, 1] \approx (0, 1)$$

(Intuitively, this says that attaching the two endpoints to the open interval has no effect on the "number" of elements present.) The Schröder–Bernstein theorem tells us that to verify the claim, it suffices to construct an injection from each of the given intervals to the other. First notice that

[*]For a highly readable version see P. R. Halmos, *Naive Set Theory* (New York: Springer-Verlag, 1974).

since $(0, 1) \subseteq [0, 1]$, the *inclusion mapping* $(0, 1) \rightarrow [0, 1]$ is a readily available injection. (Recall Example 3.3(a).) In the other direction, we map $[0, 1]$ into $(0, 1)$ according to the following scheme:

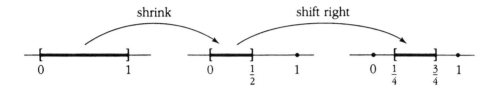

More formally, define $f : [0, 1] \rightarrow (0, 1)$ by the formula

$$f(x) = \frac{x}{2} + \frac{1}{4}$$

and check that f is injective. It follows that $[0, 1] \approx (0, 1)$, by the Schröder–Bernstein theorem. Notice that the theorem tells us that *there exists* a bijection between the two intervals, but it does not spell out an explicit formula for such a bijection (and neither of the injections we have mentioned is surjective). Suggestion: try to construct a bijection from $[0, 1]$ to $(0, 1)$. (We'll come back to this in Exercise 4 at the end of this section.)

4.30 Theorem. Let A, B, and C be sets. Then

(a) $\#A < \#B < \#C \quad \Rightarrow \quad \#A < \#C$
(b) $\#A < \#B \leq \#C \quad \Rightarrow \quad \#A < \#C$
(c) $\#A \leq \#B < \#C \quad \Rightarrow \quad \#A < \#C$

[If the sets in the theorem are not all finite, then these alleged inequalities are *not* numerical inequalities of the high-school variety. (They just *look* like them.) Instead, they are assertions about the existence and nonexistence of certain functions, as spelled out in Theorem 4.26 and Definition 4.27. So there really is something to prove here.]

PROOF OF (a). The hypothesis and the fact that the composition of two injections is an injection give $\#A \leq \#C$. So it remains to prove that $A \not\approx C$, and we do this by contradiction.

If in fact $A \approx C$ then there is a bijection $C \rightarrow A$; and the hypothesis $\#B < \#C$ provides an injection $B \rightarrow C$. Then the composition $B \rightarrow C \rightarrow A$ is injective, so $\#B \leq \#A$. But the hypothesis $\#A < \#B$ implies the weaker statement $\#A \leq \#B$, and therefore the Schröder–Bernstein theorem gives

$A \approx B$. This contradicts the hypothesis $\#A < \#B$. So the assumption $A \approx C$ must be discarded, and the inequality is strict: $\#A < \#C$. Proofs of (b) and (c) are similar and are left as exercises.   □

The careful comparison of infinite sets is outside the range of our childhood experience, and our intuition is no longer completely reliable. For example, it might seem as though all infinite sets are equipotent, because of our vague sense that there are always enough elements in one infinite set to accommodate the needs of another; but this is *not* the case, as the next theorem shows. This theorem was proved by Georg Cantor (1845–1918), whom we first encountered in Chapter 3 (see Example 3.19). Cantor's results on infinite sets in the last quarter of the nineteenth century startled the mathematical world and infuriated much of it, and led to a reexamination and reconstruction of the foundations of mathematics.* Recall from Chapter 2 that the **power set** $P(S)$ of a set S is the set of all subsets of S; so "member of $P(S)$" and "subset of S" are synonymous expressions.

4.31 Cantor's Theorem (I). Let S be a set with power set $P(S)$. Then

$$\#S < \#P(S)$$

PROOF.   First note that if $S = \emptyset$ then $P(S) = \{\emptyset\}$, so $\#S = 0$ and $\#P(S) = 1$, and the inequality is valid.

Now suppose $S \neq \emptyset$. To prove the theorem, the definition of "$<$" requires that we show the existence of an injection and the nonexistence of a bijection from S to $P(S)$. Define a function $g: S \rightarrow P(S)$ by setting $g(x) = \{x\}$ for each $x \in S$. Then g is injective, since

$$g(x_1) = g(x_2) \quad \Rightarrow \quad \{x_1\} = \{x_2\} \quad \Rightarrow \quad x_1 = x_2$$

This proves that $\#S \leq \#P(S)$.

It remains to prove that there is no bijection from S to $P(S)$. Suppose, to the contrary, that there *is* such a bijection f. Then for each $x \in S$ we have $f(x) \in P(S)$; that is, $f(x)$ is a subset of S. Thus either $x \in f(x)$ or $x \notin f(x)$. Define

$$E = \{x \in S \mid x \notin f(x)\}$$

---

*David Hilbert (1862–1943), another great mathematician, later called set theory "a paradise created by Cantor from which nobody will ever expel us."

Then E is a subset of S; that is, $E \in P(S)$. Since f is onto $P(S)$ (remember, f is a bijection), there is an element $z \in S$ such that $f(z) = E$. Now, is the statement "$z \in E$" true or false? Observe:

$$z \in E \quad \Leftrightarrow \quad z \notin f(z) \qquad \text{(from the definition of } E\text{)}$$
$$\Leftrightarrow \quad z \notin E \qquad \text{(since } f(z) = E\text{)}$$

This is madness. That is, the assumption that f is a bijection has led to an impossibility: a statement that is equivalent to its negation. Therefore no such bijection can exist. $\square$

The following astonishing result is a corollary of Cantor's theorem: Not only are there infinite sets (for example, $\mathbb{N}$), but *there are higher and higher levels of infinity*. In particular:

4.32 Corollary. $\#\mathbb{N} < \#P(\mathbb{N}) < \#P(P(\mathbb{N})) < \#P(P(P(\mathbb{N}))) < \cdots$

Exercises

1. (a) Supplement Lemma 4.25 by showing that the "empty function"

$$\emptyset : \emptyset \to A$$

   is surjective if and only if $A = \emptyset$.

   (b) Show that for any set A, the empty function is the *only* function from $\emptyset$ to A.

2. Someone deduces that the following statement is a consequence of the Schröder–Bernstein theorem: "If there are injections $f : A \to B$ and $g : B \to A$, then each of these injections is a bijection." Either *show* that this is a consequence of the theorem or give a counterexample to the statement.

3. Prove Theorem 4.30(b).

4. In Example 4.29 we deduced the equipotence $[0, 1] \approx (0, 1)$ by invoking the Schröder–Bernstein theorem, but we didn't actually construct a bijection $[0, 1] \to (0, 1)$.

   (a) Verify that the function h given by the following scheme is such a bijection:

$$0 \overset{h}{\longmapsto} \frac{1}{2}$$
$$\frac{1}{n} \longmapsto \frac{1}{n + 2} \qquad \text{for each integer } n \geq 1$$
$$x \longmapsto x \qquad \text{otherwise}$$

(b) The function h in part (a) acts on $[0, 1]$ in a way that resembles the strategy of the hotel manager at the start of the chapter. How?

5. Let A, B, and C be sets. For each of the following, either prove the statement or give a counterexample.

   (a) $\#(A - B) \leq \#A$

   (b) $\#A \leq \#B \implies \#(A \times C) \leq \#(B \times C)$

   (c) $\#(A - B) \leq \#B$

6. Show that if $\#A \leq \#B$ then $\#P(A) \leq \#P(B)$.

7. Let I denote the closed unit interval $[0, 1]$; then $I \times I$ is the closed unit square. (Here "closed" means that the boundary points are included.)

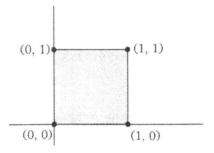

Show that $I \times I \approx I$. You may use (without proof) the fact that every nonzero real number can be written in a unique way as a nonterminating decimal, that is, a decimal without an infinite string of zeros on its right end. (For example, we can write $.38000\ldots = .37999\ldots$.) Suggestion: In mapping $I \times I$ to I as part of the solution, "shuffle" the decimal representations of the two coordinates.

8. (a) Use Cantor's theorem to deduce that $n < 2^n$ for every nonnegative integer n.

   (b) Prove that $n < 2^n$ for every nonnegative integer n, using mathematical induction instead of Cantor's theorem.

4.3 Countable and Uncountable Sets

4.33 Definition.   A set S is said to be **countably infinite** if $\mathbb{N} \approx S$; that is, if there is a bijection from $\mathbb{N}$ to S. And a set is said to be **countable** or **denumerable** if it is finite or countably infinite.* A set that is not countable is called **uncountable, uncountably infinite**, or **nondenumerable**.

---

*Terminology varies slightly from book to book. Some authors use "countable" or "denumerable" to mean what we have called "countably infinite."

In the language of Chapter 3, a set S is countable if there is a finite or infinite sequence whose terms are the elements of S. Thus, to show that a set is countable, it suffices to exhibit a procedure for listing its elements, and for this it is sufficient to start the list and to exhibit a method for picking the successor of any element on the list. (See the material on definition of sequences by recursion in Section 3.2.)

4.34 EXAMPLE. Show that the set $\mathbb{Z}$ of integers is countably infinite.

PARTIAL SOLUTION. The set $\mathbb{Z}$ is infinite because it contains the infinite set $\mathbb{N}$. (See Theorems 4.12(b) and 4.13.) To show that $\mathbb{Z}$ is countable, we will first informally list its elements, then determine a function that makes our listing process precise. It's easy to start such a list: 0, 1, −1, 2, −2, 3, −3, and so on. In more detail:

Position on list	Listed element
1	0
2	1
3	−1
4	2
5	−2
6	3
7	−3

The relation between the left column and the right column is formally described by the function $f : \mathbb{N} \to \mathbb{Z}$ defined by

$$f(n) = \begin{cases} n/2 & \text{if } n \text{ is even} \\ -(n-1)/2 & \text{if } n \text{ is odd} \end{cases}$$

Checking that f is a bijection will complete the solution.

The following theorem explains the "always room for one more" principle in the hotel-with-infinitely-many-rooms discussion.

4.35 Theorem. If A is finite and B is countable then $A \cup B$ is countable.

PROOF. First notice that if B is finite then $A \cup B$ is finite (by 4.16) and hence countable.

Now suppose B is countably infinite. Observe that $A \cup B = (A - B) \cup B$. Here is a corresponding Venn diagram:

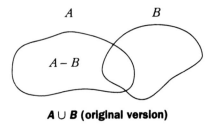

A ∪ B (original version)

The set $A - B$ is finite because it is a subset of the finite set A. Moreover, $A - B$ is disjoint from B. If we now relabel by writing A instead of $A - B$, we see that our proof will be complete if we verify the following statement: If A is finite and B is countably infinite and $A \cap B = \emptyset$, then $A \cup B$ is countably infinite.

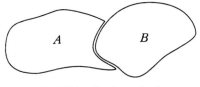

A ∪ B (revised version)

For this it suffices to show that there is a bijection $A \cup B \to \mathbb{N}$. Since A is finite and B is countably infinite, there are bijections

$$f : A \to \mathbb{N}_n \quad \text{for some } n \geq 0, \qquad \text{and} \qquad g : B \to \mathbb{N}$$

Now define $h : A \cup B \to \mathbb{N}$ by

$(*)$
$$h(x) = \begin{cases} f(x) & \text{if } x \in A \\ n + g(x) & \text{if } x \in B \end{cases}$$

Intuitively we sense that h shifts the image of g to the right on the real line in order to make room for the image of f, just as the guests filling the rooms of the infinite hotel moved down the hall to accommodate a new arrival.

We claim that h is the desired bijection. First note that since A and B are disjoint, there is no ambiguity about which line of definition $(*)$ applies to any given element x. (We say that h is *well defined* by the given formula.)

Injectivity. For all $x_1, x_2 \in B$, we must verify the implication

$$h(x_1) = h(x_2) \quad \Rightarrow \quad x_1 = x_2$$

Case (1). Suppose $x_1, x_2 \in A$. Then

$$h(x_1) = h(x_2) \quad \Rightarrow \quad f(x_1) = f(x_2) \quad \text{(by definition of } h)$$
$$\Rightarrow \quad x_1 = x_2 \quad \text{(since } f \text{ is injective)}$$

Case (2). Suppose $x_1, x_2 \in B$. Then

$$h(x_1) = h(x_2) \quad \Rightarrow \quad n + g(x_1) = n + g(x_2) \quad \text{(by definition of } h)$$
$$\Rightarrow \quad g(x_1) = g(x_2)$$
$$\Rightarrow \quad x_1 = x_2 \quad \text{(since } g \text{ is injective)}$$

Case (3). Suppose $x_1 \in A$ and $x_2 \in B$ (so $x_1 \neq x_2$). Here $h(x_1) = f(x_1) \leq n$, while $h(x_2) = n + g(x_2) \geq n + 1$, and so $h(x_1) \neq h(x_2)$.

Surjectivity. Let $k \in \mathbb{N}$. If $1 \leq k \leq n$ then

$$k = f(x) = h(x)$$

for some $x \in A$, since $f : A \to \mathbb{N}_n$ is surjective. If $k \geq n+1$ then $k = n+t$ for some $t \in \mathbb{N}$. Therefore $k = n + g(x) = h(x)$ for some $x \in B$, because $g : B \to \mathbb{N}$ is surjective. □

Before proceeding with the discussion, let's touch again on the adjective "well defined" introduced in the preceding proof. Suppose A is the set of all living people, and we try to define a function $f : A \to \mathbb{N}$ by

$$f(x) = \begin{cases} 1 & \text{if } x\text{'s name is Daniel} \\ 2 & \text{if } x \text{ weighs} \geq 150 \text{ pounds} \\ 3 & \text{otherwise} \end{cases}$$

Then f is *not* well defined, since the formula pairs someone named Daniel who weighs ≥ 150 pounds with more than one element of $\mathbb{N}$.

The following two-part theorem is useful in the study of infinite sets. We leave the proof for a later course in set theory.

4.36 Theorem. (a) Every subset of a countable set is countable. (b) Every infinite set contains a countably infinite subset.

Proofs of bijectivity are at the heart of most counting arguments, no matter how informal they may seem: injectivity guarantees that nothing is counted more than once, and surjectivity guarantees that everything is counted. Nevertheless, as the proof of Theorem 4.35 shows, the arguments can be long and they tend to have many cases, corresponding to different sections of the underlying Venn diagram. From now on most proofs of bijectivity will be omitted or only informally sketched. In each instance, supplying the details is a worthwhile exercise.

Now we will prove the countable analogues of some of our earlier results on finite sets.

4.37 Theorem.   If A and B are countable sets then $A \cup B$ is countable.

PROOF. As in the proof of Theorem 4.35, we can write $A \cup B = (A - B) \cup B$. Notice that $A - B$ is countable, by Theorem 4.36(a). Also, we can assume that $A - B$ and B are both infinite, since otherwise Theorem 4.16 completes the proof for us. Now relabel by writing A instead of $A - B$. We sum up this groundwork as follows: without loss of generality, it suffices to prove that if A and B are disjoint countably infinite sets, then $A \cup B$ is countably infinite.

We know (from Examples 4.5 and 4.34) that the set E of even integers is countably infinite. Similarly, if E' denotes the set of odd integers, the bijectivity of the mapping $\mathbb{Z} \to E'$ given by $n \mapsto 2n - 1$ shows that E' is countably infinite. Our hypothesis that A and B are countably infinite therefore guarantees the existence of bijections $A \xrightarrow{f} E$ and $B \xrightarrow{g} E'$. Now take the union of f and g as sets of ordered pairs.* Because the function f pairs the elements of A with elements of E, and g pairs the elements of B with elements of E', then the function $f \cup g$ pairs the elements of $A \cup B$ with elements of $E \cup E'$ (which is $\mathbb{Z}$). Moreover, since $A \cap B = \emptyset$, there is no ambiguity about the image of each element of $A \cup B$. Explicitly, the function

$$f \cup g : A \cup B \to E \cup E' = \mathbb{Z}$$

is given by the formula

$$(f \cup g)(x) = \begin{cases} f(x) & \text{if } x \in A \\ g(x) & \text{if } x \in B \end{cases}$$

or pictorially by

*See Exercise 14 in Section 3.3 for further exploration of the properties of functions obtained as unions of given functions.

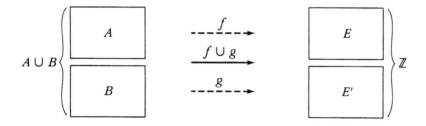

Since f and g are bijections onto E and E', respectively, and $E \cap E' = \emptyset$, it follows that $f \cup g$ is a bijection. Therefore, since $\mathbb{Z}$ is countably infinite, so is $A \cup B$. □

From Theorem 4.37, a short induction argument yields the following.

4.38 Corollary. If $A_1, \ldots, A_n$ are countable sets, then $\cup_{i=1}^{n} A_i$ is countable.

To facilitate the reading of the next proof, recall that a **prime number** is an integer $p > 1$ having no factorization of the form $p = ab$, where $a > 1$ and $b > 1$ are integers. (Examples: 2, 3, 5, 7, 11, 13, 17, 19, 23 are the first few primes.) The *Fundamental Theorem of Arithmetic* is the following statement: *Every integer $n > 1$ can be written in exactly one way as a product of prime numbers.* (We proved part of this in Theorem 2.74, and we will complete the proof in Chapter 6.) That is, if $n = p_1 p_2 \cdots p_r = q_1 q_2 \cdots q_s$, where the p's and q's are primes, then $r = s$ and the p's and q's are equal (though perhaps listed in different order).

4.39 Theorem. (a) $\mathbb{N} \times \mathbb{N}$ is countably infinite.

(b) If A and B are countable then $A \times B$ is countable.

PROOF. (a) The function $\mathbb{N} \to \mathbb{N} \times \mathbb{N}$ constructed in Example 3.18 is a bijection, from which the result follows. Here's another proof. Define $f : \mathbb{N} \times \mathbb{N} \to \mathbb{N}$ by

$$f(m, n) = 2^m 3^n$$

By the Fundamental Theorem of Arithmetic, it follows that f is injective; so, since $f(\mathbb{N} \times \mathbb{N})$ is an infinite subset of the countable set $\mathbb{N}$, it is countably infinite by Theorem 4.36(a). Hence there is a bijection g from $f(\mathbb{N} \times \mathbb{N})$ to $\mathbb{N}$, and the composition $g \circ f$ is a bijection from $\mathbb{N} \times \mathbb{N}$ to $\mathbb{N}$. Therefore $\mathbb{N} \times \mathbb{N}$ is countably infinite.

(b) If A and B are finite, we're through by Theorem 4.17. If $A = \{a_1, \dots, a_n\}$ and B is countably infinite, then

$$A \times B = (\{a_1\} \times B) \cup \cdots \cup (\{a_n\} \times B)$$

Since $\{a_i\} \times B \approx B$ [via the bijection with action $(a_i, b) \mapsto b$], each set $\{a_i\} \times B$ is countably infinite, so invocation of 4.38 completes the proof. Finally, suppose A and B are both countably infinite; then there are bijections $f : A \to \mathbb{N}$ and $g : B \to \mathbb{N}$. It follows that the mapping $A \times B \to \mathbb{N} \times \mathbb{N}$ given by

$$(a, b) \mapsto (f(a), g(b))$$

is also a bijection (check this), so $A \times B \approx \mathbb{N} \times \mathbb{N}$. But $\mathbb{N} \times \mathbb{N}$ is countable, and therefore $A \times B$ is countable also.   □

Notation. The symbol $\aleph_0$ is often used to denote the cardinality of a countably infinite set. ($\aleph$ is *aleph*, the first letter of the Hebrew alphabet; and $\aleph_0$ is read "aleph naught.") That is, the statement "A is a countable set" is symbolically represented by

$$\#A = \aleph_0$$

With this notation, the infinite cases of Theorems 4.37 and 4.39(b) become this:

If $\#A = \#B = \aleph_0$, then $\#(A \cup B) = \aleph_0$ and $\#(A \times B) = \aleph_0$

(Compare this with the properties of *finite* sets in 4.16 and 4.17!)

Before you read the next theorem, draw two copies of the real line, mark off the positive integers on one of them and the rational numbers on the other (the rationals will constitute a "fuzz" seeming to fill up most of the line), and consider which set is larger. Meditation on this theme will add to your appreciation of the theorem, which tells us that there is actually a one-to-one correspondence between the two sets. (Also see Example 3.25 for some related discussion.)

4.40 Theorem.   The set $\mathbb{Q}$ of rational numbers is countable.

PROOF.   First write $\mathbb{Q} = \mathbb{Q}^+ \cup \{0\} \cup \mathbb{Q}^-$, where $\mathbb{Q}^+$ and $\mathbb{Q}^-$ denote the sets of positive and negative rationals, respectively. Clearly $\mathbb{Q}^+ \approx \mathbb{Q}^-$ (the mapping $x \longmapsto -x$ does the job), so by 4.38 it will suffice to show that $\mathbb{Q}^+$ is countable.

Every positive rational number can be written in exactly one way in the form a/b, where a and b are positive integers with no common prime factors. (We say the number is "in lowest terms.") With this notation, we define $f: \mathbb{Q}^+ \to \mathbb{N} \times \mathbb{N}$ by $a/b \longmapsto (a, b)$. This function is injective, so $\mathbb{Q}^+ \approx f(\mathbb{Q}^+)$. By Theorems 4.39(a) and 4.36(a) we know that $f(\mathbb{Q}^+)$ is countable, and therefore so is $\mathbb{Q}^+$. $\square$

An explicit listing of $\mathbb{Q}$ can be carried out as follows. First imagine $\mathbb{Q}^+$ displayed in a rectangular array as shown here, omitting fractions that are not in lowest terms (so each rational number appears only once).

$$\begin{array}{cccccccc}
\frac{1}{1} & \frac{1}{2} & \frac{1}{3} & \frac{1}{4} & \frac{1}{5} & \frac{1}{6} & \frac{1}{7} & \frac{1}{8} & \cdots \\
\frac{2}{1} & & \frac{2}{3} & & \frac{2}{5} & & \frac{2}{7} & & \cdots \\
\frac{3}{1} & \frac{3}{2} & & \frac{3}{4} & \frac{3}{5} & & \frac{3}{7} & \frac{3}{8} & \cdots \\
\frac{4}{1} & & \frac{4}{3} & & \frac{4}{5} & & \frac{4}{7} & & \cdots \\
\frac{5}{1} & \frac{5}{2} & \frac{5}{3} & \frac{5}{4} & & \frac{5}{6} & \frac{5}{7} & \frac{5}{8} & \cdots \\
\vdots & \vdots & \vdots & \vdots & \vdots & \vdots & \vdots & \vdots
\end{array}$$

Then $\mathbb{Q}^+$ can be listed by moving down the diagonals in succession. Now take a similar list for $\mathbb{Q}^-$ (just negate each entry in the listing of $\mathbb{Q}^+$), merge the two lists by alternately choosing from one list and then from the other, and precede the whole business with zero. This produces a listing of $\mathbb{Q}$:

$$0, 1, -1, \tfrac{1}{2}, -\tfrac{1}{2}, 2, -2, \tfrac{1}{3}, -\tfrac{1}{3}, 3, -3, \tfrac{1}{4}, -\tfrac{1}{4}, \tfrac{2}{3}, -\tfrac{2}{3}, \tfrac{3}{2}, -\tfrac{3}{2}, \cdots$$

We conclude this section with a proof of the uncountability of the real numbers. The proof is very close to the proof of 3.19, in that Cantor's *diagonalization method* again provides the key. We will also need to accept (without proof) the following fact about real numbers:

Every nonzero real number has a unique representation as a nonterminating decimal. (If a number has a decimal representation of finite length, reduce the last nonzero digit by 1 and append an infinite string of 9s. For example, $2.38 = 2.37999\ldots$.)

4.41 Cantor's Theorem (II). The set $\mathbb{R}$ of real numbers is uncountable.

PROOF.   It suffices to show that the open unit interval

$$I = \{x \in \mathbb{R} \mid 0 < x < 1\}$$

is uncountable, since we saw earlier (in 4.6) that $\mathbb{R} \approx I$; and we will achieve that by showing that there is no surjection $\mathbb{N} \to I$. (Otherwise stated: every list of numbers from I is incomplete.)

Let $f: \mathbb{N} \to I$ be any function. Then f determines a list of nonterminating decimals:

$$f(1) = .a_{11}a_{12}a_{13}a_{14}\ldots$$
$$f(2) = .a_{21}a_{22}a_{23}a_{24}\ldots$$
$$f(3) = .a_{31}a_{32}a_{33}a_{34}\ldots$$
$$\vdots$$

Here a_{ij} is the jth decimal digit of $f(i)$. Now define a number $m = .m_1 m_2 m_3 \ldots$ as follows:

$$m_i = \begin{cases} 2 & \text{if } a_{ii} = 1, \\ 1 & \text{if } a_{ii} \neq 1. \end{cases}$$

Then $m \in I$; and for each $i \in \mathbb{N}$ we notice that $f(i) \neq m$, since $f(i)$ and m differ in the ith decimal place. (That is, the decimal expansion of m nowhere intersects the diagonal of the array.) Therefore $m \notin f(\mathbb{N})$; that is, f is not surjective.   □

4.42 Corollary.   The set of irrational numbers is uncountable.

PROOF.   Let S denote the set of irrational numbers; then $\mathbb{R} = \mathbb{Q} \cup S$. If S were countable then $\mathbb{R}$ would also be countable, in contradiction to Theorem 4.41.   □

4.43 EXAMPLE.   Since $\mathbb{Q}$ is countable, the set $\mathbb{Q} \times \mathbb{Q}$, consisting of all the points in the xy-plane that have rational coordinates, is also countable. We will use this fact to sketch a proof of the following remarkable geometric fact:

If A and B are distinct points in the xy-plane and not in $\mathbb{Q} \times \mathbb{Q}$, then A and B can be connected by a path that contains no points in $\mathbb{Q} \times \mathbb{Q}$.

PROOF. Let L denote the perpendicular bisector of the line segment AB. It is easy to believe (and prove) that $L \approx \mathbb{R}$. Now for each point $X \in L$ let P_X denote the path $AX \cup XB$ connecting A to B.

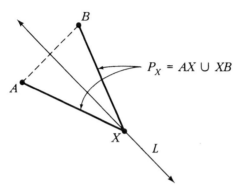

We claim: Some path P_X contains no points in $\mathbb{Q} \times \mathbb{Q}$. Suppose, to the contrary, that for each $X \in L$ we have $(\mathbb{Q} \times \mathbb{Q}) \cap P_X \neq \emptyset$. Then we can define a function $f : L \to \mathbb{Q} \times \mathbb{Q}$ by assigning to each $X \in L$ a point in $(\mathbb{Q} \times \mathbb{Q}) \cap P_X$. Notice that if X and Y are different points on L, then A and B are the only points shared by the paths P_X and P_Y. It follows from this that f is injective. But this is impossible, because L is uncountable and $\mathbb{Q} \times \mathbb{Q}$ is countable. $\square$

Exercises

1. Express the set $\mathbb{Z}$ of integers as the union of three countably infinite subsets that are pairwise disjoint.

2. Imagine a hotel with infinitely many rooms. One stormy night a countably infinite crowd of weary travellers arrives, seeking shelter. They are also seeking privacy: no two of them will share a room. Upon arriving at the hotel, they learn that the rooms are full. Can the hotel manager accommodate this mass of would-be guests? Explain in detail.

3. This exercise presents a pair of pigeonhole principles for infinite sets.
   (a) Show that if a countably infinite set is partitioned into a finite number of blocks, then at least one of the blocks is countably infinite.
   (b) Repeat (a), but with "countably infinite" replaced by "uncountable."

4. Answer *true* or *false*, and justify: If A is countable and B is a finite subset of A, then $A - B$ is countable.

5. Show that the integers that are 3 more than a multiple of 7 constitute a countable set.

6. Prove Corollary 4.38.

7. (a) Show that the set $\mathbb{N} \times \mathbb{N}$ can be expressed as the union of a countably infinite family of countably infinite sets.

   (b) Use part (a) to prove that a union of countably many pairwise disjoint countably infinite sets is countably infinite.

8. Without attempting to supply all the details, argue convincingly that the union of a countably infinite family of countable sets is countable. Do *not* assume the sets to be pairwise disjoint. (A reasonable solution to this exercise would be to outline a procedure for listing the elements of the union under consideration.)

9. Show that on the real line $\mathbb{R}$, the collection of all closed intervals with rational endpoints is a countable set.

10. Suppose a pairwise disjoint family of intervals on the real line is given. Assume that none of the intervals is just a single point. (For instance, the degenerate interval $[5, 5] = \{5\}$ does not belong to the given family.) A partial picture:

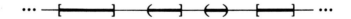

Outline a proof of the fact that this family of intervals is a countable family.

11. Here's an opportunity for you to give another proof of the fact that $\mathbb{N} \times \mathbb{N}$ is countably infinite. Define $g: \mathbb{N} \times \mathbb{N} \to \mathbb{N}$ by

$$g(m, n) = 2^{m-1}(2n - 1)$$

and use the Fundamental Theorem of Arithmetic to show that g is a bijection.

12. (For readers who have had calculus) If you try to mark all the points on the real line that correspond to rational numbers, and thereby draw a "picture" of $\mathbb{Q}$, you will find yourself marking so many points that they will seem to fill up most of the line. (For instance if you were to mark all the points corresponding to rationals with denominator 1,000,000, the line would appear virtually completely marked.) The purpose of this exercise is to show that this impression is dramatically false.

Since $\mathbb{Q}$ is countable, its members can be listed:

$$\mathbb{Q} = \{q_1, q_2, q_3, \ldots\}$$

(a) Surround q_1 by an interval I_1 of length $1/2$. (The precise location of I_1 is not important.) Then surround q_2 by an interval I_2 of length $1/2^2 = 1/4$. Continue in this manner, covering each q_n by an interval I_n of length $1/2^n$. (Some of the intervals will overlap, and that is acceptable.) What is the "total" of the lengths of all these intervals, and what does this tell you about the size of $\mathbb{Q}$ as a geometric object?

(b) Now let ϵ denote a small positive number (the smaller the better), and again cover the rationals by intervals; but this time cover each q_n by an interval of length $\epsilon/2^n$. Again find the "total" of the lengths of all these intervals. *Now* what do you conclude about the size of $\mathbb{Q}$ as a geometric object?

(c) Why have there been quotation marks around the word "total" in this exercise?

13. (Refer to the result of Exercise 12.) Imagine that you are going to throw a dart at the xy-plane; in this fantasy include the assumption that the tip of the dart will hit exactly one point P. Peer pressure demands that you bet on one of the following three possibilities:

(a) Neither coordinate of P will be rational.

(b) Exactly one coordinate of P will be rational.

(c) Both coordinates of P will be rational.

What is your best bet? Explain.

14. Prove that in the xy-plane there is a circle centered at the origin that passes through no points whose coordinates are both rational numbers.

15. Prove that there is a line in the xy-plane that passes through no points whose coordinates are both rational. (Suggestion: Let P be a point with at least one irrational coordinate. Consider the lines through P.)

4.4 More on Infinity

The purpose of this brief section is to give another characterization of infinite sets. History tells us that infinite sets were the source of considerable confusion and anxiety among nineteenth century mathematicians. Perhaps the reader has experienced a similar response to the subject. Why should this be? Probably because we grow up counting finite sets, and when we leave that realm we are at a loss for where to begin. Our definition of an infinite set earlier in this chapter reflected that despair by saying, in effect: A set is infinite if no natural number has the "strength" to measure its size.

Now let's seek a more positive description of infinity. We have seen that a finite set cannot be put into one-to-one correspondence with a proper subset. On the other hand, we have exhibited examples of infinite sets for which the opposite is true, and it turns out that this is exactly the property needed to characterize infinite sets. We remark that the following theorem's statement was used as the *definition* of an infinite set by R. Dedekind and C. S. Pierce in the 1880s.

4.44 Theorem. Let S be a set. Then

$$S \text{ is infinite} \quad \Leftrightarrow \quad S \approx S' \text{ for some } S' \subset S.$$

PROOF. First assume $S \approx S'$ for some $S' \subset S$; we must show S is infinite. If S were finite we would have

$$\mathbb{N}_n \approx S \approx S' \approx \mathbb{N}_m$$

for some $m < n$. But this is impossible, by Theorem 4.8, so S must be infinite.

Conversely, assume S is infinite. Then by Theorem 4.36(b), S contains a countably infinite subset $C = \{c_1, c_2, c_3, \ldots\}$. Define $f: S \rightarrow S$ by

$$f(c_i) = c_{2i} \qquad \text{for all } c_i \in C$$
$$f(x) = x \qquad \text{for all } x \notin C$$

Then f is a bijection of S onto the proper subset

$$S' = S - \{c_1, c_3, c_5, \ldots\} \qquad \square$$

4.5 Languages and Finite Automata

Languages are used by people and computers, and perhaps also by porpoises and other creatures. Computer programs, solutions of mathematical problems, and proofs of theorems are finite lists of statements in a language; and statements are suitably designed finite lists of symbols. If we want to understand what kinds of problems are solvable, and perhaps have a means of measuring the complexity of those problems before seeking a solution, we had better have a clear understanding of the nature and limitations of the language in which we are working. This is a matter of great importance in mathematics and computer science, as well as in psychology and linguistics.

Mathematical modeling of real-world phenomena is often an enormously difficult task. We begin by extracting some essential features of the subject under study and ignoring others. Thus, for example, we may find ourselves studying feathers falling in a vacuum, apples twirling from weightless strings, and balls rolling over frictionless surfaces. Similarly, a simplest possible mathematical definition of "language" must ignore matters of pronunciation, style, grammar, and nearly everything else that makes a language interesting. What's left? Just this: a language is a collection of strings of symbols from some alphabet. The purpose of this section is to formulate this idea in the mathematical framework required by theoretical computer science and to have a brief look at a procedure for specifying languages by means of *finite automata*. At the heart of all this material are sets and functions, which play a key role in mathematical modeling. And the relevance of infinite sets and countability makes the subject of languages and automata especially appropriate for inclusion in this chapter.

4.45 Definition. An **alphabet** Σ is a finite nonempty set.

4.46 Examples. $\{ \text{\textcent} \}$, $\{a, b, c, \ldots, z\}$, and $\{0, 1\}$ are alphabets.

4.47 Definition. Let n be a nonnegative integer. A **word** or **string** w of **length** n over the alphabet Σ is a function $w: \mathbb{N}_n \to \Sigma$.

If w is given by $i \overset{w}{\longmapsto} a_i$, for $1 \leq i \leq n$, then w is usually written as a string of symbols:

$$w = a_1 \ldots a_n$$

On the other hand, if $n = 0$ then $w = \emptyset$. (To see this, recall that $\mathbb{N}_0 = \emptyset$ and review the first part of the proof of Lemma 4.25.) In this case w is called the **empty string**, and we will denote it by ϵ (epsilon). Our intuition is that ϵ denotes a string of *no* symbols. Thus, if we are waiting for printed output from a computer but the printer remains silent, instead of saying "no output" we say "output ϵ."

4.48 EXAMPLES. Words of length three over the alphabets in 4.46 are, respectively,

$$\text{\maltese\maltese\maltese}, \qquad \text{zap}, \qquad 001$$

The empty string is the only string of length zero (no matter what alphabet is in use).

The set of all words over Σ, including the empty word, is denoted Σ^* (pronounced "sigma star"). If $w \in \Sigma^*$, the symbol $|w|$ denotes the length of w.

4.49 Theorem. If Σ is an alphabet then Σ^* is countably infinite.

PROOF OUTLINE. Let $\Sigma = \{s_1, \ldots, s_t\}$. Then Σ^* contains the countably infinite subset $\{s_1, s_1 s_1, s_1 s_1 s_1, \ldots\}$, and therefore $\#(\Sigma^*) \geq \aleph_0$. Now we can give a method for listing Σ^*. Just as our English alphabet comes equipped with an ordering (a precedes b, and b precedes c, and so on), we can impose an ordering on Σ by declaring that s_1 precedes s_2, and s_2 precedes s_3, and so on. Call this the **lexicographic ordering** of Σ. We now list Σ^* as follows: we start with ϵ, then list words of length 1 (think of these as the symbols in Σ) in lexicographic order, then the words of length 2 in lexicographic order, then the words of length 3, and so on. This produces the list

$$\underbrace{\epsilon, s_1, s_2, \ldots, s_t,}_{\text{length 1}} \underbrace{s_1 s_1, s_1 s_2, \ldots, s_1 s_t, \ldots, s_t s_1, s_t s_2, \ldots, s_t s_t,}_{\text{length 2}}$$

$$\underbrace{s_1 s_1 s_1, s_1 s_1 s_2, \ldots, s_t s_t s_t, \ldots}_{\text{length 3}}$$

If the words are read in this order, then any given word in Σ^* will eventually be reached. Therefore Σ^* is countable. $\square$

4.50 Definition. Let Σ be an alphabet. A subset $L \subseteq \Sigma^*$ is called a **language** over Σ.

4.51 Theorem. Let Σ be any alphabet. Then there are uncountably many languages over Σ.

PROOF. The set of all languages over Σ is just the power set $P(\Sigma^*)$. By Cantor's theorem (4.31) we know that $\#(\Sigma^*) < \#P(\Sigma^*)$. But $\#(\Sigma^*) = \aleph_0$ by 4.49, and this completes the proof. $\square$

How can we describe a language? There are many ways to do this, but each of these ways can be transcribed into a succession of statements made up of symbols from the world's typewriters; and each such succession of statements can be viewed as a word (perhaps a very long word) over this finite set T of typewriter symbols, that is, as an element of T^*. But T^* is countable. Thus there are only countably many possible descriptions of languages and uncountably many languages. The philosophical conclusion: *Not all languages are describable.* Therefore the best we can do is to describe *some* languages, with the hope that we can describe some useful ones. This is a central topic in computer science (and linguistics). For instance, if we are to design a computer that acts in accordance with the instructions we provide it, we must have a precise way of specifying the language of those instructions.

Is the expression

(∗)   *Celui fromage de la parce que maintenant*

a legitimate French sentence? If the reader knows no French, then an approach to this question might start by determining that the alphabet of the expression is the correct one, that the words are listed in a reputable French dictionary, and that they are organized in accordance with the rules of French grammar. (This last step may be no picnic.) There is a simpler way to investigate: take it to someone fluent in French, and ask whether the expression is acceptable.

Similarly, given a language L, suppose that a computer can be constructed that will accept a statement if and only if that statement is in L. Then a symbol string alleged to be in L can be tested by putting it into the machine and seeing whether it is accepted. Conversely, suppose we take a computer and tinker with it (perhaps by modifying its hardware in a haphazard way, or by infecting its memory with a bizarre program), in effect obtaining a new machine M; then we can *define* a language $L(M)$ to be the set of all strings that M will accept.

Our approach to languages in this section will be that of the previous paragraph, emphasizing the linkage between languages and machines; except instead of an actual computer we will use a primitive mathematical *model* of a computer, designed to "read" strings over a given alphabet Σ and "accept" them or not according to whether they satisfy certain criteria. (The quotation marks reflect our initial discomfort in attributing human activity to a mathematical construction; from now on they will be omitted.)

Let's write down the essential features of a machine designed for the purpose of language recognition. Picture yourself sitting in front of a computer. There is a keyboard filled with symbols; we call that collection of symbols the *alphabet* Σ. The overall condition of the machine's components at a particular time (including, for example, the configuration of data in the memory and the display on the monitor) is called the *state* of the machine at that time; thus the machine has a finite set S of states. When the machine is turned on and prepared to receive its first piece of input, we say that the machine is in its *initial state* $q_0 \in S$. In general, typing in a symbol from Σ may change the state (perhaps modifying what is in the memory, or altering the display on the monitor), depending on what is typed and the state just before typing. This change occurs in a deterministic way; that is, for every state $q \in S$ and symbol $\sigma \in \Sigma$, the ordered pair (q, σ) determines a unique new state, which we will denote by $\delta(q, \sigma)$. (We know the machine is not working properly if an ordered pair (q, σ) determines different states at different times.) For the purpose of language recognition, there must be a subset F of S such that whenever the machine is in a state in F, we can say that the machine has *accepted* the data we have just entered.

Now we can give the formal definition that ties all this together into a single mathematical package. Notice that the definition is unencumbered by any connection with physical reality and depends only on the basic notions of set theory. (We need no electricity, no disks, and no incomprehensible 750-page manual.)

4.52 Definition.   A **finite automaton** (or **finite-state machine**) is a five-tuple

$$M = (S, \Sigma, \delta, q_0, F)$$

where

   S is a finite nonempty set (the set of **states**);

   Σ is a finite nonempty set (the **alphabet**);

   δ is a function from $S \times \Sigma$ to S (the **transition function**);

   $q_0 \in S$ (the **initial state**);

   F is a subset of S (the set of **final states**).

4.53 EXAMPLES.   (a) Consider an automaton M that reads the alphabet $\Sigma = \{a, b\}$, and suppose there are two states: $S = \{q_0, q_1\}$. Let q_0

be the only final state (that is, $F = \{q_0\}$), as well as the initial state. Assume that reading a always causes a state to change [more formally: $\forall q \in S$, $\delta(q, a) \neq q$], while reading b has no effect. The transition function δ corresponding to this response pattern can be represented by a table, which follows. The rows are labeled (on the left) by the states of S, and the columns (on top) by the symbols from Σ. The state appearing at the intersection of row q and column σ is $\delta(q, \sigma)$.

σ q	a	b
q_0	q_1	q_0
q_1	q_0	q_1

(b) David wakes up in the morning and checks the weather. If it is sunny he goes fishing; if it is rainy he goes to the movies. He is happy if he sees a good movie or if he finds that the fish are biting; otherwise he is sad. Not every input condition will change David's state; for example, if he has gone to the movies or if he has just awakened, then he is unaffected by the activities of the fish. Once David's mood is set, it doesn't change. His criterion for "accepting" the day is that the events make him happy. We represent David's situation by the automaton $M = (S, \Sigma, \delta, q_0, F)$, where

$S = \{$wakeup, fishing, movies, happy, sad$\}$

$\Sigma = \{$sunny, rainy, biting, not biting, good movie, poor movie$\}$

$q_0 = $ wakeup

$F = \{$happy$\}$

and the transition function δ is given by the following table:

σ q	sunny	rainy	biting	not biting	good movie	poor movie
wakeup	fishing	movies	wakeup	wakeup	wakeup	wakeup
fishing	fishing	fishing	happy	sad	fishing	fishing
movies	movies	movies	movies	movies	happy	sad
happy	happy	happy	happy	happy	happy	happy
sad	sad	sad	sad	sad	sad	sad

Remember: an alphabet can be any finite nonempty set. So, for instance, "biting" is a symbol in our alphabet in this example.

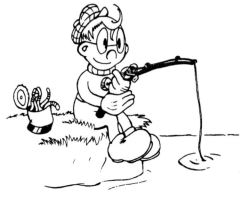

A finite automaton in one of its states

It is hard to get an intuitive feeling for the operation of an automaton M by looking at the table of its transition function. It is usually more insightful to represent M by a graph called a **transition diagram** or **state graph**. The graph is a collection of points (called **vertices** or **nodes**), one for each state in S, together with a set of *directed* arcs (called **edges**), each labeled by a symbol from Σ. If q_1 and q_2 are states of M and $\sigma \in \Sigma$, then an edge

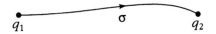

in the diagram indicates that M goes from state q_1 to state q_2 upon reading σ; that is, $\delta(q_1, \sigma) = q_2$. The vertex of each final state is circled in the diagram. For example, the automaton in 4.53(a) has the following state graph:

(4.54)

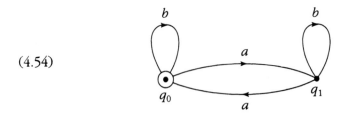

And here is a state graph for 4.53(b):

(4.55)

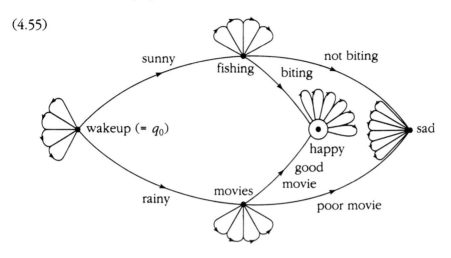

To avoid congestion in this diagram, we have omitted the labels on edges corresponding to inputs that don't cause a state change. (These are the unmarked loops at each vertex.)

Up to now our automata have been able to read only one-symbol words, and it is time to correct this reading disability. (We are viewing the elements of Σ as one-symbol words, so that $\Sigma \subseteq \Sigma^*$.) More formally, we want to extend the transition function δ to a function

$$S \times \Sigma^* \to S$$

Let $w \in \Sigma^*$; say, $w = \sigma_1 \ldots \sigma_n$. How should we teach M to read w when M is in state q? The answer: First read σ_1, which takes M into state $\delta(q, \sigma_1)$. Then read σ_2, which produces state $\delta(\delta(q, \sigma_1), \sigma_2)$; call the resulting state $\delta(q, \sigma_1\sigma_2)$. In general, having defined $\delta(q, \sigma_1 \ldots \sigma_k)$, define

(4.56) $\qquad \delta(q, \sigma_1 \ldots \sigma_k\sigma_{k+1}) = \delta(\delta(q, \sigma_1 \ldots \sigma_k), \sigma_{k+1})$

This recursion tells M how to read every string of length 1 or greater, starting in any state q. Finally, define

$$\delta(q, \epsilon) = q \quad \forall q \in S$$

(That is, the state of M doesn't change if we give it no input.) This completes the extension of our original transition function δ to a new function, also denoted δ, from $S \times \Sigma^*$ to S; so *we have taught M to read any element of Σ^**. From now on, the symbol δ will always denote the extended transition function that we have defined here.

Now that each of our automata can read any word over its associated alphabet, we can endow each of them with the ability to accept some of what it reads.

4.57 Definition.   Let $M = (S, \Sigma, \delta, q_0, F)$ be a finite automaton, and let $w \in \Sigma^*$. We say that M **accepts** w if $\delta(q_0, w) \in F$. (In words: M accepts w if M goes from its initial state to some final state upon reading w.) Define the **language accepted by M** to be the language

$$L(M) = \{w \in \Sigma^* \mid M \text{ accepts } w\}$$

4.58 EXAMPLES.   (a) Let M be the automaton represented by diagram 4.54. Then $L(M)$ is the set of all words over the alphabet $\{a, b\}$ that have an even number of a's.

(b) With M as represented by 4.55, an element of $L(M)$ is a string over Σ satisfying one of the following sets of conditions:

1. There is an occurrence of "sunny" that has no occurrence of "rainy" anywhere preceding it; and "biting" occurs somewhere after that "sunny," without "not biting" in between.

2. There is an occurrence of "rainy" that has no occurrence of "sunny" anywhere preceding it; and "good movie" occurs somewhere after that "rainy," without "poor movie" in between.

(c) Some automata are completely tasteless, and others are impossible to please. To be precise, let $M = (S, \Sigma, \delta, q_0, F)$. If $F = S$ then $L(M) = \Sigma^*$; if $F = \emptyset$ then $L(M) = \emptyset$.

(d) Let $\Sigma = \{a, b\}$, and let M have the following platypus-like transition diagram:

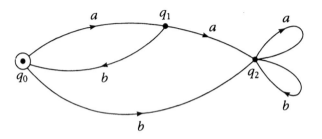

Then $L(M)$ consists of the empty string together with all strings of even length whose symbols alternate between a and b, starting with *a* and ending with *b*. Thus,

$$ababab \ldots ab \in L(M)$$

(e) Now let's construct an automaton M that excludes the empty string but otherwise accepts the same language as the one in (d). We can insist on an initial "syllable" ab by making the following modification of the preceding automaton:

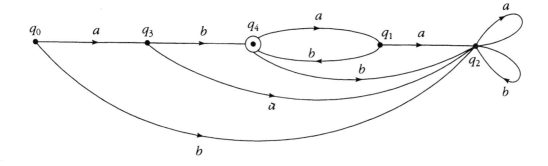

(f) We seek an automaton M such that

$$L(M) = \{w \in \{a, b\}^* \mid \text{no two consecutive letters in } w \text{ are the same}\}$$

The following diagram gives an appropriate M:

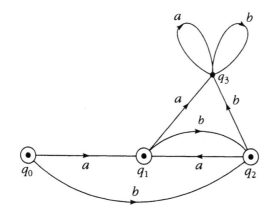

Notice that in every completed state graph, each vertex has exactly one edge emanating from it corresponding to each alphabet symbol. For if *no* edge from q were marked with σ, then $\delta(q, \sigma)$ would not be defined by the graph; and if *two* edges from q were marked with σ, then δ would not be well-defined. (That is, $\delta(q, \sigma)$ would have two different values, which is taboo because δ is a function.)

We are likely to find that networks of long and multi-claused sentences result from an attempt to describe a complex language verbally. And if such a description is all we have for a language, it can be a real challenge to check a particular string to see whether it satisfies the criteria for membership. But once we know a transition diagram for the language, it is a triviality to test a particular string's membership credentials.

4.59 Definition.   A language L is **regular** if $L = L(M)$ for some finite automaton M.

The preceding examples display several regular languages, without formally proving regularity. *Proving* that a particular language is or is not regular can be a difficult matter, and we will only touch briefly on the subject here. It can be shown that every finite language is regular. (We omit the details, but to get the flavor of the argument try this exercise: draw the graph of a finite automaton M with alphabet $\Sigma = \{a, b, c\}$, having the property that $L(M) = \{cab\}$. Then do Exercise 5 at the end of this section.)

The situation for infinite languages is considerably more complicated. The *Pumping Lemma*, which we are about to examine, is an important tool for proving that certain languages are not regular. First we need some notation and terminology. If Σ is an alphabet and x and y are words in Σ^*, then the **concatenation** of x and y, denoted xy, is the word obtained upon following x by y. Thus if $x = $ cat and $y = $ nips, then $xy = $ catnips. Concatenation of a word with itself is usually abbreviated with exponential notation; so with x and y as just given, the concatenation denoted x^2y^3x is shorthand for

catcatnipsnipsnipscat

4.60 Pumping Lemma. Let Σ be an alphabet, and let $L \subseteq \Sigma^*$ be an infinite regular language. Then there are strings x, y, z in Σ^*, with $y \neq \epsilon$, such that for every $n \in \mathbb{N}$ the string xy^nz belongs to L.

PROOF OUTLINE.   Because L is regular, there is a finite automaton M such that $L = L(M)$, and let's suppose that M has exactly k states. Since L is infinite, there is a word $w \in L$ of length greater than k. Now, when M reads the symbols of w, it shifts from state to state; and, since w has more letters than M has states, there must be some state q that M enters twice during the reading (by the pigeonhole principle).

Thus there are strings x, y, z, with $y \neq \epsilon$, such that $w = xyz$ (so the strings x, y, z can be viewed as "syllables" of w) and such that M is in state q before and after reading y. Then M also accepts the longer word $xyyz$; for, after reading the middle section yy, the machine is in state q, and then reading z takes M into an accepting state. (We know this from the fact that M accepts w.) More generally, an induction argument shows that M accepts every word of the form xy^nz for $n \in \mathbb{N}$. Therefore every such word belongs to L (since L consists of precisely those words accepted by M), and the argument is complete. $\square$

4.61 EXAMPLES. (a) Consider the language $L \subseteq \{a, b\}^*$ consisting of all strings formed by following a string of a's with a string of b's of the same length:

$$L = \{a^n b^n \mid n > 0\}$$

We assert that L is not regular. If we suppose otherwise, then by the Pumping Lemma there exist strings $x, y, z \in \{a, b\}^*$, with $y \neq \epsilon$, such that $xy^nz \in L$ for all $n > 0$. But y cannot be a string of a's, since otherwise when $n > 1$ the string xy^nz would have more a's than b's and hence not belong to L. Similarly, y cannot be a string of b's. Finally, if y were to have both a's and b's, then the string xy^2z would not have the form $a^n b^n$, and therefore it could not belong to L. So the assumption that L is regular has led to a contradiction, and the assertion is verified.

In this example our intuition is that no finite automaton has enough memory to keep count of an arbitrarily large number of a's in order to check that each string of a's is followed by a string of b's of the same length. To accept L, a more sophisticated piece of "hardware" called a *pushdown automaton* is used. Roughly speaking, this is an automaton with an expandable memory modeled after the plate-stacking devices used by cafeterias.

(b) Consider the patterns of parentheses used in arithmetic expressions. For instance, the expression

$$((a + b)c + d(ab))f + (g)(ac + b)$$

has the parentheses pattern

$$(()())()()$$

and can be understood; whereas

$$a + (c + d)) + f(g + c(d((}$$

has the parentheses pattern

$$( )) (((($$

and leaves us confused. Define L to be the set of acceptable parentheses patterns. (We won't write a formal definition.) So

$$L \subseteq \{),(\}^*$$

It can be shown that L is not regular; therefore no finite automaton has the capacity to scan *every* arithmetic expression and check whether its parenthesization is legitimate. As in part (a), a pushdown automaton can do the job. Alternatively, we can use an automaton with a countably infinite number of states, diagrammed as follows:

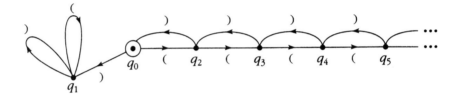

If an upper bound on the expression lengths is given in advance, then a *finite* automaton can be constructed that will accept the legitimate parenthesizations.

In addition to their work as language acceptors, automata also have important applications in other aspects of computer science, particularly in the analysis of algorithms and in the study of the field called *computational complexity*.

Exercises

1. Let $x = a_1 \ldots a_m$ and $y = b_1 \ldots b_n$ be strings over the alphabet Σ. Then the concatenation xy is the string $a_1 \ldots a_m b_1 \ldots b_n$. Give a more formal definition of the concatenation xy as a kind of function, in the manner of Definition 4.47.

2. Suppose $\Sigma = \{a, \ldots, z\}$, our usual alphabet with its standard lexicographic order. In the listing for Σ^* given in the proof outline for Theorem 4.49, in what position on the list will we find the word *dog*? (Note: Remember to start your list with the empty word.)

3. If L_1 and L_2 are languages, define the **concatenation** L_1L_2 of L_1 and L_2 to be the language consisting of all words of the form w_1w_2 with $w_i \in L_i$.

(a) Describe the concatenation LL of a language L with itself.

(b) Give an example of a language L having the property that $L \subseteq LL$.

(c) Assume that L_1 and L_2 are regular languages; say $L_i = L(M_i)$. Show that the concatenation L_1L_2 is also regular. Your argument needn't include all the technical details. Just give an informal verbal description of how one can use M_1 and M_2 to construct an automaton M such that $L_1L_2 = L(M)$.

4. Describe the language accepted by the automaton with this state diagram:

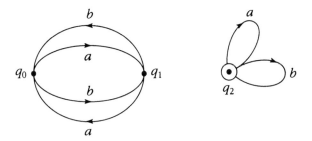

Explain briefly. Then go on to assert (without proof) some general principle that this example supports.

5. Imagine that the rectangle in this figure

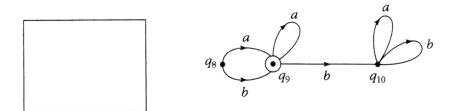

covers up the transition graph for a finite-state machine M, and assume that q_8, q_9, q_{10} are not states of M. Now consider a new machine N whose transition graph consists of the hidden graph together with the visible graph in the figure. How are the languages $L(M)$ and $L(N)$ related? Explain.

6. Under what condition(s) on a finite automaton M is the empty string accepted by M?

7. Suppose L_1 and L_2 are regular languages over the alphabet $\Sigma = \{a, b\}$; say, $L_1 = L(M_1)$ and $L_2 = L(M_2)$, where M_1 and M_2 are finite automata. Assume that every string in L_1 starts with a, and every string in L_2 starts with b. Without proof, but with some explanation, give a way to use the transition diagrams of M_1 and M_2 to construct a transition diagram for an automaton M such that

$$L(M) = L_1 \cup L_2$$

8. In each case, describe the language accepted by the automaton with the given transition diagram.

(a)

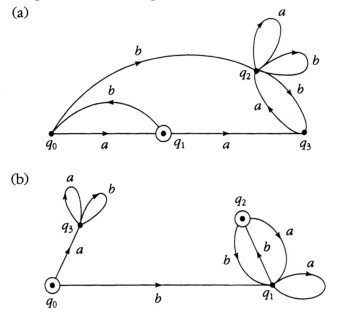

(b)

9. In each of the following parts, give a state graph for a finite automaton that accepts the described language in $\{a, b\}^*$.

   (a) The set of all words that start with a (as we read from left to right).

   (b) The set of all words that end with b.

   (c) The set of all words that have exactly one b.

   (d) The set of all words that have exactly two b's.

   (e) All the words with an even number of a's.

   (f) All the words in which three consecutive b's don't occur.

10. In the proof of Theorem 4.49, we gave a procedure for listing the elements of Σ^* based on a given ordering for Σ. The resulting ordering

of Σ^* is called the *lexicographic ordering* of Σ^*. For the purpose of this exercise, think of Σ as our standard alphabet:

$$\Sigma = \{a, b, c, \ldots, z\}$$

(a) The words in a dictionary are listed in what we will call *alphabetic order*. Explain the difference between alphabetic order and lexicographic order as the terms are being used here.

(b) Could the proof of Theorem 4.49 have been carried out by listing the words in alphabetic order?

PERMUTATIONS AND COMBINATIONS

Let me count the wheys.

LITTLE MISS MUFFET

5.1 Combinatorial Problems

Imagine that you are gathering data for a major report on the government's economic policies. An influential friend arranges for your access to the most up-to-date files in the Bureau of the Census. Because the report is due in a few days, you are hoping that these files will give you the information you need to complete your report. Unfortunately, the files contain raw data that has not been organized or cross-referenced in any way; there is no way you can extract enough coherent information in the available time. You lose your job. Moral: *having* a set is not enough for most purposes; we must understand its *structure*.

In this chapter our focus will be on topics from the branch of mathematics known as *combinatorics*, a subject concerned with counting, selection, and arrangement. These are processes by which we organize sets so that we can interpret and apply the data they contain. Generally speaking, combinatorial questions ask whether a subset of a given set can be chosen and arranged in a way that conforms with certain constraints and, if so, in how many ways it can be done. As we proceed we will extend and refine the counting procedures introduced in Chapter 4, but our concern here will be almost entirely with finite sets. As we have seen, counting the elements of a set can be a difficult task. While we can all count a tubful of marbles, given the time and the will, it is another matter to count a set that has not presented itself to our senses.

We have already discussed some combinatorial topics: we counted the subsets of finite sets in Chapter 2; we chose systems of distinct representatives in Chapter 3; and we considered the product rule and countability questions in Chapter 4. (Showing that a set is countable can amount to giving a procedure for arranging the elements of that set in a line.) Combinatorics also includes the theory of permutations and combinations and probability theory. These topics have an enormous range of applications in pure and applied mathematics and computer science. For example, combinatorial methods can be used to estimate the time and storage requirements of complex computer programs. Combinatorics also deals with questions about *configurations* of sets: families of finite sets that overlap according to some prescribed numerical or geometrical conditions.

Here are some representative combinatorial problems.

5.1 EXAMPLES. (a) Ten people are seated in a ten-seat row in a movie theater, one person per seat: say p_1 is in seat 1, p_2 is in seat 2, and so on. Trouble begins when p_1 is offended by p_2 and insists that p_2 move to seat 10. Meanwhile p_3 falls in love with p_8 and demands to sit on p_8's right. A few other such needs are expressed, and after some heated discussion a configuration is agreed upon that will make everyone happy. Someone offers a valid plan whereby the rearrangement can be carried out in 14 steps, where each step consists of two adjacent people getting up and switching seats. Then someone offers a second plan in which only 11 such switches are needed to achieve the same result, but there isn't time to check the details before the movie begins. Should they try the second plan?

(b) A standard checkerboard has eight rows and eight columns of squares, and the squares are alternately black and white. Suppose we remove the two diagonally opposite white corners from the board. Can we cover the remaining squares with dominoes? (Assume that each domino is a rectangle that covers exactly two squares, and also assume that dominoes are not allowed to overlap.) This one is easy, so we give the answer immediately: Each domino will cover a white square and a black square, therefore any distribution of dominoes will cover the same number of squares of both colors. But because we have removed the two white corners, there are more black squares than white ones to be covered, hence we cannot achieve the desired coverage.

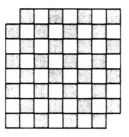

(c) Now picture a complete checkerboard, but ignore the colors and view the lines (including those along the outer border) as streets and the little squares as city blocks. How many routes are there from the southwest corner to the northeast corner, assuming that the only allowable directions of travel are east and north? Once we view the situation from the appropriate perspective, we will use an elementary computation to show that there are 12,870 acceptable routes.

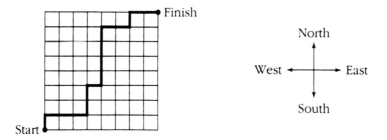

(d) A whiz at Rubik's Cube wants to obtain a certain configuration. Rubik's Cube appears to be constructed by slicing a given cube into 27 little cubes; these are called the **cubies**.* There are three kinds of cubies with at least one visible face: corner cubies, center cubies, and edge cubies. (We can also imagine an invisible cubie in the middle of the Cube, but that won't enter our discussion.) The visible faces of

*We are using the terminology in A. H. Frey, Jr., and D. Singmaster, *Handbook of Cubik Math* (Hillside, N.J.: Enslow. 1982).

the cubies are **facelets**. Question: can the whiz manipulate a Cube, without disassembling it, into a configuration that differs from the original one only in that a single edge cubie has been flipped around?

? 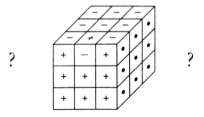 ?

(e) Ten joyful music lovers meet on December 16 to celebrate Beethoven's birthday. They raise their glasses in a toast, and each insists upon clinking his or her glass with everyone else's. How many clinks occur? Later in the evening they will select from among them the best possible team of three people to represent them in the National Three-Person Minuet Championships. How many teams must they consider?

(f) Here is a famous problem that was posed by W. S. B. Woolhouse in *The Ladies' and Gentlemen's Diary* in 1844 and solved (affirmatively) by Rev. P. T. Kirkman in 1850. It is referred to as "Kirkman's schoolgirls problem," and it is a nice representative of the subject of combinatorial configurations (or *designs*). Suppose a teacher has a class of 15 girls that she wants to take out walking on seven consecutive days. She wants the girls to walk in five rows, with three girls per row. Unfortunately, by the end of a day's walk the girls in each row no longer get along. Here's the problem: Is it possible to reorganize the girls every day so that no two girls share the same row more than once?

Among the preceding examples, (a) has a quick solution when formulated in the language of *permutations*. The solution to example (d) also follows from basic properties of permutations, although the formulation of it has some subtleties. Examples (c) and (e) also have quick solutions, but they use *combinations*, not permutations. We'll see solutions to all of these; but Kirkman's schoolgirl problem, (f), is best handled as part of a general study of combinatorial designs, which we leave for more advanced courses.*

*For a solution to the problem, see Richard A. Brualdi, *Introductory Combinatorics*, 2nd ed. (Englewood Cliffs, NJ: Prentice-Hall, 1992); especially p. 368.

5.2 The Addition and Product Rules (review)

We will be making a great many choices in this chapter, so we will restate the two fundamental rules of selection that were developed in Chapter 4. The first is an interpretation of 4.15; the second is a copy of 4.22.

Addition Rule. If an element is to be chosen from one of n pairwise disjoint finite sets that contain $m_1, \ldots, m_n$ elements, respectively, then there are altogether $m_1 + \cdots + m_n$ possibilities for that choice.

Product Rule. Suppose that n consecutive choices are to be made. Suppose further that there are m_1 possibilities for the first choice and, for each k satisfying $2 \le k \le n$, that there are m_k possibilities for the kth choice, no matter how the first $k - 1$ choices have been made. Then there are exactly $m_1 m_2 \cdots m_n$ possibilities for the sequence of n choices.

Before moving into new material, it may be helpful to see these rules in action again, so here is an example for that purpose.

5.2 EXAMPLE. Determine the number of odd three-digit positive integers that have no repeated digits.

SOLUTION 1. The idea is to represent the selection of such an integer as a succession of choices, each from a set whose size is independent of the preceding choices. Then we can invoke the product rule. We do this in three steps. First we choose the units digit: there are five possibilities, since it must be odd. Next we choose the hundreds digit: there are eight possibilities, because it must be nonzero and different from the units digit. Last we choose the tens digit: there are eight possibilities, because it must not be one of the two digits already chosen. Therefore the answer, by the product rule, is $5 \cdot 8 \cdot 8 = 320$.

SOLUTION 2. We proceed in a way similar to Solution 1, but we first choose the units digit, then the tens digit, then the hundreds digit. As before, there are five possibilities for the units digit. After that there are nine possibilities for the tens digit. Finally, how many possibilities are left for the hundreds digit? That depends on whether the tens digit was zero, so the conditions are not appropriate for application of the product rule. We resolve this difficulty by separating the selections into two families: those numbers with zero for the tens digit, and those with a nonzero tens digit. In the first family there are five possible units digits, then one choice for tens digit (zero), and eight possible hundreds digits; in all,

$5 \cdot 1 \cdot 8 = 40$ possibilities, by the product rule. In the second family there are five possible units digits, then eight choices for tens digits (zero and the units digit are unavailable), and seven possible hundreds digits; in all, $5 \cdot 8 \cdot 7 = 280$ possibilities. Since the two families are disjoint, the addition rule yields a grand total of $40 + 280 = 320$ possibilities.

OTHER PROCEDURES. If we choose the digits from left to right, the number of choices available for the units digit will depend on the *parities* (the oddness or evenness) of the first two choices. Once again it is necessary to separate the entire collection into pairwise disjoint batches. The details are left to the reader.

The crudest way to proceed is to list all the possibilities,

$$103, 105, 107, 109, 123, 125, 127, 129, 135, 137, 139, \ldots, 987$$

and count them.

Exercises

1. An **n-bit string** is an n-tuple of 0s and 1s. Prove that for each $n \geq 1$, exactly half the n-bit strings have an even number of 1s. (Use induction on n.)

2. In each of the following cases, determine the number of four-digit integers that satisfy the given condition.
   (a) Unrestricted.
   (b) The digits are all even.
   (c) There are no repeated digits.
   (d) No two consecutive digits are equal.
   (e) The integer is even and no two consecutive digits are equal.

3. If a and b are integers, a is said to be a **divisor** of b if $b = ac$ for some integer c. The number $n = 15,246,000$ has the prime factorization

$$2^4 \cdot 3^2 \cdot 5^3 \cdot 7 \cdot 11^2$$

   (a) How many positive divisors does n have? (Use the Fundamental Theorem of Arithmetic.)
   (b) How many positive divisors does n have that are not divisible by 10?

4. A host offers his party guests five varieties of crackers, six cheeses, and three jams. Regrettably one of the cheeses (a great delicacy) has the property that when combined with two or more jams, it produces a

lethal result. How many nonlethal snacks are possible? [Assume that a snack consists of a cracker with at most one cheese and any combination of jams (possibly none).]

5. Twelve horses are in a race. The only results that matter are the first three finishers. How many possibilities are there?

5.3 Introduction to Permutations

5.3 Definition. Let A be a nonempty set. A **permutation** of A is a bijection from A to A.

5.4 EXAMPLE. Let $A = \{1, 2, 3, 4\}$. Then the mapping $\sigma: A \rightarrow A$ given by the table

i	1	2	3	4
$\sigma(i)$	4	1	3	2

is a permutation of A.

If $A = \{a_1, \ldots, a_n\}$, then we usually write

$$(5.5) \qquad \sigma = \begin{pmatrix} a_1 & a_2 & \cdots & a_n \\ \sigma(a_1) & \sigma(a_2) & \cdots & \sigma(a_n) \end{pmatrix}$$

for the permutation $\sigma: A \rightarrow A$ that takes a_i to $\sigma(a_i)$, for $1 \leq i \leq n$. For instance, in this notation the permutation σ in Example 5.4 is written

$$\begin{pmatrix} 1 & 2 & 3 & 4 \\ 4 & 1 & 3 & 2 \end{pmatrix}$$

(So we are really just giving the table for σ when we use this notation.) Here we have followed the standard custom of listing the domain elements in ascending order in the top row. This is not essential; for instance, according to 5.5, the symbol

$$\begin{pmatrix} 3 & 1 & 4 & 2 \\ 3 & 4 & 2 & 1 \end{pmatrix}$$

also represents σ.

The set of all permutations of a set A is called the **symmetric group** on A, denoted S_A. If $A = \mathbb{N}_n = \{1, 2, \ldots, n\}$ we write S_n instead of $S_{\mathbb{N}_n}$. Finally, a set with n elements is called an **n-set**.

5.6 Theorem. If A and B are n-sets, then there are exactly $n!$ bijections from A to B. In particular, $\#S_n = n!$.

PROOF 1. Let $A = \{a_1, \ldots, a_n\}$ and $B = \{b_1, \ldots, b_n\}$. A bijection pairs a_1 with one of the n elements of B. Once we choose that element of B, there remain $n - 1$ elements of B from which we can choose an element to pair with a_2, and then $n - 2$ candidates for pairing with a_3, and so on. Altogether there are $n(n - 1)(n - 2) \cdots 2 \cdot 1 = n!$ possibilities, by the product rule.

The second statement follows from the first by taking $A = B = \mathbb{N}_n$.

PROOF 2. We use induction on n. (The product rule will not be needed.) If $n = 1$, there is only one bijection (in fact, only one function) from $\{a_1\}$ to $\{b_1\}$, and $1! = 1$. Now assume there are $k!$ bijections from one k-set to another, and suppose $\#A = \#B = k + 1$; say $A = \{a_1, \ldots, a_{k+1}\}$ and $B = \{b_1, \ldots, b_{k+1}\}$. Let J_1 be the set of all bijections from A to B that take a_1 to b_1. Then each $\sigma \in J_1$ is completely determined by the images $\sigma(a_2), \ldots, \sigma(a_{k+1})$, that is, by σ's restriction to $\{a_2, \ldots, a_{k+1}\}$. Because that restriction is a bijection from the k-set $\{a_2, \ldots, a_{k+1}\}$ to the k-set $\{b_2, \ldots, b_{k+1}\}$, the induction hypothesis tells us that there are $k!$ possibilities for it. Thus $\#J_1 = k!$. Similarly, if J_i denotes the set of all bijections from A to B that take a_1 to b_i, with $2 \le i \le k + 1$, then $\#J_i = k!$. Notice that the set of bijections from A to B is equal to $\cup_{i=1}^{k+1} J_i$, a union of pairwise disjoint sets; therefore by Theorem 4.15 the union has $(k + 1) \cdot k! = (k + 1)!$ elements, completing the induction argument. $\square$

5.7 EXAMPLE. For every $n \ge 1$, the identity mapping on $\mathbb{N}_n$ is an element of S_n. When $n = 1$ there are no other mappings, so

$$S_1 = \left\{ \begin{pmatrix} 1 \\ 1 \end{pmatrix} \right\}$$

We have

$$S_2 = \left\{ \begin{pmatrix} 1 & 2 \\ 1 & 2 \end{pmatrix}, \begin{pmatrix} 1 & 2 \\ 2 & 1 \end{pmatrix} \right\}$$

and the symmetric group S_3 consists of the following six permutations:

$$\begin{pmatrix} 1 & 2 & 3 \\ 1 & 2 & 3 \end{pmatrix} \quad \begin{pmatrix} 1 & 2 & 3 \\ 2 & 1 & 3 \end{pmatrix} \quad \begin{pmatrix} 1 & 2 & 3 \\ 3 & 2 & 1 \end{pmatrix}$$

$$\begin{pmatrix} 1 & 2 & 3 \\ 1 & 3 & 2 \end{pmatrix} \quad \begin{pmatrix} 1 & 2 & 3 \\ 2 & 3 & 1 \end{pmatrix} \quad \begin{pmatrix} 1 & 2 & 3 \\ 3 & 1 & 2 \end{pmatrix}$$

From Theorem 5.6 we know that $\#S_3 = 3! = 6$, so this list is complete. (Without 5.6 it would take careful bookkeeping to assure that all the permutations of $\{1, 2, 3\}$ have been included.)

If σ and λ are in S_A, then so is their composition, $\sigma \circ \lambda$, since the composition of two bijections from A to A is again a bijection from A to A. The permutation $\sigma \circ \lambda$ is usually written $\sigma\lambda$; we call it a **product**, and we say we have **multiplied** σ and λ. (As you might expect, σ and λ are called the **factors** of the product $\sigma\lambda$.) Thus $\sigma\lambda(x) = \sigma(\lambda(x))$ for all $x \in A$. To illustrate, consider these two permutations in S_4:

$$\sigma = \begin{pmatrix} 1 & 2 & 3 & 4 \\ 3 & 1 & 4 & 2 \end{pmatrix} \quad \text{and} \quad \lambda = \begin{pmatrix} 1 & 2 & 3 & 4 \\ 4 & 1 & 3 & 2 \end{pmatrix}$$

Then

$$\sigma\lambda = \begin{pmatrix} 1 & 2 & 3 & 4 \\ 2 & 3 & 4 & 1 \end{pmatrix}$$

In detail:

and hence

In practice we don't write all these arrows to compute $\sigma\lambda$. We write

$$\sigma\lambda = \underbrace{\begin{pmatrix} 1 & 2 & 3 & 4 \\ 3 & 1 & 4 & 2 \end{pmatrix}}_{\sigma}\underbrace{\begin{pmatrix} 1 & 2 & 3 & 4 \\ 4 & 1 & 3 & 2 \end{pmatrix}}_{\lambda} = \begin{pmatrix} 1 & 2 & 3 & 4 \\ & & & \end{pmatrix}$$

Then we think, "1 goes to 4 (by means of λ), and then 4 goes to 2 (by means of σ)," and we write 2 in the blank space under the 1. Then we proceed similarly with the other elements. Since a permutation is a bijection, every entry of the top row will appear exactly once in the bottom row after a computation of this kind. For example,

$$\begin{pmatrix} 1 & 2 & 3 & 4 \\ 2 & 1 & 4 & 2 \end{pmatrix}$$

does *not* denote a permutation, since the simultaneous actions $1 \longmapsto 2$ and $4 \longmapsto 2$ defy injectivity. Also remember: *to compute $\sigma\lambda$, first apply λ, then σ.*

5.8 EXAMPLE. With

$$\sigma = \begin{pmatrix} 1 & 2 & 3 & 4 \\ 3 & 1 & 4 & 2 \end{pmatrix} \quad \text{and} \quad \lambda = \begin{pmatrix} 1 & 2 & 3 & 4 \\ 4 & 1 & 3 & 2 \end{pmatrix}$$

as before, we have

$$\lambda\sigma = \begin{pmatrix} 1 & 2 & 3 & 4 \\ 4 & 1 & 3 & 2 \end{pmatrix}\begin{pmatrix} 1 & 2 & 3 & 4 \\ 3 & 1 & 4 & 2 \end{pmatrix} = \begin{pmatrix} 1 & 2 & 3 & 4 \\ 3 & 4 & 2 & 1 \end{pmatrix} \neq \sigma\lambda$$

Therefore, *the result of multiplying permutations can be expected to depend on the order in which the permutations are listed.* (We say that permutation multiplication is not a **commutative** operation.) Notice, however, that sometimes the order doesn't matter. For instance,

$$\begin{pmatrix} 1 & 2 & 3 & 4 \\ 4 & 2 & 3 & 1 \end{pmatrix}\begin{pmatrix} 1 & 2 & 3 & 4 \\ 1 & 3 & 2 & 4 \end{pmatrix} = \begin{pmatrix} 1 & 2 & 3 & 4 \\ 4 & 3 & 2 & 1 \end{pmatrix}$$

$$= \begin{pmatrix} 1 & 2 & 3 & 4 \\ 1 & 3 & 2 & 4 \end{pmatrix}\begin{pmatrix} 1 & 2 & 3 & 4 \\ 4 & 2 & 3 & 1 \end{pmatrix}$$

5.9 Remark. Some authors write functions to the *right* of the domain elements on which they act: $(x)\sigma$ instead of $\sigma(x)$. With that notation the product $\sigma\lambda$ has the action $(x)\sigma\lambda = ((x)\sigma)\lambda$; that is, *first σ then λ.* If you encounter permutation computations in other books or papers, check to see whether products should be read from right to left, as we do here, or from left to right. (*It matters*, as Example 5.8 shows.) Suggestion: start by locating a couple of worked examples and multiplying them for yourself, and then compare your results with the author's.

In the expression

$$\sigma = \begin{pmatrix} 1 & 2 & 3 & \cdots & n \\ \sigma(1) & \sigma(2) & \sigma(3) & \cdots & \sigma(n) \end{pmatrix}$$

the bottom row of the symbol is just a rearrangement of the top row. Conversely, every arrangement of the integers from 1 to n in a row can be viewed as the bottom row of a permutation symbol. Hence there is a one-to-one correspondence between S_n and the collection of all linear arrangements of the numbers from 1 to n. For this reason, permutations are often described as "ordered arrangements" in the mathematical literature.

Permutations appear in a variety of mathematical contexts and in the modelling of physical phenomena. In general, permutations arise when the essential data in the description of an event can be summarized by observing how n objects shift among n locations, one object per location. If the locations are numbered from 1 to n, a process that moves the object in location i to location j can be associated with a permutation σ that takes i to j.

5.10 EXAMPLE. A major athletic competition has contests in five water sports, six running events, four bicycling events, and seven varieties of self-defense.

(a) Each participant chooses one event from each of the four categories. In how many ways can the selections be made?

SOLUTION. This is a straightforward application of the product rule: altogether there are $5 \cdot 6 \cdot 4 \cdot 7 = 840$ possibilities.

(b) Now suppose that besides selecting events, each participant also must specify the order in which he will engage in the events (perhaps bicycling first, then a water sport, and so on). How many possibilities are there for an individual's event program?

SOLUTION. After a participant has selected his four events, he must then specify an ordering of the events. But each such ordering corresponds to an element of S_4, so there are $4! = 24$ possible orderings. Therefore, by the product rule, there are $840 \cdot 24 = 20{,}160$ program possibilities.

5.11 EXAMPLE. (a) In how many ways can eight indistinguishable rooks be placed on a chess board so that none of them can attack another? To answer this question, first recall that a rook can attach any other piece located in its row or column. (Rows are horizontal, and row 1 is on top; columns are vertical, and column 1 is at the left.) To say that two rooks are indistinguishable means that given any configuration of rooks on the board, if any two rooks are interchanged, then the new configuration is viewed as the same as the original.

Note that there is at least one solution: position all the rooks on the main diagonal, as pictured.

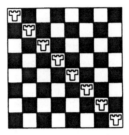

Also note that if there were nine or more rooks there could be no solution, because some row would have at least two rooks, by the pigeonhole principle.

In an arrangement of eight rooks satisfying the given conditions, each row contains a rook, and so does each column. (If all eight rooks were situated in seven or fewer rows, then two would be in the same row, again by the pigeonhole principle; similarly for columns.) With each such arrangement we associate a permutation as follows: for each i satisfying $1 \le i \le 8$, let $\sigma(i)$ be the number of the column occupied by the rook in row i. So, for instance, the arrangement

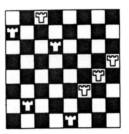

corresponds to the permutation

$$\sigma = \begin{pmatrix} 1 & 2 & 3 & 4 & 5 & 6 & 7 & 8 \\ 3 & 1 & 4 & 8 & 7 & 6 & 2 & 5 \end{pmatrix}$$

This procedure gives a one-to-one correspondence between the set of acceptable rook configurations and the symmetric group S_8. (Check this.) Therefore there are $8! = 40{,}320$ such configurations.

(b) Now let's revise the conditions of part (a) and suppose that the rooks *are* distinguishable; for example, suppose they are all differently colored. Again we ask for the number of ways in which the rooks can be arranged on the board in a nonattacking mode. Each such arrangement can be viewed as the result of two successive choices: first we decide which squares will hold the rooks, then we decide the pattern of colors for the rooks on those squares. By the first part of this example, there are 8! ways to choose an acceptable configuration of squares. Then, having fixed such a configuration, there are 8! ways of distributing the eight colors among those squares. Therefore, by the product rule, there are altogether $(8!)^2 = 1,625,702,400$ possibilities.

It is sometimes difficult to apply the product rule directly to a given combinatorial construction. In that event, it may be helpful to regard the construction as a part of a larger process to which the product rule *does* apply. The following example illustrates this approach.

5.12 EXAMPLE. A necklace is made by stringing seven differently colored beads on a cord and then tying the ends of the cord together. The knot will be small enough to slide through the holes in the beads. Determine the number of different necklaces that can be made in this way from a given set of beads, assuming that necklaces are called "different" if their color patterns are different.

SOLUTION 1. The temptation is to blurt out a fast answer: "The ordered strings of seven beads are in one-to-one correspondence with S_7, hence there are $7! = 5040$ possibilities." But, for example, the untied beaded strings in the figure (see page 218) will all produce the same necklace once the cord is tied, so we need to count more carefully.

The statement of the example is concerned with the construction of necklaces from beaded strings. On the other hand, given a collection of necklaces, we can produce and display a beaded string like the ones in the figure by first choosing a necklace, then cutting it, and then displaying the result. For the latter two parts of the construction, we first decide which of the necklace's seven beads is going to be on the left in the final display, and then we decide (before we cut) which of that bead's two neighbors is going to be on the right in the display. As we have already discussed, there are 7! possible results. Thus by the product rule we have

$$7! = (\text{number of necklaces}) \cdot 7 \cdot 2$$

and therefore the number of necklaces is $7!/14 = 360$.

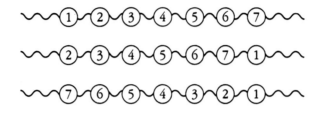

SOLUTION 2. There are 7! ways of ordering seven beads from left to right. Call two such strings of beads *equivalent* if they yield the same necklace. This is an equivalence relation, and we assert that each equivalence class has 14 strings in it. For, given any string, removing the bead from the right end and putting it on the left produces an equivalent string. Iterating (repeating again and again) this maneuver produces seven equivalent strings. Moreover, reversing the bead order of these seven strings produces seven more equivalent strings. Thus we have 14 left-to-right strings in the equivalence class of the given string. We leave it to the reader to determine that these constitute the entire equivalence class (that is, no other strings produce the same necklace). We have 7! strings altogether and 14 strings in each equivalence class, where each equivalence class corresponds to a necklace. Therefore

$$7! = 14 \cdot (\text{numbers of necklaces})$$

which gives the same result as Solution 1.

Exercises

1. Which of the following functions are permutations? Explain briefly.
   (a) The identity function on the set $\mathbb{Z}$ of integers.
   (b) The function on the unit circle that shifts each point on the circle clockwise by an angle of $\pi/16$ radians.
   (c) The function from the closed interval $[0, 8]$ to itself given by the formula $x \mapsto x/3$.
   (d) The function from the open interval $(0, 8)$ to itself given by the formula $x \mapsto x/3$.
   (e) The function from $\mathbb{R}$ to $\mathbb{R}$ given by $x \mapsto x/3$.

2. Use the language of functions to explain why

$$\begin{pmatrix} 1 & 2 & 3 & 4 \\ 3 & 4 & 1 & 3 \end{pmatrix} \quad \text{and} \quad \begin{pmatrix} 1 & 2 & 3 & 4 & 5 \\ 3 & 1 & 4 & 6 & 2 \end{pmatrix}$$

do not represent permutations.

3. List the members of S_4.

4. Compute the indicated products:

(a) $\begin{pmatrix} 1 & 2 & 3 & 4 & 5 \\ 3 & 1 & 5 & 2 & 4 \end{pmatrix} \begin{pmatrix} 1 & 2 & 3 & 4 & 5 \\ 4 & 1 & 5 & 2 & 3 \end{pmatrix}$

(b) $\begin{pmatrix} 1 & 2 & 3 & 4 \\ 2 & 4 & 1 & 3 \end{pmatrix} \begin{pmatrix} 1 & 2 & 3 & 4 \\ 3 & 4 & 1 & 2 \end{pmatrix}$

5. Suppose m and n are positive integers, with $m < n$. Strictly speaking, if $\lambda = S_m$ and $\sigma \in S_n$, then the product $\sigma\lambda$ is not defined.

   (a) Suggest a reasonable way to view S_m as a subset of S_n in such a way that the product $\sigma\lambda$ makes sense.

   (b) Use the idea in part (a) to obtain the product of $\sigma\lambda$, where

$$\sigma = \begin{pmatrix} 1 & 2 & 3 & 4 & 5 \\ 5 & 3 & 1 & 2 & 4 \end{pmatrix} \quad \text{and} \quad \lambda = \begin{pmatrix} 1 & 2 & 3 \\ 3 & 1 & 2 \end{pmatrix}$$

6. Suppose $\sigma, \lambda, \mu \in S_n$. Cite a theorem in Chapter 3 that justifies the assertion

$$(\sigma\lambda)\mu = \sigma(\lambda\mu)$$

and explain briefly.

7. It can be shown that the assertion in Exercise 6 can be extended to lengthier products of permutations. Thus, given $\sigma_1, \ldots, \sigma_t \in S_n$, no matter how parentheses are inserted in the expression

$$\sigma_1\sigma_2 \cdots \sigma_t$$

to create a meaningful product, the results will be the same. For example,

$$(\sigma_1(\sigma_2\sigma_3))\sigma_4 = (\sigma_1\sigma_2)(\sigma_3\sigma_4) = \sigma_1((\sigma_2\sigma_3)\sigma_4)$$

Therefore it is customary to omit parentheses from products of this kind, unless there is a special reason to prescribe the order in which the products are to be performed. Now define

$$\sigma_1 = \begin{pmatrix} 1 & 2 & 3 & 4 & 5 \\ 3 & 5 & 4 & 1 & 2 \end{pmatrix}$$

$$\sigma_2 = \begin{pmatrix} 1 & 2 & 3 & 4 & 5 \\ 2 & 4 & 1 & 5 & 3 \end{pmatrix}$$

$$\sigma_3 = \begin{pmatrix} 1 & 2 & 3 & 4 & 5 \\ 5 & 4 & 3 & 2 & 1 \end{pmatrix}$$

Compute each of the following products.

(a) $\sigma_1\sigma_2\sigma_3$ (b) $\sigma_1\sigma_3\sigma_2$ (c) $\sigma_2\sigma_2\sigma_3$ (d) $\sigma_3\sigma_3\sigma_3$

8. Let $\sigma \in S_n$. Define σ^0 to be the identity permutation:

$$\sigma^0 = \begin{pmatrix} 1 & 2 & \cdots & n \\ 1 & 2 & \cdots & n \end{pmatrix}$$

For $k > 0$ define

$$\sigma^k = \underbrace{\sigma\sigma\cdots\sigma}_{k \text{ factors}} \qquad \text{(the } k\text{th \textbf{power} of } \sigma\text{)}.$$

Now let

$$\sigma = \begin{pmatrix} 1 & 2 & 3 & 4 & 5 \\ 3 & 5 & 4 & 1 & 2 \end{pmatrix}$$

(a) Determine all the members of S_5 that are powers of σ, and explain your reasoning.

(b) Compute σ^{268}, and explain.

9. Consider the permutations

$$\sigma = \begin{pmatrix} 1 & 2 & 3 & 4 & 5 & 6 & 7 & 8 \\ 7 & 2 & 4 & 1 & 5 & 6 & 3 & 8 \end{pmatrix}$$

$$\text{and} \qquad \lambda = \begin{pmatrix} 1 & 2 & 3 & 4 & 5 & 6 & 7 & 8 \\ 1 & 6 & 3 & 4 & 5 & 8 & 7 & 2 \end{pmatrix}$$

By discussing how each of these permutations acts on the set $\mathbb{N}_8$, give an intuitive explanation for why, without actually multiplying, you would expect that

$$\sigma\lambda = \lambda\sigma$$

(While you're at it, verify that this equation is true.)

10. Imagine that you have made it your mission to reduce eyestrain among students of mathematics. Use this as a base for arguing that functions should be written to the *right* of their domain elements. (See Remark 5.9.) Include the function diagram

$$A \xrightarrow{f} B \xrightarrow{g} C \xrightarrow{h} D$$

as part of your discussion.

11. How many permutations are there in S_{10} that hold the numbers 2 and 8 fixed?

12. How many permutations σ are there in S_{10} having the property that the restriction $\sigma|_{\mathbb{N}_4}$ belongs to S_4?

13. The ten winners of the Great American Pet Contest, 7 dogs and 3 cats, are to be arranged in a line in front of the TV cameras for a national audience. In each of the following cases, determine the number of possible arrangements of the ten beasts under the given conditions.

    (a) unrestricted

    (b) The three cats are at one end of the line.

    (c) The three cats are in adjacent positions (but not necessarily at the end).

    (d) No two cats are next to each other in line.

    (e) Both end positions are occupied by dogs.

14. How many seven-letter "words" can be obtained by arranging the letters of the word "anagram"? (You may use the fact that a set of seven elements has 35 three-element subsets.)

15. A riverboat gambler has five inverted cups, with a bean hidden under one of them. A *move* is an interchange of two cups, and a *repositioning* is the result of a finite sequence of moves.

    (a) Associate the gambler's actions with elements of S_5.

    (b) How many moves are there?

    (c) How many repositionings are there?

    (d) How many repositionings are there that take the bean from the position on the gambler's far left to the position on his far right?

16. Four married couples are to form one large circle for a folk dance. How many circles can be formed under each of the following conditions?

    (a) Each woman's husband is on her immediate right.

    (b) The people in the circle alternate by sex.

    (c) There are no restrictions.

    (d) There are two men who loathe each other and refuse to hold each other's hand.

17. A necklace is to be made with seven differently colored beads, as in Example 5.12. Unfortunately the string is quite thick, and the knot will be too large to pass through the holes in the beads and too ugly to be worn where it can be seen. (It will be worn behind the neck, under the collar.) How many different necklaces are there?

5.4 Permutations and Geometric Symmetry

> Symmetry...is one idea by which man through the ages has tried to comprehend and create order, beauty, and perfection.
>
> HERMANN WEYL
> *Symmetry*

What makes a daisy beautiful? We cannot answer this here beyond saying that there is something about the balance, harmony, and regularity of the daisy's structure that we find at once startling, mysterious, and glorious. What we *can* do is describe certain aspects of the "regularity" of a daisy's structure. The idealized daisy has 16 identically shaped petals. Here we have inscribed the daisy in a circle, so its petal tips mark the vertices of a regular 16-gon, that is, a polygon with 16 sides of equal length. Now if the whole plane is rotated by the angle of $2\pi/16 = \pi/8$ radians around the center of the floral design, the daisy is carried onto itself. Such a rotation is called a **symmetry** of the daisy. Repeated applications of this rotation continue to carry the daisy onto itself. Thus if σ denotes the rotation by $\pi/8$, then σ^n, meaning the composition

$$\underbrace{\sigma\sigma\cdots\sigma}_{n}$$

is also a symmetry of the daisy.

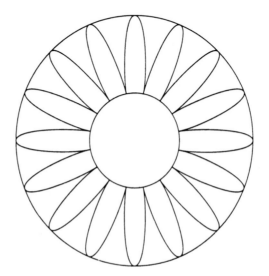

Now consider the following two five-petalled flowers:

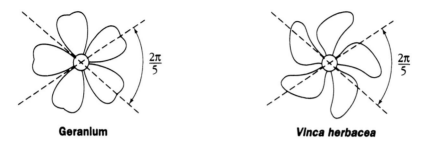

Geranium   **Vinca herbacea**

Here a rotation by $2\pi/5$ radians about either flower's center is a symmetry of the flower. But the geranium has more symmetry than the *Vinca herbacea*. For, if L is a line that passes through the geranium's center and splits one of the petals in half, then the flower is carried onto itself by a **reflection** through L. (This reflection is the function from the plane to itself that carries each point to its "mirror image" on the other side of L.) But *Vinca herbacea* has no such reflective property, because of the irregularity of its petal shape.

A symmetry of a daisy acts as a permutation on the vertex set of the corresponding regular polygon. Moreover, if we know the symmetry's action on the vertices, then we know what this symmetry does to the flower, and indeed to the whole plane. This observation allows us to study the geometric concept of symmetry by studying certain families of permutations.[*]

5.13 Definition. A **geometric figure** is a subset of the plane or of ordinary three-dimensional space. A **symmetry** of a geometric figure F is a bijection s of the plane or space to itself such that $s(F) = F$ and such that *distances are preserved.* In other words, for any two points x and y, the distance between $s(x)$ and $s(y)$ is equal to the distance between x and y. More briefly, we say that a symmetry of F is a **rigid motion** that carries F onto F.

A **polygon** is a geometric figure in the plane consisting of a finite sequence of points (the **vertices**) $v_1, v_2, \ldots, v_n$, together with the line segments (the **edges** or **sides**) connecting v_i and v_{i+1}, for $1 \le i \le n$. (Here it is understood that $v_{n+1} = v_1$.)

Now consider the symmetries of a polygon. We leave to your geometric intuition these facts: a symmetry of a polygon takes vertices to vertices,

[*]For an extensive treatment of this topic, see Hermann Weyl, *Symmetry* (Princeton: Princeton University Press, 1952).

and we know what it does to every point if we know its action on the vertices.

If a polygon P has n vertices in locations numbered 1 through n, then a symmetry of P determines a permutation $\sigma \in S_n$ as follows: for each $i \in \mathbb{N}_n$, the number $\sigma(i)$ is the location to which the symmetry carries the vertex that started in location i. A polygon with n vertices is an **n-gon**.

5.14 EXAMPLE. Let P be the equilateral triangle with vertices at locations labelled 1, 2, 3 in the accompanying figure.

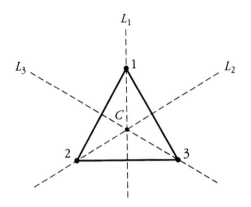

In this figure, each line L_i is the perpendicular bisector of the edge opposite the vertex at location i. A counterclockwise rotation of $2\pi/3$ radians about the center C is a symmetry of the triangle, and it sends the vertex initially at location 1 to location 2, the one at location 2 to location 3, and so on. Thus the corresponding permutation in S_3 is

$$\begin{pmatrix} 1 & 2 & 3 \\ 2 & 3 & 1 \end{pmatrix}$$

Similarly, reflecting the triangle through the line L_2 corresponds to the permutation

$$\begin{pmatrix} 1 & 2 & 3 \\ 3 & 2 & 1 \end{pmatrix}$$

Altogether, we have the following correspondence between symmetries of the triangle and permutations in S_3.

(5.15)	Symmetry	Corresponding permutation
	s_1: identity function	$\begin{pmatrix} 1 & 2 & 3 \\ 1 & 2 & 3 \end{pmatrix} = \sigma_1$
	s_2: reflection through L_1	$\begin{pmatrix} 1 & 2 & 3 \\ 1 & 3 & 2 \end{pmatrix} = \sigma_2$
	s_3: reflection through L_2	$\begin{pmatrix} 1 & 2 & 3 \\ 3 & 2 & 1 \end{pmatrix} = \sigma_3$
	s_4: reflection through L_3	$\begin{pmatrix} 1 & 2 & 3 \\ 2 & 1 & 3 \end{pmatrix} = \sigma_4$
	s_5: counterclockwise rotation by $2\pi/3$	$\begin{pmatrix} 1 & 2 & 3 \\ 2 & 3 & 1 \end{pmatrix} = \sigma_5$
	s_6: counterclockwise rotation by $4\pi/3$	$\begin{pmatrix} 1 & 2 & 3 \\ 3 & 1 & 2 \end{pmatrix} = \sigma_6$

We have listed six distinct permutations in Table 5.15. Since $\#S_3 = 3! = 6$ and every symmetry of the triangle corresponds to an element of S_3, we know that we have found *all* the symmetries of the triangle.

From our association of symmetries of an n-gon with elements of S_n, we conclude that an n-gon can have at most $n!$ symmetries. Moreover, if s_1 and s_2 are symmetries corresponding to permutations σ_1 and σ_2, respectively, then the composition $s_2 \circ s_1$ corresponds to the permutation $\sigma_2\sigma_1$. (To check this, use the fact that a symmetry and its associated permutation both have essentially the same action. More precisely, if a symmetry takes the vertex at location i to location j, then the associated permutation takes i to j.) It follows that we can determine the effect of applying a succession of symmetries by computing the product of the corresponding permutations. So once we establish the correspondence between symmetries and permutations, we can answer geometric questions of the form, "What is the effect of successively applying the symmetries $s_1, s_2, \ldots, s_l$?" by computing permutation products.

5.16 EXAMPLE. With the symmetries $s_1, \ldots, s_6$ as in Table 5.15, compute the composition

$$s_4 \circ s_6 \circ s_2 \circ s_5 \circ s_3$$

while keeping your mind free of geometric thoughts.

SOLUTION. We take the corresponding product of permutations:

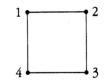

$$\sigma_4\sigma_6\sigma_2\sigma_5\sigma_3 = \begin{pmatrix} 1 & 2 & 3 \\ 2 & 1 & 3 \end{pmatrix}\begin{pmatrix} 1 & 2 & 3 \\ 3 & 1 & 2 \end{pmatrix}\begin{pmatrix} 1 & 2 & 3 \\ 1 & 3 & 2 \end{pmatrix}\begin{pmatrix} 1 & 2 & 3 \\ 2 & 3 & 1 \end{pmatrix}\begin{pmatrix} 1 & 2 & 3 \\ 3 & 2 & 1 \end{pmatrix}$$

$$= \begin{pmatrix} 1 & 2 & 3 \\ 3 & 2 & 1 \end{pmatrix} = \sigma_3$$

Therefore the given composition of symmetries is equal to s_3.

Example 5.16 illustrates an important reason to represent symmetries by permutations: it allows us to compute symmetry compositions in a purely mechanical fashion, without having to struggle with the complexities of geometric imagery. This is very much in the spirit of the quotation from Whitehead on page 54.

The symmetries of a square correspond to permutations in S_4.

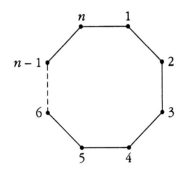

But notice that no symmetry of the square corresponds to the permutation $\begin{pmatrix} 1 & 2 & 3 & 4 \\ 1 & 3 & 2 & 4 \end{pmatrix}$, since a symmetry that holds the vertex at location 1 fixed can't take the vertex at location 2 to location 3. More generally, each symmetry of the **regular** n-gon (an equilateral and equiangular n-gon) takes the vertex initially at location 1 to one of the n vertex locations, call it $\sigma(1)$. Then, because a symmetry is distance-preserving, it must take the vertex initially at location 2 to one of the two neighboring locations of $\sigma(1)$. Once $\sigma(1)$ and $\sigma(2)$ have been fixed, the other $\sigma(i)$ are uniquely determined by the geometry (in particular, by the "rigidity" of the motion). It follows from the product rule that there are precisely $2n$ symmetries of the regular n-gon, and these correspond to a set of $2n$ permutations in S_n.

5.17 EXAMPLE. A regular 9-gon has 18 symmetries. If the vertices are at locations numbered clockwise from 1 to 9, then there are exactly two symmetries that take the vertex at location 1 to the vertex at location 5, namely, those associated with the following permutations in S_9:

$$\begin{pmatrix} 1 & 2 & 3 & 4 & 5 & 6 & 7 & 8 & 9 \\ 5 & 6 & 7 & 8 & 9 & 1 & 2 & 3 & 4 \end{pmatrix}$$

and $$\begin{pmatrix} 1 & 2 & 3 & 4 & 5 & 6 & 7 & 8 & 9 \\ 5 & 4 & 3 & 2 & 1 & 9 & 8 & 7 & 6 \end{pmatrix}$$

The first of these corresponds to a clockwise rotation of the 9-gon by $8\pi/9$ radians. The second corresponds to a reflection through the line that passes through the center of the 9-gon and the vertex at location 3. (Suggestion: Draw and label the regular 9-gon to check these two assertions.)

The set of permutations associated with the symmetries of the regular n-gon is usually denoted D_n; it is called the **dihedral group of degree n**. Our discussion here shows that working with symmetries of the regular n-gon is essentially the same as computing with permutations in D_n. The collection of symmetries of the n-gon and the dihedral group D_n are said to be *isomorphic* structures. (From the Greek: *iso* means equal and *morphē* means form.)

We have seen that, with the help of permutations, the geometry of polygonal symmetries can be analyzed by tracking the paths of vertices as they move from one location to another. It turns out that the movie theater problem and the Rubik's Cube problem from Example 5.1 can also be formulated (and then solved) as permutation problems. In the movie theater problem, the locations are the seats. (They hold people instead of vertices, but otherwise we proceed as in the geometric setting.) A permutation

$$\sigma = \begin{pmatrix} 1 & 2 & \cdots & 10 \\ \sigma(1) & \sigma(2) & \cdots & \sigma(10) \end{pmatrix}$$

corresponds to the rearrangement in which the person in seat i ends up in seat $\sigma(i)$, for $1 \le i \le 10$. As for Rubik's Cube, each of the Cube's six faces is partitioned into nine facelets. An operation on the Cube consists of a succession of face rotations, and we can describe the effect of an operation by judiciously recording the position of each facelet before and after the operation. When we looked at symmetries of the n-gon, we saw that not every permutation of vertex positions corresponds to a symmetry. Similarly, not every permutation of the set of facelet positions corresponds to a Cube operation. For instance, a facelet on a corner cubie cannot be moved to the center of a face. We'll return to both of these problems later in this chapter.

Exercises

1. A **scalene** triangle is a triangle that is not isosceles. Show that the identity function is the only symmetry of a scalene triangle.

2. Let X be the set of all symmetries of the unit circle. Without proof, give a geometric description of the members of X. Also, is X finite, countably infinite, or uncountable?

3. (a) List the members of the dihedral group D_4 (which corresponds to the set of symmetries of the square).

   (b) List the members of D_6 (corresponding to the symmetries of the regular hexagon), and give a geometric explanation of a way in which D_3 can be viewed as a subset of D_6.

   (c) Show (without all the details) how for each $n \geq 2$, the dihedral group D_n can be viewed as a subset of the set of symmetries of the unit circle.

4. Let F be a geometric figure.

   (a) Prove that if s_1 and s_2 are symmetries of F, then so is the composition $s_2 \circ s_1$.

   (b) Prove that if s is a symmetry of F, then so is s^{-1}.

5. In each case describe the set of all symmetries of the given geometric figure in the coordinatized plane. Include the cardinality of the symmetry set as part of your description.

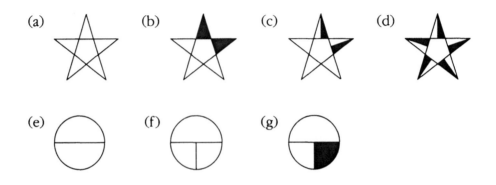

(h) $\mathbb{N} \times \mathbb{N}$ (i) $\mathbb{Z} \times \mathbb{Z}$ (j) $\mathbb{Z}$ (k) $\mathbb{R}$

(l) ⋯ 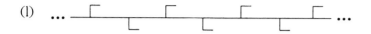 ⋯

6. Describe the symmetries of each of the following figures in three-dimensional space, and determine the number of symmetries.

   (a) A regular tetrahedron

   (b) A pyramid (with a square base and four sides, each an equilateral triangle)

   (c) A regular octahedron (formed by gluing together the bases of two pyramids of the same size)

   (d) A cube

   (e) A rectangular noncubic solid

   (f) A sphere

7. Let $Q = (a, b)$ be a point in the coordinatized xy-plane $\mathbb{R}^2 = \mathbb{R} \times \mathbb{R}$. For each point $P \in \mathbb{R}^2$, let $R_Q(P)$ denote the mirror image of P on the other side of Q. The function $R_Q : \mathbb{R}^2 \to \mathbb{R}^2$ is called **reflection in Q**.

   (a) Give a precise formula for R_Q (that is, give the coordinates of $R_Q(P)$ in terms of those of Q and P).

   (b) Prove that R_Q preserves distances. (See Definition 5.13.)

   (c) Prove that R_Q is a symmetry of any circle centered at Q.

8. The notation in this exercise is that of Table 5.15. Use permutations (and not geometry) to determine the result of applying the symmetry composition $s_6 \circ s_3 \circ s_5$ a total of 787 times.

5.5 Decomposition into Cycles

In this section and the next, we will see how to decompose elements of S_n into products of especially simple kinds of permutations called *cycles*, and we will consider some applications. But first consider this: in focusing on S_n, the set of permutations of $\{1, \ldots, n\}$, aren't we neglecting the study of permutations of *other* finite sets? The response to this is that a typical

n-set $A = \{a_1, \ldots, a_n\}$ has permutations of the form

(*)
$$\begin{pmatrix} a_1 & a_2 & \cdots & a_n \\ a_{i_1} & a_{i_2} & \cdots & a_{i_n} \end{pmatrix}$$

where the subscripts in the bottom row are some arrangement of $1, 2, \ldots, n$. Properties of such a permutation are completely determined by the corresponding permutation of the subscripts:

(**)
$$\begin{pmatrix} 1 & 2 & \cdots & n \\ i_1 & i_2 & \cdots & i_n \end{pmatrix}$$

(If you like, view (**) as an abbreviation for (*) obtained by erasing all the a's.) Thus we can focus our attention on S_n with the knowledge that our results will carry over to S_A for any n-set A. In the terminology introduced near the end of the preceding section, if A has n elements then the symmetric groups S_A and S_n are *isomorphic*.

From now on we let e denote the identity permutation:

$$e = \begin{pmatrix} 1 & 2 & \cdots & n \\ 1 & 2 & \cdots & n \end{pmatrix}$$

Strictly speaking, there is a different identity permutation for each value of n, but it will always be clear which identity is relevant.

A permutation is a bijection and therefore has an inverse that is also a bijection. That is,

$$\sigma \in S_n \quad \Rightarrow \quad \sigma^{-1} \in S_n$$

and σ^{-1} takes each element $\sigma(i)$ back to i. The standard permutation notation displays $\sigma(i)$ directly below i, and therefore σ^{-1} can be obtained by interchanging the two rows of σ. For example, if

$$\sigma = \begin{pmatrix} 1 & 2 & 3 & 4 \\ 3 & 1 & 4 & 2 \end{pmatrix} \quad \text{then} \quad \sigma^{-1} = \begin{pmatrix} 3 & 1 & 4 & 2 \\ 1 & 2 & 3 & 4 \end{pmatrix} = \begin{pmatrix} 1 & 2 & 3 & 4 \\ 2 & 4 & 1 & 3 \end{pmatrix}$$

Here the right-hand equality reflects the standard practice of listing the top row in ascending order, a visual aid in computations.

Alternatively, σ^{-1} can be obtained by writing $\sigma^{-1} = \begin{pmatrix} 1 & 2 & \cdots & n \\ & & & \end{pmatrix}$ and then writing below each number in σ^{-1} the number that appears *above* it in σ.

5.18 EXAMPLE. Let

$$\sigma = \begin{pmatrix} 1 & 2 & 3 & 4 & 5 & 6 & 7 & 8 \\ 3 & 7 & 1 & 6 & 4 & 8 & 2 & 5 \end{pmatrix}$$

Check the equation

$$\sigma^{-1} = \begin{pmatrix} 1 & 2 & 3 & 4 & 5 & 6 & 7 & 8 \\ 3 & 7 & 1 & 6 & 8 & 4 & 5 & 6 \end{pmatrix}$$

SOLUTION 1. Compute σ^{-1} directly and compare it with the candidate:

$$\sigma^{-1} = \begin{pmatrix} 3 & 7 & 1 & 6 & 4 & 8 & 2 & 5 \\ 1 & 2 & 3 & 4 & 5 & 6 & 7 & 8 \end{pmatrix} = \begin{pmatrix} 1 & 2 & 3 & 4 & 5 & 6 & 7 & 8 \\ 3 & 7 & 1 & 5 & 8 & 4 & 2 & 6 \end{pmatrix}$$

$$\neq \begin{pmatrix} 1 & 2 & 3 & 4 & 5 & 6 & 7 & 8 \\ 3 & 7 & 1 & 6 & 8 & 4 & 5 & 6 \end{pmatrix}$$

Therefore the equation is false.

SOLUTION 2. The permutation σ^{-1} must satisfy the equation $\sigma\sigma^{-1} = e$; so the strategy is to multiply the two given permutations and observe whether the answer is e:

$$\begin{pmatrix} 1 & 2 & 3 & 4 & 5 & 6 & 7 & 8 \\ 3 & 7 & 1 & 6 & 4 & 8 & 2 & 5 \end{pmatrix}\begin{pmatrix} 1 & 2 & 3 & 4 & 5 & 6 & 7 & 8 \\ 3 & 7 & 1 & 6 & 8 & 4 & 5 & 6 \end{pmatrix}$$

$$= \begin{pmatrix} 1 & 2 & 3 & 4 & 5 & 6 & 7 & 8 \\ 1 & 2 & 3 & 8 & 5 & 6 & 4 & 8 \end{pmatrix} \neq e$$

False again.

SOLUTION 3. Notice that our given candidate for σ^{-1} has two appearances of 6 in the bottom row, and it is therefore not a permutation. In particular, it is not σ^{-1}.

If $\sigma \in S_n$ and $t \geq 0$, we define σ^t recursively by

(5.19)
$$\begin{cases} \sigma^0 = e, \\ \sigma^{k+1} = \sigma^k\sigma \end{cases}$$

Thus $\sigma^1 = \sigma$ and, more generally, if $t > 0$ then

$$\sigma^t = \underbrace{\sigma\sigma\cdots\sigma}_{t}$$

We also can define negative powers of σ: if $t > 0$ define

(5.20)
$$\sigma^{-t} = (\sigma^{-1})^t$$

5.21 Example. If

$$\sigma = \begin{pmatrix} 1 & 2 & 3 & 4 & 5 \\ 3 & 5 & 1 & 2 & 4 \end{pmatrix}$$

then

$$\sigma^2 = \begin{pmatrix} 1 & 2 & 3 & 4 & 5 \\ 1 & 4 & 3 & 5 & 2 \end{pmatrix}$$

$$\sigma^{-1} = \begin{pmatrix} 1 & 2 & 3 & 4 & 5 \\ 3 & 4 & 1 & 5 & 2 \end{pmatrix}$$

$$\sigma^{-2} = \begin{pmatrix} 1 & 2 & 3 & 4 & 5 \\ 1 & 5 & 3 & 2 & 4 \end{pmatrix}$$

A quick computation shows that in Example 5.21 we have $\sigma^{-2} = (\sigma^2)^{-1}$. Perhaps this is not a surprise; it is a special case of the next theorem, whose statement will seem plausible because of our previous experience in multiplying real numbers. The complete proofs are unexpectedly technical (for instance, there are special cases according to the signs of the exponents), and we'll give only a partial proof. Notice that part (c) is a special case of part (b).

5.22 Theorem (Laws of Exponents). If $\sigma \in S_n$, then for all $s, t \in \mathbb{Z}$,

(a) $\sigma^s \sigma^t = \sigma^{s+t}$
(b) $(\sigma^s)^t = \sigma^{st}$
(c) $(\sigma^s)^{-1} = \sigma^{-s}$

Partial Proof of (a). We will prove that $\sigma^s \sigma^t = \sigma^{s+t}$ when s and t are natural numbers. Fix $s \in N$; the proof will be by induction on t. For $t = 1$ we have, by 5.19,

$$\sigma^s \sigma^1 = \sigma^s \sigma = \sigma^{s+1}$$

Now assume that $\sigma^s \sigma^k = \sigma^{s+k}$ for some $k \in \mathbb{N}$, and remember that permutation product is actually composition of functions. We have

$$\sigma^s\sigma^{k+1} = \sigma^s(\sigma^k\sigma) \qquad \text{(by 5.19)}$$

$$= (\sigma^s\sigma^k)\sigma \qquad \text{(by the associative law for composition of functions)}$$

$$= (\sigma^{s+k})\sigma \qquad \text{(by the induction hypothesis)}$$

$$= \sigma^{(s+k)+1} \qquad \text{(by 5.19)}$$

$$= \sigma^{s+(k+1)}$$

This completes the proof of the assertion. □

We can associate a graph with each permutation $\sigma \in S_n$ as follows. Represent each element $i \in \{1, 2, \ldots, n\}$ by a point; these are the vertices of the graph. Then, for each i, draw a directed edge from vertex i to vertex $\sigma(i)$. So, for instance, the permutation

$$\sigma = \begin{pmatrix} 1 & 2 & 3 & 4 & 5 & 6 & 7 & 8 & 9 & 10 \\ 5 & 8 & 7 & 10 & 3 & 4 & 1 & 2 & 9 & 6 \end{pmatrix}$$

has this graph:

(5.23)

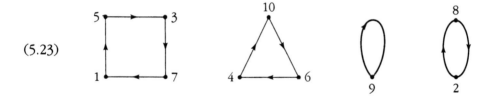

An application of σ then corresponds to moving each vertex in the direction of the arrow to the location of the next vertex. Each vertex has only one edge leading *away* from it, because a permutation is a function, and so takes each point in its domain to a unique image. Also, each vertex has exactly one edge leading *into* it, because a permutation is bijective. Thus, graphs like the following three do not represent permutations:

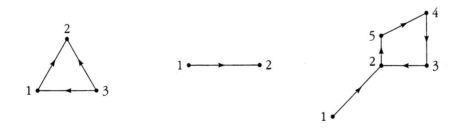

5.24 Definition. Suppose $1 \leq r \leq n$. A permutation $\sigma \in S_n$ is called a **cycle of length r** or an **r-cycle** if there are r different numbers $a_1, \ldots, a_r$ in $\mathbb{N}_n$ such that

$$\sigma(a_i) = \begin{cases} a_{i+1} & \text{if } 1 \leq i \leq r - 1 \\ a_1 & \text{if } i = r \end{cases}$$

and $\sigma(x) = x$ for all $x \notin \{a_1, \ldots, a_r\}$. The set $\{a_1, \ldots, a_r\}$ is called the **orbit** of σ (and of each a_i), denoted **orb σ**.

A cycle that fits the description in 5.24 is usually denoted by

$$\sigma = (a_1 \quad a_2 \quad \cdots \quad a_r)$$

and its graph can be drawn as an r-gon with directed edges:

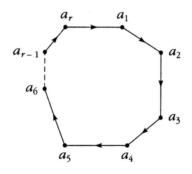

Here we have not bothered to write the little loops like

3

that correspond to fixed points. We will continue to omit them in future permutation graphs in order to avoid clutter.

5.25 EXAMPLE. The permutation

$$\sigma = \begin{pmatrix} 1 & 2 & 3 & 4 & 5 & 6 & 7 \\ 7 & 3 & 5 & 4 & 1 & 6 & 2 \end{pmatrix}$$

is a 5-cycle, namely, $\sigma = (1 \quad 7 \quad 2 \quad 3 \quad 5)$. Its graph looks like this:

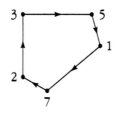

5.26 Remarks. (a) In writing the symbol for a cycle of length $r \geq 2$, the list inside the parentheses can start with any element in the orbit. For instance, in Example 5.25 we can also write $\sigma = (7 \quad 2 \quad 3 \quad 5 \quad 1) = (2 \quad 3 \quad 5 \quad 1 \quad 7)$. (The underlying intuition: the description of a wheel can begin at any of its spokes.)

(b) Consider a 1-cycle, say, $\sigma = (a_1)$. Careful reading of Definition 5.24 shows that σ is actually the identity permutation.

(c) If σ is an r-cycle, so is σ^{-1}. In fact, it is easily checked that if $\sigma = (a_1 \quad a_2 \quad \cdots \quad a_r)$, then $\sigma^{-1} = (a_r \quad a_{r-1} \quad \cdots \quad a_1)$. If σ corresponds to a clockwise movement on a polygon, then σ^{-1} corresponds to a counterclockwise movement of the same magnitude on the same polygon.

5.27 Definition. A family of cycles is **disjoint** if their orbits are pairwise disjoint; that is, no cycle in the family moves any element moved by another cycle in the family.

5.28 Example.

$$\alpha = \begin{pmatrix} 1 & 2 & 3 & 4 & 5 & 6 & 7 \\ 1 & 6 & 3 & 5 & 2 & 4 & 7 \end{pmatrix} \quad \text{and} \quad \beta = \begin{pmatrix} 1 & 2 & 3 & 4 & 5 & 6 & 7 \\ 1 & 2 & 7 & 4 & 5 & 6 & 3 \end{pmatrix}$$

are disjoint cycles, since $\alpha = (2 \quad 6 \quad 4 \quad 5)$ and $\beta = (3 \quad 7)$, and $\{2, 6, 4, 5\} \cap \{3, 7\} = \emptyset$.

The formal statement and proof of the following theorem is technical, but the underlying idea is easily stated and easily believed: If Frank moves objects from one position to another in his backyard A, and George moves objects around in his backyard B, and neither moves anything in the other person's yard, then the result is independent of the order in which they act. (If there were a common region on which both men acted, then the result *might* depend on the order in which they acted.)

5.29 Theorem. Let A and B be nonempty sets. Suppose f and g are functions from $A \cup B$ to $A \cup B$ satisfying

$$f(A) \subseteq A \qquad \text{and} \qquad f(x) = x \quad \forall x \in B$$

$$g(B) \subseteq B \qquad \text{and} \qquad g(x) = x \quad \forall x \in A$$

Then $g \circ f = f \circ g$.

PROOF. We must show that $(g \circ f)(x) = (f \circ g)(x)$ for all $x \in A \cup B$. If $x \in A$ then $(g \circ f)(x) = g(f(x)) = f(x)$, since $f(x) \in A$; also, $(f \circ g)(x) = f(g(x)) = f(x)$, since $g(x) = x$ for all $x \in A$. This shows that $(g \circ f)(x) = (f \circ g)(x)$ for all $x \in A$. The same equation holds for all $x \in B$ by a similar argument (check this), and hence for all $x \in A \cup B$. $\square$

5.30 Corollary. If α and β are disjoint cycles, then $\alpha\beta = \beta\alpha$. (More briefly: disjoint cycles commute.)

PROOF. Let A and B be the orbits of α and β, respectively. Since α and β are disjoint, we have $A \cap B = \emptyset$; so $\alpha(x) = x$ for all $x \in B$ and $\beta(x) = x$ for all $x \in A$. Now apply Theorem 5.29. $\square$

5.31 EXAMPLE. In S_{10} we have

$$(3 \ 1 \ 5 \ 7 \ 9)(2 \ 8 \ 6) = (2 \ 8 \ 6)(3 \ 1 \ 5 \ 7 \ 9)$$

$$= \begin{pmatrix} 1 & 2 & 3 & 4 & 5 & 6 & 7 & 8 & 9 & 10 \\ 5 & 8 & 1 & 4 & 7 & 2 & 9 & 6 & 3 & 10 \end{pmatrix}$$

This permutation can be graphed as follows:

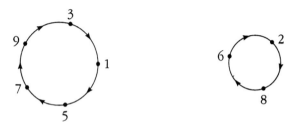

(Following our convention, vertices corresponding to the fixed values 4 and 10 are omitted from our graph.)

The action of a product of disjoint cycles is easy to picture. Is *every* permutation in S_n a product of disjoint cycles? (A single cycle is viewed as such a product.) We claim that the answer is yes. Although our examples may make the claim seem evident, we need a proof to be sure that our examples were not atypical. In fact, at first glance the action of an arbitrary permutation $\sigma \in S_n$ on the set $\mathbb{N}_n = \{1, 2, \ldots, n\}$ might appear to be too chaotic for such a controlled description. Our goal is to make sense of this situation.

5.32 Definition. Let $\sigma \in S_n$. The **order** of σ, denoted **ord** σ, is the smallest positive integer k such that $\sigma^k = e$.

5.33 EXAMPLE. Let

$$\sigma = \begin{pmatrix} 1 & 2 & 3 & 4 & 5 \\ 5 & 3 & 4 & 2 & 1 \end{pmatrix}$$

Then

$$\sigma^2 = \begin{pmatrix} 1 & 2 & 3 & 4 & 5 \\ 1 & 4 & 2 & 3 & 5 \end{pmatrix} \qquad \sigma^3 = \begin{pmatrix} 1 & 2 & 3 & 4 & 5 \\ 5 & 2 & 3 & 4 & 1 \end{pmatrix}$$

$$\sigma^4 = \begin{pmatrix} 1 & 2 & 3 & 4 & 5 \\ 1 & 3 & 4 & 2 & 5 \end{pmatrix} \qquad \sigma^5 = \begin{pmatrix} 1 & 2 & 3 & 4 & 5 \\ 5 & 4 & 2 & 3 & 1 \end{pmatrix}$$

and $\sigma^6 = e$. Therefore ord $\sigma = 6$.

We claim that every $\sigma \in S_n$ has an order. To see this, first note that the powers $e, \sigma, \sigma^2, \sigma^3, \ldots$ are not all different, since S_n is finite. So we have $\sigma^i = \sigma^j$ for some i and j satisfying $0 \le i < j$. Multiplication by σ^{-i} then gives $e = \sigma^{j-i}$. Thus $e = \sigma^k$ for some $k > 0$, and the smallest such k is ord σ.

5.34 Theorem. If ord $\sigma = k$ then the permutations $e, \sigma, \ldots, \sigma^{k-1}$ are all different, and every power (positive, negative, or zero) of σ is equal to one of these k permutations.

PROOF. First a reminder of the *division algorithm* from grade school arithmetic: Given any two positive integers, one will divide into the other, yielding a quotient and a remainder that is strictly less than the divisor. More generally, in Section 6.3 we will show that if k and s are integers and $k > 0$, then we can write $s = kq + r$ for some integers q and r, with $0 \le r < k$. With this notation, if σ^s is an arbitrary power of σ and $k = \text{ord}\,\sigma$, then

$$\sigma^s = \sigma^{kq+r} = (\sigma^k)^q \sigma^r \qquad \text{(by the laws of exponents)}$$

$$= \sigma^r \qquad \text{(since } \sigma^k = e\text{)}$$

where $0 \le r \le k - 1$. Therefore every power of σ is equal to one of $e, \sigma, \ldots, \sigma^{k-1}$.

If the permutations $e, \sigma, \ldots, \sigma^{k-1}$ were not all different, then there would be integers i, j satisfying $0 \le i < j \le k - 1$ such that $\sigma^i = \sigma^j$. Multiplication of this equation by σ^{-i} would then yield a contradiction of the minimality of k.   □

5.35 Cycle Decomposition Theorem. Every permutation in S_n is a product of disjoint cycles.

PROOF. We begin by following the trail of an element in $\mathbb{N}_n$ under repeated action by σ. Consider the sequence

$$1 = \sigma^0(1), \quad \sigma(1), \quad \sigma^2(1), \quad \sigma^3(1), \ldots$$

Since $\mathbb{N}_n$ is finite this list must contain repetitions. Suppose the first repetition is

(∗) $$\sigma^r(1) = \sigma^{t_1}(1)$$

where $0 \le r < t_1$ and t_1 is minimal. If r were positive, then applying σ^{-r} to both sides of (∗) would produce an earlier repetition, which would contradict the minimality of t_1. Therefore $r = 0$, so we have shown that σ acts as a t_1-cycle on the elements $1, \sigma(1), \ldots, \sigma^{t_1-1}(1)$.

If σ moves no other elements of $\mathbb{N}_n$, then σ is equal to the t_1-cycle $\gamma_1 = (1 \quad \sigma(1) \cdots \sigma^{t_1-1}(1))$, and we are finished. But if σ *does* move other elements, choose some element b moved by σ but not by γ_1 and consider the sequence $b, \sigma(b), \sigma^2(b), \ldots$. By the same argument as before, this yields a t_2-cycle $\gamma_2 = (b \quad \sigma(b) \cdots \sigma^{t_2-1}(b))$.

We claim that γ_1 and γ_2 are disjoint cycles. To see this, suppose we had $\sigma^i(1) = \sigma^j(b)$ for some integers i and j. Then application of σ^{-j} to both sides of this equation yields $\sigma^{i-j}(1) = b$. But by Theorem 5.34, $\sigma^{i-j} = \sigma^r$ for some r satisfying $0 \le r < \text{ord}\,\sigma$. Therefore $b = \sigma^r(1)$, contradicting the fact that $b \notin \{1, \sigma(1), \ldots, \sigma^{t_1-1}(1)\}$. Thus γ_1 and γ_2 must be disjoint.

Now, if no other elements of $\mathbb{N}_n$ are moved by σ, then $\sigma = \gamma_2 \gamma_1$. Otherwise we repeat the preceding argument on the remaining elements moved by σ. Eventually we get a factorization $\sigma = \gamma_m \cdots \gamma_2 \gamma_1$, where γ_i is a t_i-cycle and the cycles $\gamma_1, \ldots, \gamma_m$ are disjoint. ☐

5.36 Remarks. (a) The cycles in the disjoint cycle decomposition of σ correspond to the connected components in the graph of σ.

(b) The proof of Theorem 5.35 actually gives an algorithm for factoring a permutation σ into disjoint cycles: Start with any element $x \in \mathbb{N}_n$ and keep applying σ until x reappears; this gives the first cycle. Repeat this process on any element that is not in the first cycle, and continue until all elements of $\mathbb{N}_n$ have appeared in cycles.

(c) As noted in 5.26, a 1-cycle is just the identity permutation, e. In expressing a nontrivial permutation as a product of cycles, it is customary to list only cycles of length 2 or more, since factors equal to e have no effect on the product. For instance, instead of

$$(1)(2 \quad 3 \quad 4)(5)(7)(6 \quad 8)$$

we write

$$(2 \quad 3 \quad 4)(6 \quad 8)$$

(d) How unique is the factorization of a permutation into disjoint cycles? For one thing, the cyclic factors can be listed in any order, in view of the fact that disjoint cycles commute (see Corollary 5.30). Also, a cycle of length 2 or more can be written in more than one way. For instance,

$$(1 \quad 2 \quad 3) = (3 \quad 1 \quad 2) = (2 \quad 3 \quad 1) = \begin{pmatrix} 1 & 2 & 3 \\ 2 & 3 & 1 \end{pmatrix}$$

Thus we have

$$(1 \ 2 \ 3)(4 \ 5)(6 \ 7 \ 8 \ 9) = (7 \ 8 \ 9 \ 6)(5 \ 4)(3 \ 1 \ 2)$$
$$= (5 \ 4)(2 \ 3 \ 1)(9 \ 6 \ 7 \ 8)$$

But except for these minor variations, we claim that the factorization into disjoint cycles is unique. To see this, suppose $\sigma = \gamma_1 \cdots \gamma_m = \lambda_1 \cdots \lambda_t$, two factorizations into disjoint cycles; we claim that the λs are the γs, but possibly listed in a different order. Fix $a_1 \in$ orb γ_1. Then a_1 is in the orbit of exactly one λ_j, say $a_1 \in$ orb λ_1, and so $\gamma_1(a) = \sigma(a) = \lambda_1(a)$. An induction argument shows that $\gamma_1^r(a) = \lambda_1^r(a)$ for every $r \geq 0$. Therefore $\gamma_1 = \lambda_1$. (From 5.24 it follows that two cycles are equal if they have the same orbit and the same action on each element of that orbit.) Similarly, *every* γ_i is one of the λ_j, and so $\{\gamma_1, \ldots, \gamma_m\} \frown \{\lambda_1, \ldots, \lambda_l\}$. The opposite inclusion is proved the same way.

(e) By the *orbits* of a permutation σ we mean the orbits of the disjoint cycles in its decomposition. The orbits of σ are the paths followed by the elements of its domain under repeated applications of σ. Each orbit corresponds to a closed polygon in the graph of σ.

5.37 EXAMPLE.

(a) $\begin{pmatrix} 1 & 2 & 3 & 4 & 5 & 6 & 7 & 8 & 9 \\ 4 & 9 & 2 & 5 & 1 & 7 & 6 & 8 & 3 \end{pmatrix} = (1 \quad 4 \quad 5)(2 \quad 9 \quad 3)(6 \quad 7)$

(b) $\begin{pmatrix} 1 & 2 & 3 & 4 & 5 & 6 & 7 & 8 & 9 & 10 & 11 & 12 \\ 9 & 6 & 8 & 7 & 2 & 5 & 4 & 1 & 3 & 10 & 12 & 11 \end{pmatrix}$

$\qquad = (1 \quad 9 \quad 3 \quad 8)(2 \quad 6 \quad 5)(11 \quad 12)(4 \quad 7)$

(c) Let $\sigma = \alpha\beta$, with $\alpha = (1 \quad 2 \quad 3)$ and $\beta = (2 \quad 3 \quad 4)$. Express σ as a product of disjoint cycles.

SOLUTION.   As in parts (a) and (b), we follow the algorithm of the cycle decomposition theorem. The only variation here is that σ is now given as a product of two cycles. We must remember to apply the right-hand cycle first.

$$\left. \begin{array}{c} 1 \overset{\beta}{\longmapsto} 1 \overset{\alpha}{\longmapsto} 2 \\ 2 \overset{\beta}{\longmapsto} 3 \overset{\alpha}{\longmapsto} 1 \end{array} \right\} \quad \text{This yields the 2-cycle } (1 \quad 2).$$

$$\left. \begin{array}{c} 3 \overset{\beta}{\longmapsto} 4 \overset{\alpha}{\longmapsto} 4 \\ 4 \overset{\beta}{\longmapsto} 2 \overset{\alpha}{\longmapsto} 3 \end{array} \right\} \quad \text{This yields the 2-cycle } (3 \quad 4).$$

Therefore $\sigma = (1 \quad 2)(3 \quad 4)$. Once this process is mastered, the answer can be written directly (without all the arrows).

Exercises

1. Compute the inverse of each of the following permutations.

   (a) $\begin{pmatrix} 1 & 2 & 3 & 4 & 5 & 6 & 7 \\ 3 & 1 & 7 & 4 & 6 & 5 & 2 \end{pmatrix}$

   (b) e

   (c) $\begin{pmatrix} 1 & 2 & 3 & 4 \\ 3 & 1 & 4 & 2 \end{pmatrix}^{-1}$

2. Suppose

$$\sigma^5 = \begin{pmatrix} 1 & 2 & 3 & 4 & 5 \\ 5 & 1 & 4 & 3 & 2 \end{pmatrix} \quad \text{and} \quad \sigma^3 = \begin{pmatrix} 1 & 2 & 3 & 4 & 5 \\ 1 & 2 & 4 & 3 & 5 \end{pmatrix}$$

   Compute each of the following permutations, and try to keep the amount of computation to a minimum. Show your methods.

   (a) σ^{-5}

   (b) σ^8

   (c) σ^{-15}

   (d) σ^{23}

   (e) σ

3. Let $\sigma = \begin{pmatrix} 1 & 2 & 3 & 4 & 5 \\ 3 & 1 & 5 & 2 & 4 \end{pmatrix}$.

   (a) Compute σ^{34} by performing at most six permutation products. (Use nothing more than the standard procedure for multiplying permutations.)

   (b) Compute σ^{-32}. [After part (a) has been completed, this should require only the technique for finding inverses.]

4. Draw the graph of the permutation

$$\begin{pmatrix} 1 & 2 & 3 & 4 & 5 & 6 & 7 & 8 & 9 & 10 & 11 \\ 5 & 3 & 7 & 11 & 1 & 10 & 4 & 6 & 9 & 8 & 2 \end{pmatrix}$$

5. How does the graph of a permutation compare with the graph of its inverse?

6. Prove that if $\sigma \in S_n$ then

$$(\sigma^s)^t = \sigma^{st} \quad \forall s, t \in \mathbb{N}.$$

   (You may use Theorem 5.22(a) in your proof. Proceed by induction on t. Because this is a special case of 5.22(b), do not *assume* that result in your proof.)

7. (a) Does the cycle notation $\sigma = (1 \quad 3 \quad 7 \quad 5 \quad 2)$ tell us the domain of σ? Explain.

(b) Compute the indicated products.

$$(1 \ 3 \ 5)\begin{pmatrix} 1 & 2 & 3 & 4 & 5 & 6 & 7 \\ 3 & 1 & 4 & 2 & 7 & 5 & 6 \end{pmatrix} = \begin{pmatrix} 1 & 2 & 3 & 4 & 5 & 6 & 7 \\ & & & & & & \end{pmatrix}$$

$$(3 \ 2 \ 1 \ 5)^{-1}(1 \ 7 \ 3 \ 4)^2 (1 \ 2) = \begin{pmatrix} 1 & 2 & 3 & 4 & 5 & 6 & 7 & 8 \\ & & & & & & & \end{pmatrix}$$

8. Let σ be an r-cycle. Without proof, obtain formulas showing the following.

(a) If r is even then σ^2 is a product of two disjoint $(r/2)$-cycles.

(b) If r is odd then σ^2 is an r-cycle.

[Suggestion: First experiment with the cycles $(1 \quad 2 \quad 3 \quad 4)$ and $(1 \quad 2 \quad 3 \quad 4 \quad 5)$.]

9. Express each of the following permutations as a product of disjoint cycles.

(a) $\begin{pmatrix} 1 & 2 & 3 & 4 & 5 & 6 & 7 \\ 5 & 6 & 1 & 4 & 3 & 7 & 2 \end{pmatrix}$

(b) $(1 \quad 2 \quad 3 \quad 4)(4 \quad 5 \quad 6 \quad 1)(1 \quad 2)$

(c) $(1 \quad 2)^{50}(2 \quad 3 \quad 4)^{101}$

(d) $\begin{pmatrix} 1 & 2 & 3 & 4 & 5 & 6 & 7 & 8 & 9 \\ 5 & 8 & 9 & 2 & 3 & 6 & 7 & 4 & 1 \end{pmatrix}^{-1}$

10. If $\sigma \in S_n$ then $\sigma\sigma^{-1} = e$, from the definition of inverse function. Use this fact to prove the following:

(a) Each $\sigma \in S_n$ has only one inverse.

(b) If $\sigma, \lambda \in S_n$ and $\lambda^{-1} = \sigma^{-1}$, then $\lambda = \sigma$.

11. Show that if $\sigma, \tau \in S_n$ then $(\sigma\tau)^{-1} = \tau^{-1}\sigma^{-1}$.

12. Let $\sigma \in S_n$. Define a relation $\sim$ on $\mathbb{N}_n$ as follows:

$$x \sim y \quad \Leftrightarrow \quad \sigma^k(x) = y \quad \text{for some } k \in \mathbb{Z}$$

(a) Prove that $\sim$ is an equivalence relation on $\mathbb{N}_n$.

(b) Use the terminology of this section to describe the associated equivalence classes.

13. Let

$$\sigma = \begin{pmatrix} 1 & 2 & 3 & 4 \\ 3 & 1 & 4 & 2 \end{pmatrix} \qquad \text{and} \qquad \lambda = (1 \quad 2 \quad 3 \quad 4).$$

(a) Find a permutation $\alpha \in S_4$ such that $\sigma^{-1}\alpha\lambda = (2 \quad 1 \quad 4)$.

(b) Show that there is only one such permutation α.

14. Suppose $2 \le k \le n$. How many k-cycles are there in S_n?

15. Find all the values of n for which S_n consists of cycles. (Recall that the identity $e \in S_n$ can be viewed as a 1-cycle.)

5.6 Computing the Order of a Permutation; A Card-Shuffling Example

Suppose we shuffle a deck of cards, perhaps in a very intricate way, and then we perform *exactly* the same maneuver again. And again. If we continue indefinitely must the cards eventually return to their original configuration? If so, when?

Our goal in this section is to achieve a more complete understanding of permutation behavior, with particular attention to features that can simplify large-scale computations. Even with computers at our disposal, knowing how to find an answer *somehow* is often not enough. We also need to consider the *efficiency* of our procedures; therefore, any insights that reduce many steps to a few are welcome.* The cycle decomposition theorem from Section 5.5 will be an important tool in our work here. At the end of the section we'll settle the card-shuffling problem posed in the preceding paragraph.

Suppose we want to compute a high power of a given permutation. For example, suppose

$$\sigma = \begin{pmatrix} 1 & 2 & 3 & 4 & 5 & 6 & 7 & 8 & 9 \\ 4 & 9 & 2 & 5 & 1 & 7 & 6 & 8 & 3 \end{pmatrix}$$

and we want to compute $\sigma^{100,000,000}$ by hand. Is this hopeless? No, but we need a few results before we can do the computation.

5.38 Theorem. Let $\alpha, \beta \in S_n$, and suppose $\alpha\beta = \beta\alpha$. Then $(\alpha\beta)^t = \alpha^t\beta^t$ for all $t \in \mathbb{Z}$.

PROOF OUTLINE. First prove by induction on k that $\alpha\beta^k = \beta^k\alpha$ for all $k \in \mathbb{N}$. Next prove the theorem for $t \ge 0$ by induction on t. Then use Theorem 5.22(c) to complete the proof for $t < 0$. □

---

*The reader interested in computer programs that multiply permutations should see D. E. Knuth, *The Art of Computer Programming*, vol. 1, 2d ed. (Reading, Mass: Addison-Wesley, 1973), especially pages 162–172.

5.39 Corollary. If $\sigma = \gamma_1 \cdots \gamma_m$ is a factorization of σ into disjoint cycles, then $\sigma^t = \gamma_1^t \cdots \gamma_m^t$ for all $t \in \mathbb{Z}$.

PROOF OUTLINE.   Use induction on m together with 5.30 and 5.38.   □

Recall (from the previous section) what is meant by the **order** of a permutation:

$$\operatorname{ord} \sigma = \min \{k \in \mathbb{N} \mid \sigma^k = e\}$$

How should we compute $\operatorname{ord} \sigma$? (Also, *why* should we compute it? We'll illustrate the usefulness of $\operatorname{ord} \sigma$ shortly.) There is a more efficient way to compute $\operatorname{ord} \sigma$ than by squandering our days computing $\sigma^2, \sigma^3, \ldots$ and waiting until $\sigma^k = e$, and we'll now give a slick method that uses the cycle decomposition of σ.

First consider the order of a k-cycle $\gamma = (a_1 \quad \ldots \quad a_k)$. The cycle's graph makes it clear that $\operatorname{ord} \gamma = k$, since a forward movement of k positions returns each element to its initial position, while a move of less than k positions fails to do so. More formally, it follows from Definition 5.24 that if $1 \le t \le k$, then

(5.40)
$$\gamma^t(a_i) = \begin{cases} a_{i+t} & \text{if } i + t \le k \\ a_{i+t-k} & \text{if } i + t > k \end{cases}$$

(Use an induction argument to see this, or at least convince yourself by trying a few values of t.) So $\gamma^k(a_i) = a_i$ for $1 \le i \le k$, therefore $\gamma^k = e$; moreover $\gamma^t \ne e$ when $0 < t < k$. Therefore $\operatorname{ord} \gamma = k$.

5.41 EXAMPLE.   Consider the 5-cycle $\gamma = (3 \quad 1 \quad 7 \quad 2 \quad 4)$, and let's compute γ^{72}. We know that $\operatorname{ord} \gamma = 5$, by what we have just shown. Employing the division algorithm, we have $72 = 5(14) + 2$, and therefore

$$\gamma^{72} = \gamma^{5(14)+2} = (\gamma^5)^{14} \gamma^2 = \gamma^2 = (3 \quad 7 \quad 4 \quad 1 \quad 2)$$

Now we can settle a problem posed earlier.

5.42 EXAMPLE.   Compute $\sigma^{100,000,000}$ if

$$\sigma = \begin{pmatrix} 1 & 2 & 3 & 4 & 5 & 6 & 7 & 8 & 9 \\ 4 & 9 & 2 & 5 & 1 & 7 & 6 & 8 & 3 \end{pmatrix}$$

SOLUTION. From 5.37(a) we have $\sigma = (1 \quad 4 \quad 5)(2 \quad 9 \quad 3)(6 \quad 7)$, a product of disjoint cycles. Therefore

$$\sigma^{100,000,000} = (1 \quad 4 \quad 5)^{100,000,000}(2 \quad 9 \quad 3)^{100,000,000}(6 \quad 7)^{100,000,000}$$

by Corollary 5.39. But $\text{ord}(6 \quad 7) = 2$ and $100,000,000$ is divisible by 2, so $(6 \quad 7)^{100,000,000} = e$. Also, $100,000,000 = 3(33,333,333) + 1$, so $(1 \quad 4 \quad 5)^{100,000,000} = (1 \quad 4 \quad 5)$ and $(2 \quad 9 \quad 3)^{100,000,000} = (2 \quad 9 \quad 3)$. Therefore

$$\sigma^{100,000,000} = (1 \quad 4 \quad 5)(2 \quad 9 \quad 3) = \begin{pmatrix} 1 & 2 & 3 & 4 & 5 & 6 & 7 & 8 & 9 \\ 4 & 9 & 2 & 5 & 1 & 6 & 7 & 8 & 3 \end{pmatrix}$$

5.43 Definition. Let S be a set of integers that contains at least one nonzero integer. The **least common multiple** of S is the smallest positive integer that is a multiple of every member of S. The least common multiple of $\{r_1, r_2, \ldots, r_m\}$ is usually denoted $\text{lcm}(r_1, \ldots, r_m)$ or $[r_1, \ldots, r_m]$.

5.44 EXAMPLES.

$$\text{lcm}(-6, 8, 5) = 120$$

$$\text{lcm}(1, 2, 3, 4, 5, 6) = 60$$

$$\text{lcm}(32, -36) = 288$$

We will look more closely at least common multiples when we discuss *number theory* in Chapter 6. Now we can present the algorithm for determining the order of an arbitrary permutation in S_n.

5.45 Theorem. Suppose $\sigma \in S_n$ has the disjoint cycle decomposition $\sigma = \gamma_1 \cdots \gamma_m$, where γ_i is a k_i-cycle, for $1 \leq i \leq m$. Then

$$\text{ord}\,\sigma = \text{lcm}(k_1, \ldots, k_m)$$

(Therefore, *to compute the order of a permutation σ, express σ as a product of disjoint cycles and then compute the least common multiple of the orders of those cycles.*)

PROOF SKETCH. Consider the graph of σ. An application of σ corresponds to each vertex moving to the position of the next vertex in its directed polygon. Since the ith polygon has k_i vertices, after k_i applications of σ, but no fewer, the objects in the ith polygon are back in their initial position. So if $\sigma^s = e$ then s must be a multiple of k_i, and this is true for each value of i satisfying $1 \leq i \leq m$. Therefore the smallest nonnegative s for which $\sigma^s = e$ is the least common multiple of $k_1, \ldots, k_m$.

ACTUAL PROOF. We assert:

$(*)\sigma^s = e \quad \Leftrightarrow \quad s$ is a multiple of k_i, for each i satisfying $1 \leq i \leq m$.

To prove "$\Leftarrow$", assume that s is a multiple of each k_i; say, $s = q_i k_i$ for $1 \leq i \leq m$. Then

$$\sigma^s = \gamma_1^s \cdots \gamma_m^s = (\gamma_1^{k_1})^{q_1} \cdots (\gamma_m^{k_m})^{q_m} = e$$

as desired.

Now for "$\Rightarrow$". Assume that $\sigma^s = e$. Then we can write $s = k_1 q + t$, with $0 \leq t < k_1$; thus $\gamma_1^s = (\gamma_1^{k_1})^q \gamma_1^t = \gamma_1^t$. Let a_1 denote an element in the orbit of γ_1. If t were positive we would have

$$\sigma^s(a_1) = \gamma_1^s(a_1) = \gamma_1^t(a_1) \neq a_1$$

(The first equality follows from the fact that none of $\gamma_2, \ldots, \gamma_m$ moves a_1, since the cycles are disjoint, and the nonequality follows from formula 5.40.) But this contradicts our assumption that $\sigma^s = e$. Therefore $t = 0$, and so $s = k_1 q$; that is, s is a multiple of k_1. A similar argument shows that s is also a multiple of $k_2, \ldots, k_m$, so we have proved assertion $(*)$.

The theorem now follows from the "smallest" condition in the definition of ord σ, and from the definition of least common multiple. □

5.46 EXAMPLE. (a) Compute the order of

$$\sigma = \begin{pmatrix} 1 & 2 & 3 & 4 & 5 & 6 & 7 & 8 & 9 & 10 & 11 & 12 & 13 & 14 & 15 \\ 12 & 5 & 8 & 3 & 13 & 9 & 6 & 4 & 10 & 7 & 14 & 1 & 11 & 2 & 15 \end{pmatrix}$$

SOLUTION. We first write σ as a product of disjoint cycles:

$$\sigma = (1 \quad 12)(2 \quad 5 \quad 13 \quad 11 \quad 14)(3 \quad 8 \quad 4)(6 \quad 9 \quad 10 \quad 7)$$

Therefore ord $\sigma = \text{lcm}(2, 5, 3, 4) = 60$.

(b) Compute the order of

$$\sigma = (1 \ 8 \ 4 \ 3)(1 \ 4 \ 7)(1 \ 4 \ 6 \ 2)(1 \ 4 \ 6)(1 \ 4 \ 5)$$

SOLUTION. To apply Theorem 5.45, we must first express σ as a product of disjoint cycles. (We are given σ as a product of cycles, but they are not disjoint.) If we do this in the manner of Example 5.37(c), we obtain $\sigma = (1 \quad 2 \quad 3)(4 \quad 5 \quad 6 \quad 7 \quad 8)$. Therefore ord $\sigma = \text{lcm}(3, 5) = 15$.

Now we can apply all of this to the analysis of card shuffling, the topic that opened this section.

5.47 EXAMPLE. (a) Perform a "perfect shuffle" on a standard deck of 52 playing cards as follows. Cut the deck exactly in half, place one half in each hand, and then *riffle* the cards; that is, release the cards (using your thumbs) from the two half-decks in an alternating way so that they overlap, then push them together to constitute one deck. (See the picture.)

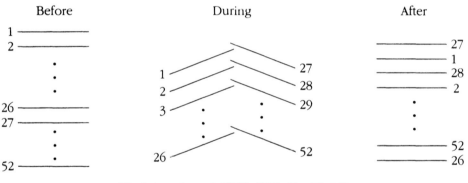

(Background song: "Riffle While You Work")

Now, with respect to this shuffle, we repeat the question from the start of this section: If a perfect shuffle is performed repeatedly, will the cards eventually return to their original order and, if so, how soon?

SOLUTION. In the shuffle, the top 26 cards go to the respective positions $2, 4, 6, 8, \ldots$, and the next 26 cards (in initial positions $26 + 1, 26 + 2, 26 + 3, \ldots$) go to the respective positions $1, 3, 5, 7, \ldots$. This position change defines a permutation $\sigma \in S_{52}$ by

$$\left. \begin{array}{r} i \mapsto 2i \\ 26 + i \mapsto 2i - 1 \end{array} \right\} \quad \text{for } 1 \le i \le 26$$

that is,

$$\sigma = \begin{pmatrix} 1 & 2 & 3 & \cdots & 26 & 27 & 28 & 29 & \cdots & 52 \\ 2 & 4 & 6 & \cdots & 52 & 1 & 3 & 5 & \cdots & 51 \end{pmatrix}$$

This has the disjoint cycle decomposition

$$\sigma = (1 \quad 2 \quad 4 \quad 8 \quad 16 \quad 32 \quad 11 \quad 22 \quad 44 \quad 35 \quad \cdots \quad 40 \quad 27)$$

(Exercise: fill in the blank.)

which is a 52-cycle!! Therefore ord σ = 52, so the cards will return to their original order after precisely 52 perfect shuffles.

(b) *Experiment.* Based on the preceding discussion you might guess that if a succession of perfect shuffles is performed on a deck of n cards, where n is any even natural number, then exactly n shuffles are required to return the cards to their original order. Test this conjecture by determining the order of the perfect shuffle for decks of 2, 4, 6, and 8 cards.

(c) Now let's return to a 52-card deck. Among all possible shuffles, does the perfect shuffle have largest order? In other words, is there a shuffle that will require *more* than 52 executions to return the deck to its original configuration?

SOLUTION. Every shuffle corresponds to a permutation in S_{52}. Each $\sigma \in S_{52}$ can be factored into disjoint cycles, and the lengths $k_1, \ldots, k_t$ of these cycles determine ord σ. Therefore, searching for a permutation of large order in S_{52} amounts to searching for positive integers $k_1, \ldots, k_t$ with these properties:

$$k_1 + k_2 + \cdots + k_t \leq 52$$

$$\text{lcm}(k_1, k_2, \ldots, k_t) \text{ is large}$$

With this in mind, consider the permutation $\sigma = \gamma_1 \gamma_2 \gamma_3 \gamma_4 \gamma_5 \gamma_6$, where

$$\gamma_1 = (1 \quad 2 \quad 3 \quad 4) \qquad \text{(4-cycle)}$$
$$\gamma_2 = (5 \quad 6 \quad \cdots \quad 9) \qquad \text{(5-cycle)}$$
$$\gamma_3 = (10 \quad 11 \quad \cdots \quad 16) \qquad \text{(7-cycle)}$$
$$\gamma_4 = (17 \quad 18 \quad \cdots \quad 25) \qquad \text{(9-cycle)}$$

$$\gamma_5 = (26 \quad 27 \quad \cdots \quad 36) \qquad (11\text{-cycle})$$

$$\gamma_6 = (37 \quad 38 \quad \cdots \quad 49) \qquad (13\text{-cycle})$$

Then

$$\text{ord } \sigma = \text{lcm}(4, 5, 7, 9, 11, 13) = 180{,}180$$

(Here we are computing the least common multiple of six numbers that have no common factors except 1, so their least common multiple is their product. We'll spend more time on this kind of thing in Section 6.3.) Thus the shuffle corresponding to the permutation σ constructed here must be performed 180,180 times before the deck returns to its original order!

Exercises

1. Give an informal definition of the notion of *order* of a permutation. (That is, say Definition 5.32 in words.)

2. Compute the order of each of the following permutations.

   (a) $\begin{pmatrix} 1 & 2 & 3 & 4 & 5 & 6 \\ 3 & 5 & 1 & 6 & 4 & 2 \end{pmatrix}$

   (b) $(1 \quad 3 \quad 5 \quad 8 \quad 2)(2 \quad 8 \quad 3 \quad 1 \quad 6)$

   (c) $\begin{pmatrix} 1 & 2 & 3 & 4 & 5 & 6 & 7 & 8 & 9 & 10 & 11 & 12 \\ 7 & 4 & 12 & 8 & 9 & 10 & 11 & 3 & 6 & 5 & 1 & 2 \end{pmatrix}$

3. Let

   $$\sigma = \begin{pmatrix} 1 & 2 & 3 & 4 & 5 & 6 & 7 \\ 2 & 1 & 4 & 5 & 3 & 7 & 6 \end{pmatrix}$$

   Compute σ^{1057}.

4. Prove that a permutation and its inverse have the same order.

5. Exhibit a permutation in S_{30} that has order 2,520. Justify your answer.

6. Exhibit a permutation in S_{10} that has the biggest possible order. Justify your answer.

7. (a) Give an example of integers m and n with $1 \le m < n$ such that the largest order of an element in S_m is equal to the largest order of an element in S_n.

   (b) If $1 \le m < n$, is it possible for S_m to have an element of larger order than that of any element of S_n? Explain.

8. The Schlimazel Truck Corporation manufactures a three-axle truck, with two wheels per axle, that also carries two spares. The company recommends that owners periodically perform an elaborate tire

interchange in order to keep the tire wear even. The pattern for the recommended maneuver is shown in the accompanying diagram. (Tires in positions 7 and 8 are the spares.)

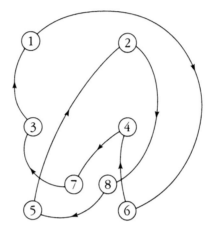

(a) Do you agree that the company's plan will keep the wear on the tires approximately uniform over many miles of driving?

(b) After how many of these tire interchanges will the tires first return to their initial configuration?

9. Suppose the "perfect shuffle" of Example 5.47 is performed with a deck of 26 cards. After how many repetitions will the deck first return to its original order?

10. Outline an algorithm for finding the least common multiple of two integers a and b (that is, the lcm of the set $\{a, b\}$).

11. Write a detailed proof of Theorem 5.38.

5.7 Odd and Even Permutations; Applications to Configurations

In this section we will classify permutations into two types, called *even* and *odd*, and we will use this classification to show the impossibility of certain rearrangement tasks. Most of our applications will involve some familiar plastic puzzles, but the underlying ideas also have a wide range of applications in mathematics and physics, and they should not be sneeringly dismissed as child's play.

Everyone instinctively knows that any rearrangement of people in a row of theater seats (one person per seat) can be carried out by a succession of two-person switches. This observation suggests another way to decompose permutations in S_n, and our next theorem will make this explicit.

First some terminology: a 2-cycle is also called a **transposition**. The transposition $\tau = (1 \quad j)$ interchanges i and j [that is, $\tau(i) = j$ and $\tau(j) = i$] and holds everything else fixed. We observe that a transposition τ satisfies $\tau^2 = e$; so $\tau^{-1} = \tau$. A transposition is the simplest possible nontrivial permutation, for if a permutation σ is not the identity, it moves some element x, say $\sigma(x) = y \neq x$. Then $\sigma(y) \neq y$, since σ is injective; so σ moves at least two elements. A transposition moves *exactly* two elements. The mathematical formulation of our theater observation in the preceding paragraph is as follows.

5.48 Theorem. If $n \geq 2$, then every permutation in S_n is a product of transpositions.

PROOF. Let $\sigma \in S_n$. If $\sigma = e$, we have $\sigma = (1 \quad 2)(1 \quad 2)$. If $\sigma \neq e$, there is a disjoint cycle decomposition $\sigma = \gamma_1 \cdots \gamma_m$, so it suffices to show that a typical r-cycle $\gamma = (a_1 \quad a_2 \quad \cdots \quad a_r)$ with $r \geq 2$ is a product of transpositions. The following formula does the job:

$$(5.49) \quad (a_1 \quad a_2 \quad \cdots \quad a_r) = (a_1 \quad a_r)(a_1 \quad a_{r-1}) \cdots (a_1 \quad a_3)(a_1 \quad a_2)$$

Check this formula by applying the permutations on both sides of the alleged equation to each of $a_1, \ldots, a_r$. □

5.50 EXAMPLE. Express

$$\sigma = \begin{pmatrix} 1 & 2 & 3 & 4 & 5 & 6 & 7 & 8 & 9 & 10 \\ 6 & 7 & 10 & 5 & 8 & 2 & 1 & 4 & 3 & 9 \end{pmatrix}$$

as a product of transpositions.

SOLUTION. We first write σ as a product of disjoint cycles, then apply 5.49 to each of those cycles:

$$\sigma = (1 \quad 6 \quad 2 \quad 7)(3 \quad 10 \quad 9)(4 \quad 5 \quad 8)$$

$$= (1 \quad 7)(1 \quad 2)(1 \quad 6)(3 \quad 9)(3 \quad 10)(4 \quad 8)(4 \quad 5)$$

5.51 Remark. Here are some observations about factorization into products of transpositions.

(a) We cannot expect the transpositions in such a product to be disjoint. For instance, a 3-cycle moves exactly three elements, whereas a product of disjoint transpositions moves an even number of elements.

(b) The inequality

$$(1 \ \ 3)(1 \ \ 2) \neq (1 \ \ 2)(1 \ \ 3)$$

shows that the order in which transpositions are listed as factors is important. [It is only when permutations are *disjoint* that we can be sure (without further checking) that their relative position doesn't matter.]

Suppose a nontrivial permutation is applied to a set of people who are waiting in line. This changes the ordering, so that now there is at least one person who is ahead of someone he used to be behind. We say that the **orientation** of these two people has been **reversed**, or that a **reversal** has occurred. Similarly, if $\sigma \in S_n$ and $\{i, j\} \subseteq \mathbb{N}_n$, with $i \neq j$, we say that σ reverses the orientation of i and j if either

$$i < j \qquad \text{and} \qquad \sigma(i) > \sigma(j)$$

or

$$i > j \qquad \text{and} \qquad \sigma(i) < \sigma(j)$$

More compactly: σ reverses i and j if

$$\frac{\sigma(i) - \sigma(j)}{i - j} < 0$$

Incidentally, notice that

$$\frac{\sigma(i) - \sigma(j)}{i - j} = \frac{\sigma(j) - \sigma(i)}{j - i}$$

so that this quotient depends only on the pair of integers under consideration, not on the way they are labelled.

For some applications we may need to know whether the total number of reversals caused by a given permutation is even or odd. (See Example 5.60.) For this purpose it is useful to define the **sign** of σ, denoted **sgn σ**, by

$$(5.52) \qquad \text{sgn}\,\sigma = \begin{cases} 1 & \text{if the number of reversals is even} \\ -1 & \text{if the number of reversals is odd} \end{cases}$$

Otherwise stated:

(5.53) sgn $\sigma = (-1)^r$, where r is the number of reversals caused by σ

The following theorem gives the basic properties of the sign function.

5.54 Theorem. (a) sgn $\sigma = \displaystyle\prod_{i<j} \frac{\sigma(i) - \sigma(j)}{i - j}$

(b) sgn $\sigma\lambda$ = (sgn σ)(sgn λ)
(c) If τ is a transposition, then sgn $\tau = -1$.
(d) If $\sigma = \tau_1 \cdots \tau_s$, where the τ_i are transpositions, then sgn $\sigma = (-1)^s$.

PROOF. (a) Here the indicated product is understood to represent the product of all the quotients of the form

$$\frac{\sigma(i) - \sigma(j)}{i - j}$$

for which the inequality $1 \le i < j \le n$ holds. From our earlier discussion we know that such a quotient is negative if and only if σ reverses i and j. Therefore, the product under scrutiny has the same sign (as a real number) as sgn σ. We will be done if we can show that the product has absolute value 1. We have

$$\left| \prod_{i<j} \frac{\sigma(i) - \sigma(j)}{i - j} \right| = \prod_{i<j} \left| \frac{\sigma(i) - \sigma(j)}{i - j} \right| = \frac{\prod |\sigma(i) - \sigma(j)|}{\prod |i - j|}$$

But the factors in the denominator on the right are all the absolute values of differences of two integers between 1 and n one factor for each integer pair; and the same is true of the numerator, since σ is a bijection. Therefore the quotient is equal to 1, which is what we wanted to show.

(b) sgn $\sigma\lambda = \displaystyle\prod_{i<j} \frac{\sigma\lambda(i) - \sigma\lambda(j)}{i - j}$

$\qquad = \displaystyle\prod_{i<j} \frac{\sigma\lambda(i) - \sigma\lambda(j)}{\lambda(i) - \lambda(j)} \cdot \frac{\lambda(i) - \lambda(j)}{i - j}$

$\qquad = \displaystyle\prod_{i<j} \frac{\sigma\lambda(i) - \sigma\lambda(j)}{\lambda(i) - \lambda(j)} \cdot \prod_{i<j} \frac{\lambda(i) - \lambda(j)}{i - j}$

$\qquad = (\text{sgn } \sigma)(\text{sgn } \lambda)$

[The last equality follows from the fact that as $\{i, j\}$ varies through the two-element subsets of $\mathbb{N}_n$, so does $\{\lambda(i), \lambda(j)\}$.]

(c) Let $\tau = (r \quad s)$, with $r < s$; we will count the reversals. Under τ's action, r reverses with respect to every element strictly between r and s, and so does s. That's two reversals for every number strictly between r and s, making an even number of reversals so far. Finally, τ reverses the orientation of r with respect to s. That makes the total number of reversals odd, so sgn $\tau = -1$.

(d) This follows immediately from parts (b) and (c), by induction on s. $\square$

5.55 Corollary. If $\sigma = \tau_1 \cdots \tau_s$ and also $\sigma = \tau_1' \cdots \tau_t'$, where each τ_i and τ_i' is a transposition, then s and t are both even or both odd.

PROOF. From the theorem we have sgn $\sigma = (-1)^s = (-1)^t$. The conclusion follows. $\square$

5.56 Definition. A permutation $\sigma \in S_n$ is **odd** if sgn $\sigma = -1$ and **even** if sgn $\sigma = 1$. The evenness or oddness of σ is called its **parity**.

A permutation $\sigma \in S_n$ ($n \geq 2$) can be written as a product of transpositions in infinitely many ways. For example, we have $e = (1 \quad 2)(1 \quad 2) = (1 \quad 2)(1 \quad 2)(1 \quad 2)(1 \quad 2)$ and so on, and such expressions can be appended to any factorization of σ to get a new factorization, or we can insert them between any two factors of a given factorization. We can also manipulate expressions in other ways; for example,

$$(2 \quad 3)(3 \quad 4) = (2 \quad 3 \quad 4) = (4 \quad 2 \quad 3) = (4 \quad 3)(4 \quad 2)$$

But however the symbols are tormented to produce a new factorization into transpositions, parity must be preserved.

The sign of a permutation can be computed directly from Equation 5.52, but it is useful to have a more explicit algorithm for the job. We'll give two.

First notice that if γ is an r-cycle then sgn $\gamma = (-1)^{r+1}$ by formula 5.49, Theorem 5.54(d), and the fact that $(-1)^{r-1} = (-1)^{r+1}$. Therefore:

(5.57)   If $\sigma = \gamma_1 \cdots \gamma_t$, where γ_i is an r_i-cycle, then

$$\text{sgn } \sigma = (-1)^{r_1 + \cdots + r_t + t}$$

For example, if

$$\sigma = \begin{pmatrix} 1 & 2 & 3 & 4 & 5 \\ 3 & 1 & 5 & 2 & 4 \end{pmatrix}$$

we have $\sigma = (1 \quad 3 \quad 5 \quad 4 \quad 2)$, and therefore $\operatorname{sgn} \sigma = (-1)^6 = 1$. And if

$$\lambda = \begin{pmatrix} 1 & 2 & 3 & 4 & 5 & 6 & 7 & 8 & 9 & 10 & 11 & 12 \\ 3 & 1 & 9 & 7 & 8 & 4 & 6 & 5 & 2 & 12 & 11 & 10 \end{pmatrix}$$

then $\lambda = (1 \quad 3 \quad 9 \quad 2)(4 \quad 7 \quad 6)(5 \quad 8)(10 \quad 12)$, and therefore

$$\operatorname{sgn} \lambda = (-1)^{4+3+2+2+4} = -1$$

Here's another method for determining the parity.

5.58 PROCEDURE. Given a permutation in its standard form

$$\sigma = \begin{pmatrix} 1 & 2 & \cdots & n \\ \sigma(1) & \sigma(2) & \cdots & \sigma(n) \end{pmatrix}$$

scan the bottom row from left to right, and determine how many times there is a number in that row with a smaller number to its right (possibly with other numbers in between). If there are t such instances, then

$$\operatorname{sgn} \sigma = (-1)^t$$

(Each occurrence of a number to the left of a smaller number corresponds to a reversal, so statement 5.53 gives the result.) Let's use this method on the permutations σ and λ to which we applied 5.57. In the bottom row of σ we find two numbers to the left of smaller numbers:

3 is to the left of 1 and 2

5 is to the left of 2 and 4

Therefore 5.58 gives $\operatorname{sgn} \sigma = (-1)^4 = 1$. The bottom row of λ has more numbers to examine, so we'll make a table.

Number	Smaller numbers to the right
3	1, 2
9	7, 8, 4, 6, 5, 2
7	4, 6, 5, 2
8	4, 6, 5, 2
4	2
6	5, 2
5	2
12	11, 10
11	10

Therefore $\operatorname{sgn} \lambda = (-1)^{23} = -1$.

We conclude this section by using the results about signs to demonstrate that certain configurations cannot be achieved.

5.59 EXAMPLE. In the theater problem (Example 5.1(a)), each neighborly seat switch corresponds to a transposition. Since 14 switches will achieve the desired rearrangement, the corresponding permutation in S_{10} is even. Therefore it *cannot* be expressed as a product of 11 transpositions, as suggested, so the second plan should be rejected.

5.60 EXAMPLE. A familiar puzzle consists of a square grid of 16 squares, with movable tiles numbered 1 through 15 occupying fifteen of those squares and the remaining square blank. A legal move involves sliding a tile onto the blank location from an adjacent location. Given the puzzle in this configuration:

1	2	3	4
5	6	7	8
9	10	11	12
13	14	15	

is it possible to rearrange the tiles into the opposite order by a sequence of legal moves?

15	14	13	12
11	10	9	8
7	6	5	4
3	2	1	■

SOLUTION. We will use permutations to solve this problem. Think of the blank location as being occupied by a black tile bearing the invisible number 16. With this intuition, our puzzle consists of sixteen tiles in sixteen locations, and a legal move interchanges the black tile with one of its neighbors, keeping all the other tiles fixed. Thus a legal move is a transposition. The attempted rearrangement corresponds to this permutation:

$$\sigma = \begin{pmatrix} 1 & 2 & 3 & 4 & 5 & 6 & 7 & 8 & 9 & 10 & 11 & 12 & 13 & 14 & 15 & 16 \\ 15 & 14 & 13 & 12 & 11 & 10 & 9 & 8 & 7 & 6 & 5 & 4 & 3 & 2 & 1 & 16 \end{pmatrix}$$

Then σ is odd, since

$$\sigma = (1 \quad 15)(2 \quad 14)(3 \quad 13)(4 \quad 12)(5 \quad 11)(6 \quad 10)(7 \quad 9)$$

Therefore any effort that produces the desired rearrangement must involve an odd number of legal moves. On the other hand, each legal move requires a horizontal or vertical move of the black tile. For that tile to return to its initial position, it must be subjected to an even number of vertical moves and an even number of horizontal moves, hence to an even number of moves altogether. Thus the desired rearrangement is impossible.

5.61 EXAMPLE. A detailed analysis of the Rubik's Cube problem (Example 5.1(d)) would take us too long here, so we will make do with a brief sketch of the argument. (For more details, including the development of more insightful notation, see the book by Frey and Singmaster cited on p. 207.) We view a Cube operation as a permutation of facelets. The flip operation in question constitutes an interchange of two facelets; that is, a transposition, which is an *odd* permutation. Now consider a 90° clockwise twist (looking down) of the upper face. To describe the corresponding permutation, we must account for the movements of all twenty-one facelets on the upper layer of the Cube.

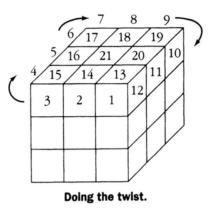

Doing the twist.

The movements of the sides of the layer are summarized by three 4-cycles:

$$(1 \quad 4 \quad 7 \quad 10)(2 \quad 5 \quad 8 \quad 11)(3 \quad 6 \quad 9 \quad 12)$$

Movements of the outer facelets of the top face are given by the product

$$(13 \quad 15 \quad 17 \quad 19)(14 \quad 16 \quad 18 \quad 20)$$

Finally, while the center facelet of the top face remains in the center, its position changes by rotation, and we record its movement by a specially denoted 4-cycle:

$$(\uparrow \quad \rightarrow \quad \downarrow \quad \leftarrow)$$

Altogether we have six disjoint 4-cycles, hence an *even* permutation. But every cube operation is a succession of face rotations. Therefore every cube operation corresponds to an even permutation, so the desired flip operation is *impossible*.

Exercises

1. Express each of the following permutations as a product of transpositions.

(a) $\begin{pmatrix} 1 & 2 & 3 & 4 & 5 & 6 & 7 & 8 \\ 3 & 1 & 7 & 5 & 2 & 4 & 8 & 6 \end{pmatrix}$

(b) $\begin{pmatrix} 1 & 2 & 3 & 4 & 5 & 6 & 7 & 8 \\ 4 & 2 & 7 & 1 & 8 & 6 & 3 & 5 \end{pmatrix}$

(c) $(1 \quad 2 \quad 3)(2 \quad 3 \quad 4)$

(d) $(3 \quad 1 \quad 4) \begin{pmatrix} 1 & 2 & 3 & 4 & 5 & 6 & 7 \\ 7 & 1 & 4 & 3 & 5 & 2 & 6 \end{pmatrix}$

(e) $(3 \quad 5 \quad 7 \quad 1 \quad 4 \quad 8)^{-1}$

2. (a) Describe the orbits of a permutation that is a product of disjoint transpositions. Use a graph to illustrate your remarks.

   (b) Let $\sigma \in S_n$, with $n \geq 2$. State a necessary and sufficient condition on the factorization of σ into disjoint cycles in order for σ to be expressible as a product of disjoint transpositions, and justify your claim.

3. In each case determine the number of reversals and then use 5.53 to compute the sign of the given permutation.

   (a) $\begin{pmatrix} 1 & 2 & 3 \\ 3 & 1 & 2 \end{pmatrix}$

   (b) $\begin{pmatrix} 1 & 2 & 3 & 4 & 5 \\ 2 & 3 & 4 & 5 & 1 \end{pmatrix}$

   (c) $\begin{pmatrix} 1 & 2 & 3 & 4 & 5 & 6 \\ 2 & 3 & 1 & 4 & 5 & 6 \end{pmatrix}$

4. The notation $(1 \quad 3 \quad 5)$ can be used to represent infinitely many cycles, one in each S_n for which $n \geq 5$. Show that all these cycles cause exactly the same reversals, so that there is no ambiguity in the phrase, "the reversals caused by $(1 \quad 3 \quad 5)$."

5. Show that for each $n \geq 2$ there is a permutation for which the number of reversals is $n(n-1)/2$. (Suggestion: First verify the assertion for $n = 2$, 3, and 4.)

6. (a) Use induction on n to prove that if $n \geq 2$ every element of S_n can be expressed as a product of transpositions from the set

$$\{(1 \quad 2), (1 \quad 3), \ldots, (1 \quad n)\}$$

   (As part of the induction step, view S_k as the subset of S_{k+1} consisting of all the permutations that fix $k + 1$. Then show that if $\sigma \in S_{k+1}$ moves $k + 1$, then there is a suitable transposition τ such that $\tau\sigma \in S_k$.)

   (b) Interpret the result in part (a) in the context of theater-seat arrangements (Example 5.1(a)).

7. The set of even permutations in S_n is called the **alternating group**, denoted A_n.

   (a) Show that if $\sigma, \lambda \in A_n$ then $\sigma\lambda \in A_n$. (We therefore say that A_n is *closed under the product operation*.)

(b) Show that if $\sigma \in A_n$ then $\sigma^{-1} \in A_n$.

(c) Show that if $\sigma \in A_n$ and $\lambda \in S_n$ then $\lambda^{-1}\sigma\lambda \in A_n$.

8. Every rearrangement of people in a row of theater seats can be achieved by successive switches of *neighbors*. Prove this assertion's mathematical formulation: If $n \geq 2$, every permutation in S_n is a product of transpositions of the form $(i \quad i+1)$. (Hint: By Theorem 5.48, it suffices to show that every *transposition* can be written as such a product. Think of how it would be done in a theater.)

9. Show that if $\sigma = \tau_1\tau_2$, where τ_1 and τ_2 are disjoint transpositions, then also $\sigma = \tau_2\tau_1$, but there is no *other* way to express σ as a product of two transpositions.

10. Suppose $n \geq 2$, and let τ be a fixed transposition in S_n. Let A_n denote the alternating group. (see Exercise 7.) Define a function $f : A_n \rightarrow S_n$ by

$$f(\sigma) = \tau\sigma \quad \forall \sigma \in A_n$$

(a) Show that f is a bijection from A_n to the set of odd permutations in S_n.

(b) Use part (a) to conclude that $\#A_n = n!/2$.

11. In each of the following cases, compute the sign of the given permutation.

(a) $\begin{pmatrix} 1 & 2 & 3 & 4 & 5 & 6 & 7 & 8 & 9 \\ 3 & 6 & 9 & 8 & 2 & 4 & 5 & 7 & 1 \end{pmatrix}$

(b) $(2 \quad 8 \quad 4)^{755}$

(c) $(1 \quad 3 \quad 8 \quad 5)^{-621}$

(d) $(3 \quad 8 \quad 7 \quad 2 \quad 1)(4 \quad 3 \quad 6 \quad 2)(5 \quad 7)(1 \quad 2 \quad 3 \quad 4 \quad 5)$

12. For which n is the cycle $(1 \quad 2 \quad 3 \quad \cdots \quad n)$ even?

13. (a) Is there a procedure that will take the puzzle in Example 5.60 from its initial configuration (the first picture in 5.60) to the following configuration in exactly 23 moves? Explain.

	1	3	4
5	2	6	8
9	10	7	11
13	14	15	12

(b) Is there a way to manipulate the puzzle into the following configuration from the initial one in 5.60? Explain.

1	2	3	4
5	14	7	■
9	10	11	8
13	6	15	12

14. Exercise 7(a) shows that the set of even permutations in S_n is closed under product. Is the set of *odd* permutations in S_n also closed under product?

15. For which values of $n \geq 3$ does the regular n-gon have a symmetry whose associated permutation is a transposition? Explain.

5.8 Binomial and Multinomial Coefficients

In Chapter 2 we learned that an n-element set has 2^n subsets. But in most contexts in which we must choose subsets, there are restrictions on the sizes of subsets to be chosen. We'll start this section by considering a question that is important in combinatorics and probability theory, as well as in algebraic computations: If $0 \leq k \leq n$, how many k-element subsets are contained in a set of n elements? Then we will obtain intriguing connections between some of the numbers (the so-called binomial coefficients) that arise in the discussion, and we will give some applications.

In what follows, a set with k elements will be called a **k-set**, as before, or a **combination** of k elements; a subset that is a k-set is a **k-subset**.

5.62 Definition. Let k and n be integers, with $0 \leq k \leq n$. The number of k-subsets of an n-set is written

$$\binom{n}{k}$$

and called the **binomial coefficient n over k**. (Other notations are $C(n, k)$ and $_nC_k$; both are pronounced "n choose k.")

5.63 Theorem.   Let n be a nonnegative integer. Then

(a) $\dbinom{n}{0} = 1$

(b) $\dbinom{n}{n} = 1$

(c) $\dbinom{n}{k} = 0$ if $k > n$

(d) $\dbinom{n}{k} = \dbinom{n}{n-k}$ if $0 \le k \le n$

(e) If $n \ge 1$ then $\dbinom{n}{1} = \dbinom{n}{n-1} = n$

(f) $2^n = \dbinom{n}{0} + \dbinom{n}{1} + \cdots + \dbinom{n}{n}$

PROOF.   (a) An n-set contains only one 0-set, namely, $\emptyset$.

(b) The only n-subset of an n-set S is S itself. (Franklin Roosevelt was widely acclaimed for a statement something like this.)

(c) If $k > n$ then an n-set contains no k-subsets.

(d) Given an n-set S, complementation gives a bijection between the collection of k-subsets of S and the collection of $(n - k)$-subsets of S. Alternatively stated, the number of ways of choosing a k-subset of S is equal to the number of ways of choosing the complement of a k-subset of S.

(e) The fact that $\binom{n}{1} = n$ is clear from the definition, and the equality $\binom{n}{1} = \binom{n}{n-1}$ follows from (d).

(f) We know (from Theorem 2.71) that if S is an n-set then $\#P(S) = 2^n$. On the other hand, $P(S)$ has as its members $\emptyset$, the 1-subsets of S, the 2-subsets of S, and so on. Counting all these subsets gives

$$\#P(S) = \binom{n}{0} + \binom{n}{1} + \binom{n}{2} + \cdots + \binom{n}{n}$$

and this yields the desired equation.   □

The next theorem provides an explicit formula for the binomial coefficients, and we will give two very different proofs. The strategy of the first proof is to count something two different ways, then to equate the results and deduce the conclusion. The second proof is by induction.

5.64 Theorem.   If $0 \leq k \leq n$, then

$$\binom{n}{k} = \frac{n!}{k!\,(n-k)!}$$

PROOF 1.   First consider how many repetition-free sequences of length k can be chosen from a given set of n elements. There are n possibilities for the first element, then $n-1$ possibilities for the second element, and so on; eventually there are $n - (k-1)$ possibilities for the kth element. Altogether there are

(∗)
$$n(n-1)\cdots(n-k+1)$$

sequences, by the product rule.

Now let's make the selection in another way. First choose k elements from the given n-set: there are $\binom{n}{k}$ ways to do this, by definition of the symbol $\binom{n}{k}$. Then, having chosen these k elements, there are $k!$ ways to arrange them in a sequence of length k. Thus the product rule yields a total of

(∗∗)
$$\binom{n}{k} \cdot k!$$

repetition-free sequences of length k.

Since (∗) and (∗∗) both count the same set, they are equal; therefore

(∗∗∗)
$$\binom{n}{k} = \frac{n(n-1)\cdots(n-k+1)}{k!}$$
$$= \frac{n(n-1)\cdots(n-k+1)}{k!} \cdot \frac{(n-k)!}{(n-k)!}$$
$$= \frac{n!}{k!\,(n-k)!}$$

This completes the first proof.

PROOF 2.   We will use induction on n. If $n = 0$ then also $k = 0$; and $\binom{0}{0} = 1$ because the empty set is the only 0-set. On the other hand,

$$\frac{0!}{0!\,(0-0)!} = 1$$

because $0! = 1$ by definition. This establishes the basis step of the induction. Now suppose the theorem is true for $n = t$. That is, assume

$$\binom{t}{k} = \frac{t!}{k!(t-k)!} \quad \text{for } 0 \le k \le t$$

To complete the induction we must verify that the theorem holds for $t + 1$; that is, that

$$\binom{t+1}{k} = \frac{(t+1)!}{k!(t+1-k)!} \quad \text{for } 1 \le k \le t+1$$

Let S be a $(t + 1)$-set, and fix an element $x \in S$. Then we can write $S = \{x\} \cup S_0$, where S_0 is a t-set. Now, a k-subset of S is either a k-subset of S_0 or has the form $A \cup \{x\}$ for some $(k - 1)$-subset $A \subseteq S_0$. But from the definition of binomial coefficient, there are $\binom{t}{k}$ of the former and $\binom{t}{k-1}$ of the latter. Thus

$$(5.65) \quad \binom{t+1}{k} = \binom{t}{k} + \binom{t}{k-1} \quad \text{(by the addition rule)}$$

$$= \frac{t!}{k!(t-k)!} + \frac{t!}{(k-1)!(t-k+1)!} \quad \text{(by the induction hypothesis)}$$

$$= \frac{t!(t-k+1) + t!\,k}{k!(t-k+1)!} \quad \text{(we have found a common denominator)}$$

$$= \frac{t!(t+1)}{k!(t-k+1)!} \quad \text{(factor } t! \text{ out of both numerator terms)}$$

$$= \frac{(t+1)!}{k!(t+1-k)!} \quad \square$$

Formula (∗∗∗) in Proof 1 of Theorem 5.64 is useful for computational purposes. It has fewer multiplications than the formula in the statement of the theorem.

5.66 Corollary (Pascal's Formula). If n and k are integers satisfying $1 \le k \le n$, then

$$\binom{n}{k} = \binom{n-1}{k} + \binom{n-1}{k-1}$$

PROOF. Substitute $t = n - 1$ in Equation 5.65. □

Pascal's formula gives a recurrence relation for the computation of binomial coefficients, given the initial data $\binom{n}{0} = \binom{n}{n} = 1$ for all n. Notice that no multiplication is needed for this computation (unlike the formula in Theorem 5.64). The recursion yields the following table, known as **Pascal's triangle**. To reproduce it, write 1s in the left column and in the diagonal inside the table. Then, from top to bottom, plug each hole in the triangle with the sum of the number directly above the hole and the number to the upper left of the hole.

Binomial Coefficients (Pascal's Triangle)

k \ n	0	1	2	3	4	5	6	7	8	$\cdots$
0	1									
1	1	1								
2	1	2	1							
3	1	3	3	1						
4	1	4	6	4	1					
5	1	5	10	10	5	1				
6	1	6	15	20	15	6	1			
7	1	7	21	35	35	21	7	1		
8	1	8	28	56	70	56	28	8	1	
$\vdots$	$\vdots$	$\vdots$	$\vdots$	$\vdots$	$\vdots$	$\vdots$	$\vdots$	$\vdots$	$\vdots$	$\ddots$

5.67 EXAMPLE. Now we can quickly settle a couple of the problems posed at the start of the chapter.

SOLUTION TO 5.1(e). The number of clinks is equal to the number of 2-sets in a 10-set, which is

$$\binom{10}{2} = \frac{10!}{2!\,8!} = 45$$

Similarly, the number of minuet teams that must be checked is

$$\binom{10}{3} = \frac{10!}{3!\,7!} = 120$$

SOLUTION TO 5.1(c). Each route from the southwest to the northeast consists of 16 one-block legs; exactly eight of these legs are easterly and eight are northerly. Each route can be represented by a string of sixteen E's and N's, using eight copies of each letter. For instance, the route shown on page 207 is represented by

NEEENNENNNNEENEE

Such a string is completely specified by indicating which eight of the sixteen positions will contain N's. Otherwise put: each route corresponds to an eight-element subset of $\mathbb{N}_{16}$. Therefore, altogether there are

$$\binom{16}{8} = \frac{16!}{8!\,8!} = \frac{16 \cdot 15 \cdot 14 \cdot 13 \cdot 12 \cdot 11 \cdot 10 \cdot 9 \cdot 8!}{8!\,8!} = 12{,}870$$

allowable routes. More generally, the same argument can be used to show that for an $n \times n$ array of city blocks, the number of allowable southwest-to-northeast routes is $\binom{2n}{n}$. [It can also be shown (by methods beyond our treatment here) that when n is large, $\binom{2n}{n}$ is approximately $4^n/\sqrt{\pi n}$. For instance, when $n = 100$, the number of routes is approximately 9×10^{58}, which is nothing to sniff at.]

If the problem setting is generalized still further, to an $m \times n$ grid, then the same reasoning as before yields $\binom{m+n}{n}$ routes.

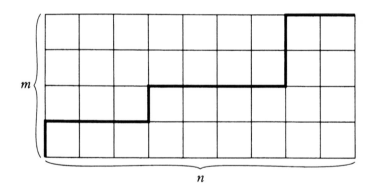

5.68 EXAMPLE. Electronically transmitted information is often coded into strings of 0s and 1s. (Each digit is called a **bit**.) The **weight** of a string is its number of 1s. Interference or mechanical problems can introduce errors into transmitted messages, and the detection and correction of errors is a major concern of the mathematical subject known as *coding theory*. Consider a code whose words are all the 16-bit strings whose weight is divisible by 4. Let's compute the number of codewords. If k is a multiple of 4 then there are $\binom{16}{k}$ codewords of weight k, since each word is determined by the set of k locations that hold 1s. So altogether the number of codewords is

$$\binom{16}{0} + \binom{16}{4} + \binom{16}{8} + \binom{16}{12} + \binom{16}{16}$$

With the help of Theorem 5.63, this simplifies to

$$\binom{16}{8} + 2\left[1 + \binom{16}{4}\right]$$

Then computing $\binom{16}{8}$ and $\binom{16}{4}$ by means of Theorem 5.64 gives 16,512 for the total number of codewords.

Incidentally, while the code described in Example 5.68 allows certain errors to be detected, it doesn't allow error *correction*. For instance, an error (a bit received as 1 when 0 was intended, or vice versa) in an odd number of bits in a transmitted word will have odd weight and hence will not be a codeword. But even though we may know a word to be wrong, we have no way to know what was intended. For this reason it is desirable for codewords to be sufficiently different from each other so that if a small number of errors are made in transmitting a word, it will be clear which codeword was intended. This is a big subject and we won't go into it (but see Exercise 13 on page 139 for the notion of *distance* between codewords). Our message in the present section is only that a thorough description of a code involves a lot of counting, and that binomial coefficients play a very active role.

5.69 Definition. Let S be a finite nonempty set. If $A \subseteq S$, define the **probability** of A (with respect to S), denoted $\Pr(A)$, to be the quotient $\#A/\#S$. (A more complete notation would be $\Pr_S(A)$, but if S has been fixed throughout a given discussion, we usually agree to remember it without writing it.)

5.70 EXAMPLES. With the notation of Definition 5.69, for any finite nonempty set S we have

$$\Pr(\emptyset) = 0, \qquad \Pr(S) = 1$$

and, in general,

$$0 \le \Pr(A) \le 1$$

The probability of a set A can be interpreted as follows. View S as the set of possible outcomes of some experiment or the set of possible choices in some decision process, with each outcome or choice equally likely. (Imagine yourself blindfolded and choosing a card from a well-shuffled deck.) Then $\Pr(A)$ represents the fraction of the time that we expect an experimental outcome or choice to be in A in a large number of trials.

5.71 EXAMPLES.   (a) What is the probability of being dealt a flush in poker?

SOLUTION.   A poker deck has 52 cards, and it is partitioned into four 13-card suits. A poker hand has five cards, so the number of possible poker hands is $\binom{52}{5}$. A flush hand consists of cards from only one suit. There are $\binom{13}{5}$ flush hands of each suit, hence $4 \cdot \binom{13}{5}$ flush hands altogether. The desired probability is therefore the fraction

$$\frac{\#(\text{flush hands})}{\#(\text{poker hands})} = \frac{4 \cdot \binom{13}{5}}{\binom{52}{5}} = \frac{5{,}148}{2{,}598{,}960} \approx \frac{1}{500}$$

(In the formal language of Definition 5.69, this is the probability of the set of flushes with respect to the set of all poker hands.)

(b) What is the probability of being dealt a full house in poker?

SOLUTION.   A full house consists of a triplet of cards of one numerical value together with a pair of cards of another value. There are 13 possibilities for the value of the triplet; having fixed that, there are $\binom{4}{3}$ ways to select three cards with that value. Then there remain 12 possibilities for the value of the pair; having chosen that value there are $\binom{4}{2}$ ways to choose the two cards. Therefore, by the product rule, we deduce that the probability of being dealt a full house is

$$\frac{\#(\text{full houses})}{\#(\text{poker hands})} = \frac{13 \cdot \binom{4}{3} \cdot 12 \cdot \binom{4}{2}}{\binom{52}{5}}$$

$$= \frac{13 \cdot 4 \cdot 12 \cdot 6}{2{,}598{,}960} \approx \frac{1}{694}$$

By comparing this with the probability of a flush, we see that the full house is less likely and hence more highly prized.

We have seen equations (in 5.63 and 5.66) that give connections between different binomial coefficients. This is to be expected. For instance, in choosing a k-subset of an n-set, along the way we will have chosen a k'-subset, for each $k' < k$, so it is natural to expect an association between $\binom{n}{k}$ and $\binom{n}{k'}$. Here are some further samples of such phenomena.

5.72 Theorem.   (a) If $1 \le k \le n$, then $\dbinom{n}{k} = \dfrac{n}{k}\dbinom{n-1}{k-1}$.

(b) If m and n are nonnegative integers, then

$$\sum_{k=0}^{n}\binom{m+k}{k} = \binom{m+n+1}{n}$$

We'll start with two different proofs of (a). The first proof will come from playing with the formula for binomial coefficients given by Theorem 5.64. It is arithmetically easy and requires no set-theoretical baggage. On the other hand, it gives no insight into the meaning of the equation in terms of decision procedures. The second proof gives that insight, but some perspiration is lost along the way. (We must not be too critical of the first proof. Once a result is discovered *somehow*, perhaps then it is possible to interpret it and mine its riches.) We will also give two proofs of (b). The first has a geometric flavor, while the second relies on arithmetic. Both proofs use our earlier results on binomial coefficients.

PROOF 1 OF (a).

$$\binom{n}{k} = \frac{n!}{k!\,(n-k)!} = \frac{n}{k}\cdot\frac{(n-1)!}{(k-1)!\,(n-k)!}$$

$$= \frac{n}{k}\cdot\frac{(n-1)!}{(k-1)!\,\big((n-1)-(k-1)\big)!} = \frac{n}{k}\binom{n-1}{k-1}$$

PROOF 2 OF (a).   Choosing a k-subset of an n-sct S can be done by first choosing an element $x \in S$ and then choosing $k-1$ elements from the remaining $n-1$ elements. Altogether there are $n\binom{n-1}{k-1}$ possibilities for this, by the product rule. But let's be careful. We have done *more* than pick a k-subset: we have also singled out one element x for special attention (as the first element chosen). More precisely, we have chosen an ordered pair (x, B), where B is a k-subset of S and $x \in B$. There is another way to do this: first choose B and *then* choose x. There are $\binom{n}{k}$ ways to choose B and, having done that, there are then k ways to choose x in B. This gives $k\binom{n}{k}$ possibilities for the choice of (x, B). We have counted something in two ways (a strategy familiar from the first proof of 5.64), and therefore the results are equal:

$$n\binom{n-1}{k-1} = k\binom{n}{k}$$

The conclusion follows.

PROOF 1 OF (b). In the labelled graph pictured here, consider all the

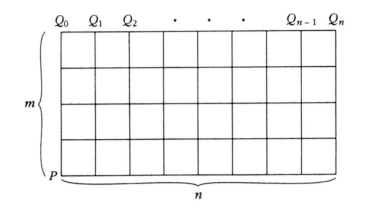

paths that start at P and end at a vertex on the upper boundary, moving up or to the right at each step. By the discussion at the end of Example 5.67, for each k satisfying $0 \leq k \leq n$, the number of paths from P to Q_k is $\binom{m+k}{k}$. Hence the total number of such paths is

(∗)
$$\sum_{k=0}^{n} \binom{m+k}{k}$$

Now extend the original diagram by adding a new row at the top. Each

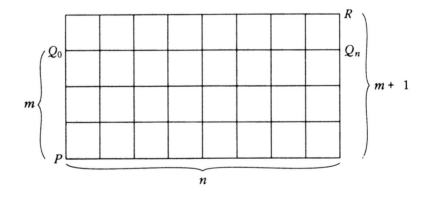

path already counted has exactly one extension to a path from P to R that touches no additional vertices on the original graph. (Move up from the original endpoint, then move right to R.) Moreover, *every* path from P to R is such an extension. Therefore the quantity (∗) is equal to the number of paths from P to R. But the number of paths from P to R is also equal to

$$\binom{m + n + 1}{n}$$

again by the argument of Example 5.67; therefore the stated equation is true.

PROOF 2 OF (b). Let m be any nonnegative integer. We must prove that the asserted equation holds for every nonnegative integer n, and we will do this by induction on n.

If $n = 0$ then the equation to be verified is

$$\binom{m + 0}{0} = \binom{m + 1}{0}$$

and this is true by Theorem 5.63(a).

Now suppose the result is true for $n = t$, and we must prove the result for the case $n = t + 1$. In other words, we must show that

$$\sum_{k=0}^{t+1} \binom{m + k}{k} = \binom{m + t + 2}{t + 1}$$

But

$$\sum_{k=0}^{t+1} \binom{m + k}{k} = \sum_{k=0}^{t} \binom{m + k}{k} + \binom{m + t + 1}{t + 1}$$

$$= \binom{m + t + 1}{t} + \binom{m + t + 1}{t + 1} \qquad \text{(by the induction hypothesis)}$$

$$= \binom{m + t + 2}{t + 1} \qquad \text{(by Pascal's formula)} \qquad \square$$

A **binomial** is an algebraic expression that is a sum of two terms. The following theorem gives us a formula for the coefficients of the terms in the expansion of a power of a binomial; hence the name **binomial coefficient**.

5.73 The Binomial Theorem. Let $a, b \in \mathbb{R}$, and let $n \in \mathbb{N}$. Then

$$(a + b)^n = \sum_{k=0}^{n} \binom{n}{k} a^k b^{n-k}$$

PREAMBLE TO PROOF. When we multiply together n factors, each equal to $a + b$, we get a sum of terms of the form $a^k b^{n-k}$. The number of times a particular $a^k b^{n-k}$ appears as a term in the product is equal to the number of times exactly k of the a's have been chosen from the n factors $a + b$ to use as a multiplier. There are $\binom{n}{k}$ ways to make this choice. Therefore, it is reasonable to believe that the coefficient of $a^k b^{n-k}$ in the product is $\binom{n}{k}$, and now we will prove it.

PROOF. We will use the following piece of notational magic: given numbers $c_0, c_1, \ldots, c_t$, then

$$(*) \qquad \sum_{k=0}^{t} c_k = \sum_{k=1}^{t+1} c_{k-1}$$

(The magic becomes believable by means of an induction argument on t. Less formally: both sides of $(*)$ are equal to $c_0 + \cdots + c_t$.)

Now we will prove the theorem by induction on n. If $n = 1$ the result is trivially true, so suppose the result is true for $n = t$; that is,

$$(a + b)^t = \sum_{k=0}^{t} \binom{t}{k} a^k b^{t-k}$$

We must prove the result for $n = t + 1$:

$$(a + b)^{t+1} = \sum_{k=0}^{t+1} \binom{t + 1}{k} a^k b^{(t+1)-k}$$

We compute:

$$(a + b)^{t+1} = (a + b)(a + b)^t$$

$$= (a + b) \sum_{k=0}^{t} \binom{t}{k} a^k b^{t-k} \qquad \text{(by the induction hypothesis)}$$

$$= \sum_{k=0}^{t} \binom{t}{k} a^{k+1} b^{t-k} + \sum_{k=0}^{t} \binom{t}{k} a^k b^{t-k+1}$$

$$= \sum_{k=1}^{t+1} \binom{t}{k - 1} a^k b^{t-k+1} + \sum_{k=0}^{t} \binom{t}{k} a^k b^{t-k+1} \qquad \text{(by } (*))$$

$$= a^{t+1} + \sum_{k=1}^{t} \binom{t}{k - 1} a^k b^{t-k+1} + \sum_{k=1}^{t} \binom{t}{k} a^k b^{t-k+1} + b^{t+1}$$

$$= a^{t+1} + \sum_{k=1}^{t} \left[\binom{t}{k-1} + \binom{t}{k} \right] a^k b^{t-k+1} + b^{t+1}$$

$$= a^{t+1} + \sum_{k=1}^{t} \binom{t+1}{k} a^k b^{t-k+1} + b^{t+1} \qquad \text{(by Pascal's formula)}$$

$$= \sum_{k=0}^{t+1} \binom{t+1}{k} a^k b^{(t+1)-k}. \qquad \square$$

5.74 Corollary. $2^n = \binom{n}{0} + \binom{n}{1} + \cdots + \binom{n}{n-1} + \binom{n}{n}$

PROOF. Let $a = b = 1$ in the binomial theorem. (This is our second proof of this fact. The first appeared in Theorem 5.63). $\square$

5.75 EXAMPLE. Suppose x is a real number. Compute the coefficient of x^6 in the expansion of $(x - 3)^{11}$.

SOLUTION. By the binomial theorem,

$$(x - 3)^{11} = (x + (-3))^{11} = \sum_{k=0}^{11} \binom{11}{k} x^k (-3)^{11-k}$$

So the term containing x^6 is $\binom{11}{6}(-3)^5 x^6$. But $\binom{11}{6} = 462$ and $(-3)^5 = -243$, therefore the answer is $-112{,}266$.

5.76 EXAMPLE. Imagine that you are at the market and that you have purchased the following items:

4 bananas (not attached)
5 cans of tuna
2 boxes of cereal
4 lemons
3 bottles of a particular classic cola
6 light bulbs.

Because some of the items are easily damaged, you care about the order in which they are put into the grocery bag, but you don't distinguish one banana from another, one cereal box from another, etc., for this purpose. In how many essentially different ways can the clerk fill the bag?

Notice that each pattern of bag loading corresponds to a sequence of length 24 of the form

$$(\text{banana}, \text{cola}, \text{cereal}, \text{bulb}, \text{bulb}, \text{tuna}, \ldots)$$

So we are really counting sequences of length 24, subject to certain conditions on the terms, with the understanding that certain sequences are equivalent. (For example, we will not interpret the interchange of two bananas, while fixing the positions of the other objects, as a different packing arrangement.)

Let's state this problem a bit more formally: We are given n elements to be listed in sequence. The elements are partitioned into t types, with k_i elements of the ith type, for $1 \le i \le t$. How many essentially different sequences are there, if we do not distinguish between two elements of the same type?

We can settle this with the help of binomial coefficients and the product rule. In a sequence of length n, there are $\binom{n}{k_1}$ ways to select the positions that will be filled by objects of the first type (say bananas). Having done this, there are $\binom{n-k_1}{k_2}$ ways to select the positions for the objects of the second type, and so on. Altogether, the product rule gives

$$\binom{n}{k_1}\binom{n-k_1}{k_2}\binom{n-k_1-k_2}{k_3}\cdots\binom{n-k_1-\cdots-k_{t-1}}{k_t}$$

different results. By the formula for binomial coefficients, this is equal to

$$\frac{n!}{k_1!(n-k_1)!} \times \frac{(n-k_1)!}{k_2!(n-k_1-k_2)!} \times \frac{(n-k_1-k_2)!}{k_3!(n-k_1-k_2-k_3)!} \times \cdots$$
$$\times \frac{(n-k_1-k_2-\cdots-k_{t-1})!}{k_t!\,0!}$$

Observe that the right-hand factor in each denominator is equal to the numerator of the next factor. So, after cancellation, the whole product dwindles to

$$\frac{n!}{k_1!\,k_2!\cdots k_t!}$$

Now we can calculate the answer to the grocery-store problem:

$$\frac{24!}{4!\,5!\,2!\,4!\,3!\,6!}$$

It is now natural to make the following definition.

5.77 Definition. Let n and $k_1, \ldots, k_t$ be nonnegative integers, with $k_1 + \cdots + k_t = n$. Define the **multinomial coefficient**

$$\binom{n}{k_1 \quad k_2 \quad \cdots \quad k_t} = \frac{n!}{k_1! \, k_2! \cdots k_t!}$$

A formal interpretation of multinomial coefficients proceeds as follows. Let A be an n-set, and suppose A is partitioned into blocks $A_1, A_2, \ldots, A_t$, where each A_i is a k_i-set, for $1 \leq i \leq t$. Consider the collection of all sequences of length n whose terms are all the elements of A. (That is, consider the set of surjections $\mathbb{N}_n \to A$.) Call two such sequences f and g *equivalent* if, for each i satisfying $1 \leq i \leq n$, the elements $f(i)$ and $g(i)$ belong to the same block. This is an equivalence relation on this collection of sequences, and the multinomial coefficient

$$\binom{n}{k_1 \quad k_2 \quad \cdots \quad k_t}$$

is the number of equivalence classes.

5.78 EXAMPLE. Consider the number of different words that can be made using all the letters of "Mississippi." (By a *word* we just mean a string of letters.) There are four i's, four s's, two p's, and one M: eleven letters in all. The solution is the multinomial coefficient

$$\binom{11}{4 \quad 4 \quad 2 \quad 1} = \frac{11!}{4! \, 4! \, 2! \, 1!} = 34{,}650$$

Like the term "binomial coefficient," the term "multinomial coefficient" comes from considering algebraic expressions. Given real numbers $x_1, x_2, \ldots, x_t$, consider the power

$$(x_1 + \cdots + x_t)^n = (x_1 + \cdots + x_t)(x_1 + \cdots + x_t) \cdots (x_1 + \cdots + x_t)$$

After performing this product but before collecting like terms, a typical term in this product has the form

$$x_1^{k_1} x_2^{k_2} \cdots x_t^{k_t}$$

The coefficient of $x_1^{k_1} \cdots x_t^{k_t}$ *after* collecting like terms is equal to the number of ways of picking k_1 factors equal to x_1, and k_2 factors equal to

x_2, and so on, as we multiply the n copies of $x_1 + x_2 + \cdots + x_t$. This is precisely the multinomial coefficient

$$\binom{n}{k_1 \quad k_2 \quad \cdots \quad k_t}$$

5.79 EXAMPLE. In the expansion of $(x_1 + x_2 + x_3 + x_4 + x_5)^7$, the coefficient of $x_1^2 x_3 x_4^3 x_5$ is

$$\binom{7}{2 \quad 0 \quad 1 \quad 3 \quad 1} = \frac{7!}{2!\,0!\,1!\,3!\,1!} = 420$$

Exercises

1. Compute the following binomial coefficients.

   (a) $\binom{9863}{1}$ (e) $\binom{63}{60}$

   (b) $\binom{805}{2}$ (f) $\binom{940}{939}$

   (c) $\binom{14}{4}$ (g) $\binom{0}{0}$

   (d) $\binom{12^{800}}{0}$ (h) $\binom{5}{8}$

2. A team of nine starting baseball players will be chosen from a group of thirteen hopefuls. The coach's child is one of the thirteen.

   (a) How many possibilities are there for the team?

   (b) Suppose the coach's child is guaranteed a position on the team. Now how many possibilities are there for the team?

3. Without referring to the text, write the top ten lines of Pascal's triangle.

4. Determine *all* the nonnegative integers n that satisfy the equation

$$\binom{n}{4} = \binom{n}{6}$$

5. A local restaurant offers a special salad lunch subject to these conditions: Each diner chooses exactly five ingredients from a menu of eight possibilities and then tops it with a blend of exactly two of the restaurant's four dressings.

   (a) How many dressed salad combinations are possible?

   (b) Jones loves the lunch, but he cannot tolerate the simultaneous inclusion of radishes (one of the eight items on the menu) and peanut butter dressing (one of the four choices), though all other possibilities are acceptable to him. How many acceptable choices does he have?

(c) In the statement of the lunch conditions, change each "exactly" to "at most." *Now* answer (a) again. (Assume that the diner chooses at least one salad ingredient, but allow for the possibility of no dressing.)

6. The definition of $\binom{n}{k}$ mentions "an n-set." Show that this definition is independent of the n-set used. That is, show that if A_1 and A_2 are both n-sets, then the number of k-subsets of A_1 is equal to the number of k-subsets of A_2.

7. Write out the expression $(x + y)^7$ as a sum of integer multiples of terms of the form $x^i y^j$.

8. What is the coefficient of y^3 in the expansion of $(2x - 5y)^6$?

9. Prove that for nonnegative integers m and n the following formula holds:

$$\sum_{k=0}^{n} \binom{k}{m} = \binom{n + 1}{m + 1}$$

Use induction on n, starting with $n = 0$. (Refer to Definition 5.62 in the case $n = 0$.) Pascal's formula may be helpful.

10. Suppose $0 \le k_1 + k_2 \le n$. Verify the equation

$$\binom{n}{k_1}\binom{n - k_1}{k_2} = \binom{n}{k_1 + k_2}\binom{k_1 + k_2}{k_1}$$

in two ways:

(a) by direct application of the formula for binomial coefficients (Theorem 5.64);

(b) by an intuitive argument similar to that used in the text to verify 5.72(a).

11. Prove the equation $\binom{n+1}{3} - \binom{n-1}{3} = (n - 1)^2$ for each $n \ge 1$.

12. Eight varieties of plant seeds are to be selected for a garden. Altogether 15 varieties of vegetables and 10 flower varieties are available. Determine the number of ways the selection can be made under each of the following conditions.

(a) Four vegetables and four flowers must be chosen.

(b) There must be more flower varieties than vegetable varieties.

(c) There must be at least two flower varieties.

13. Determine the number of paths from P to Q in the accompanying graph under each of the following conditions. (Assume each leg of the path moves either up or to the right.)

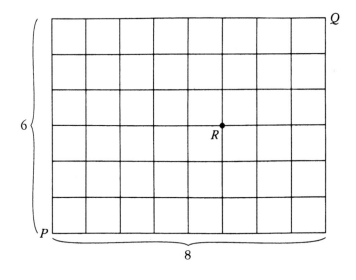

(a) The path must go through vertex R.

(b) The path must not go through vertex R.

(c) Every one-directional section of each path has even length. (An edge of a small square is one unit long.)

14. In how many ways can a collection of 25 objects be partitioned into two blocks of ten elements and one block of five elements?

15. What is the probability of being dealt four-of-a-kind in poker (that is, a five-card hand containing four cards of the same value, such as four aces or four 5s).

16. Show that if A is a nonempty finite set with subsets A_1 and A_2, then

$$\Pr(A_1 \cup A_2) = \Pr(A_1) + \Pr(A_2) - \Pr(A_1 \cap A_2)$$

17. (a) What is the probability that a fair coin will land on heads exactly four times if it is flipped seven times?

(b) What is the probability that a fair coin will land on heads either three times or four times if it is flipped seven times?

18. The menu at the fabulous Niftyburger restaurant lists 40 different varieties of burger, numbered 1 to 40. (Two burgers of the same variety are indistinguishable from one another.) There is an elementary school

near the restaurant. In each of the following cases, the named teacher comes to the restaurant with 10 easily distinguished children. Determine the number of possible outcomes for each stated procedure. (An "outcome" is an arrangement of certain people eating certain things.)

(a) Danny orders 10 burgers without specifying the variety (so they might all be of the same variety, all of different varieties, etc.) and gives one to each child.

(b) Ben wants to create a spirit of healthy competition, so he orders only 7 plain hamburgers and distributes them to 7 of his 10 children.

(c) Susan orders 7 burgers, all of different varieties, and distributes them to 7 of her students.

(d) David buys 10 burgers, all of different varieties, and arranges them in numerical order, with the lowest numbered variety on top of the pile. Then he arranges the children in alphabetical order. He gives the top burger to the first child (in alphabetical order), the next burger to the second child, and so on.

(e) Faye buys 2 soyburgers, 5 cheeseburgers, and 3 salmonburgers, and she distributes them to her children, one burger per student.

(f) Stan buys one burger of each of the first 15 varieties listed on the menu. He gives one to each child and then eats the remaining 5 burgers himself.

(g) Mozie buys 20 flaxburgers (his favorite) and distributes them to his children in a random way, not caring if some kids get none while others get more than one. (So possibly one child will get all 20 burgers.)

[Suggestion for (g): Consider keeping a record of each such burger distribution by dividing a piece of paper into 10 columns, one for each child, and marking an x in a column when the corresponding child gets a burger. Separate adjacent columns from each other with a vertical line.]

19. With words and without formulas, explain why it is that if $n = k_1 + k_2$, then

$$\binom{n}{k_1 \ k_2} = \binom{n}{k_1} = \binom{n}{k_2}$$

20. With words and without formulas, explain the equation

$$\binom{n}{1 \ 1 \ \ldots \ 1} = n!$$

21. In the setting of Example 5.76, suppose you insist that light bulbs be packed on top, just above the bananas, but the order in which the products in the lower part of the bag are put in doesn't matter. Under those conditions, determine the number of essentially different acceptable orderings in which the products can be put into the bag.

22. (a) How many different words can be constructed using (all) the letters of the word "magnesium"?

    (b) How many different words can be constructed from "magnesium" if the vowels are to remain in their original order?

23. (a) How many words can be constructed using all the letters of the word "zebratious"?

    (b) Answer the same question, except require the vowels to appear in alphabetical order.

    (c) Answer the same question, but require the vowels to appear in alphabetical order and the consonants to do likewise.

24. When the expression $(x_1 + x_2 + x_3 + x_4 + x_5)^9$ is multiplied out, what is the coefficient of $x_1^4 x_4^2 x_5^3$?

25. Determine the coefficient of $x^2 yz$ in the expansion of

$$(2x - y + z + 1)^7$$

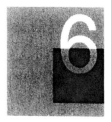

NUMBER THEORY

A peculiarity of the higher arithmetic is the great difficulty which has often been experienced in proving simple general theorems which had been suggested quite naturally by numerical evidence. "It is just this," said Gauss, "which gives the higher arithmetic that magical charm which has made it the favourite science of the greatest mathematicians, not to mention its inexhaustible wealth, wherein it so greatly surpasses other parts of mathematics."

HAROLD DAVENPORT
The Higher Arithmetic

During twenty centuries the theory of numbers has been a favorite subject of research by leading mathematicians and thousands of amateurs. Recent investigations compare favorably with the older ones. Future discoveries will far surpass those of the past.

LEONARD EUGENE DICKSON
Introduction to the Theory of Numbers

Well, anyway, the people who are making up the English language found themselves with names for every digit except "three." And, as there were three of quite a lot of things (Marx Brothers, blind mice, wishes and cent stamps) it got increasingly embarrassing not to have a word to express "three." They tried using the word "four," but it ended only in confusion, especially when addition or subtraction was at stake.

ROBERT BENCHLEY
My Ten Years in a Quandary

The subject of this chapter is number theory—the study of the integers and related structures—a subject born in prehistory, already flourishing in ancient Babylon, and still flourishing today; a subject filled with results that are beautiful and magical, and with haunting mysteries; a subject once viewed as the purest of pure mathematics—art for art's sake—but that in recent years has been applied to problems associated with the transmission, coding, and manipulation of numerical data. (Pure mathematics has become applied mathematics!) Number theory is unique in its abundance of appealing problems whose *statements* are accessible to elementary school students, but whose *solutions* have eluded mathematicians for centuries. The struggle to solve problems in number theory led to the development of much of modern algebra, which in turn is linked to an enormous range of subjects in mathematics and the other sciences. Our brief treatment here will be an introduction to some of the most basic properties of the integers. The fundamentals of the **divisibility** and **congruence** relations will be explored. A remarkable function, **Euler's φ-function**, will be introduced, and we will use it to consider this question: *Is it possible to show that a given integer is not prime without actually factoring it?* (To appreciate the difficulty of this task, think about how you might try to show that a number with, say, 50 digits is not prime, assuming that it has no *obvious* factors.)

As is our custom, we continue to use $\mathbb{N}$, $\mathbb{Z}$, and $\mathbb{R}$ for the sets of natural numbers, integers, and real numbers, respectively.

6.1 Operations

6.1 Definition.   Let S be a nonempty set. A **binary operation** on S is a function

$$* : S \times S \rightarrow S$$

(The adjective *binary*, which we will usually omit, informs us that $*$ acts on ordered *pairs* of elements.)

If $(a, b) \in S \times S$, we usually write $a * b$ instead of the more cumbersome function notation $*\big((a, b)\big)$ for the result of applying $*$ to (a, b). For instance, addition is an operation on the set $\mathbb{Z}$ of integers, and we write $3 + 5$ instead of $+\big((3, 5)\big)$.

6.2 Definition.   Let $*$ be an operation on S. Then

(i) $*$ is **commutative** if $a * b = b * a$ for every $a, b \in S$.

(ii) ∗ is **associative** if $(a * b) * c = a * (b * c)$ for every $a, b, c \in S$.

(iii) An element $e \in S$ is an **identity element** for ∗ if, for all $a \in S$,

$$e * a = a \quad \text{and} \quad a * e = a$$

6.3 EXAMPLES. (a) Ordinary addition, subtraction, and multiplication are operations on $\mathbb{R}$, with the respective actions

$$(a, b) \overset{+}{\longmapsto} a + b$$

$$(a, b) \overset{-}{\longmapsto} a - b$$

$$(a, b) \overset{\cdot}{\longmapsto} a \cdot b$$

Division, given by $(a, b) \longmapsto a \div b$, is strictly speaking *not* an operation on $\mathbb{R}$, since $a \div 0$ has no meaning. (That is, ordered pairs of the form $(a, 0)$ are not in the operation's domain.) But $\div$ *is* an operation on the set $\dot{\mathbb{R}}$ of nonzero real numbers. Addition and multiplication are commutative and associative operations, while subtraction is neither commutative nor associative. The number 0 is an identity element for addition and subtraction (but not for multiplication), while 1 is an identity for multiplication. When these operations are restricted to $\mathbb{Z}$ and $\mathbb{N}$ (more precisely, when they are restricted to $\mathbb{Z} \times \mathbb{Z}$ and $\mathbb{N} \times \mathbb{N}$) the same observations hold, except that subtraction is not an operation on $\mathbb{N}$: $3 - 5 \notin \mathbb{N}$.

(b) If A is any set, then union and intersection are commutative and associative operations on the power set $P(A)$. The empty set is an identity for $\cup$, while A is an identity for $\cap$.

(c) Consider the set Σ^* of all strings over a finite alphabet Σ, as defined in the last section of Chapter 4. The **concatenation** of two strings is the string obtained by following one by the other. More precisely: if $w_1 = a_1 \ldots a_m$ and $w_2 = b_1 \ldots b_n$, with the a's and b's in Σ, define $w_1 w_2 = a_1 \ldots a_m b_1 \ldots b_n$; if $w \in \Sigma^*$ and ϵ is the empty word, define $\epsilon w = w \epsilon = w$. So if Σ is our usual alphabet, $w_1 = $ ybar, and $w_2 = $ cand, then $w_1 w_2 = $ ybarcand and $w_2 w_1 = $ candybar. Concatenation is associative but not commutative (unless Σ has only one element); the empty word ϵ is an identity for concatenation.

(d) Let S be any nonempty set. Define an operation ∗ on S by declaring $a * b = a$ for all $a, b \in S$. (That is, ∗ takes each ordered pair to its first coordinate.) Is ∗ associative? Commutative? Is there an identity element?

(e) Define an operation $*$ on $\mathbb{R}$ by $a * b = \max\{a, b\}$, the larger of a and b. This operation is useful in "sorting" problems. For example, if $\{a_1, \ldots, a_n\}$ is a set of real numbers then

$$((((a_1 * a_2) * a_3) * \cdots) * a_{n-1}) * a_n$$

is the largest number in the set. (Check this claim by induction on n.) It follows that this operation is associative and commutative, but there is no identity element.

(f) Let A be a nonempty set, and let $F(A)$ denote the set of all functions from A to A. Then composition of functions is an operation on $F(A)$. (The operation takes each ordered pair of functions (f, g) to the associated composition $f \circ g$.)

(g) If A is a nonempty set, then the permutation product is an operation on the symmetric group S_A. (See Section 5.3 for terminology and notation.)

The issues of associativity, commutativity, and identity for function composition and permutation product were considered in Chapters 3 and 5, respectively.

An operation $*$ on a small set $A = \{a_1, a_2, \ldots, a_n\}$ can be specified by a square table with n rows and n columns, in which the entry at the intersection of row i and column j is the element $a_i * a_j$. (*Rows* are horizontal, *columns* are vertical.) We list the elements of A outside the left and top borders of the table as indices for the rows and columns, respectively; and it is customary to adorn the table further with the operation symbol at the upper left corner. For example, the table

$*$	a_1	a_2	a_3
a_1	a_3	a_1	a_2
a_2	a_2	a_3	a_1
a_3	a_1	a_2	a_1

specifies an operation $*$ on the set $A = \{a_1, a_2, a_3\}$. This table tells us that $a_3 * a_1 = a_1$, $a_2 * a_2 = a_3$, and so on. (The table represents a set of nine such equations.)

In each of the examples in 6.3 we have displayed at most one identity. The following result shows that this is not due to lack of ambition.

6.4 Theorem. An operation has at most one identity.

PROOF. If e and e_1 are identities for $*$, then

$$e * e_1 = e_1$$

since e is an identity; but also

$$e * e_1 = e$$

since e_1 is an identity. Thus $e_1 = e * e_1 = e$. □

6.5 Definition. Suppose the operation $*$ on S has identity element e, and let $a \in S$. If there is an element $b \in S$ satisfying $a * b = b * a = e$, then b is said to be an **inverse** of a with respect to $*$.

6.6 Theorem. Suppose $*$ is an associative operation on S with identity e. If an element $a \in S$ has an inverse, then it has only one inverse.

PROOF. If b and c are inverses of a, then

$$
\begin{aligned}
b &= b * e & &\text{by definition of } e\\
&= b * (a * c) & &\text{since } c \text{ is an inverse of } a\\
&= (b * a) * c & &\text{by associativity}\\
&= e * c & &\text{since } b \text{ is an inverse of } a\\
&= c & &\text{by definition of } e \quad \square
\end{aligned}
$$

Refer to Examples 6.3. With respect to addition, each $a \in \mathbb{R}$ has inverse $-a$; with respect to multiplication, each $a \neq 0$ has inverse $1/a$. If A is a nonempty set, then $\emptyset$ is the identity with respect to the operation $\cup$ on $P(A)$, but no $X \in P(A) - \{\emptyset\}$ has an inverse, since for every $Y \in P(A)$ we have $X \cup Y \neq \emptyset$. Similarly, though Σ^* has the empty word ϵ as identity, if $w \in \Sigma^* - \{\epsilon\}$ then w has no inverse with respect to concatenation, since concatenation can never decrease word length (so no word z exists satisfying $wz = \epsilon$).

Exercises

1. (a) Suppose the sum and product of integers a, b are denoted $+\big((a, b)\big)$ and $\cdot\big((a, b)\big)$, respectively. Use this notation to rewrite the familiar rule $a(b + c) = ab + ac$.

(b) Similarly, using the notation $+\big((a, b)\big)$ instead of $a + b$, write the associative law of addition.

(The purpose of Exercise 1 is to demonstrate the benefits of streamlining the operation notation as indicated just after Definition 6.1.)

2. Recall from Definition 4.47 that a string of length n over the alphabet Σ is a function $\mathbb{N}_n \rightarrow \Sigma$. Use this recollection to give a careful definition of the concatenation of two strings. (That is, define the concatenation as a *function* instead of using the intuitive phrase "by following one by the other" used in Example 6.3(c).)

3. Let n be a positive integer. How many different binary operations can be defined on a set of n elements?

4. (a) Determine all the real numbers a, b, c for which the equation $(a - b) - c = a - (b - c)$ holds.

   (b) Do the same for the equation $(a \div b) \div c = a \div (b \div c)$.

5. If S is a nonempty set and $n \in \mathbb{N}$, let S^n denote the set of n-tuples of elements of S. An **n-ary operation** on S is a function $S^n \rightarrow S$. (In particular, a binary operation is 2-ary.) Suppose $*$ is a binary operation on S. Show that $*$ can be used recursively to define an n-ary operation on S for each $n \geq 2$. (Suggestion: Start by considering the case $n = 3$.)

6. When the subtraction operation is restricted to $\mathbb{N} \times \mathbb{N}$, the result is not an operation on $\mathbb{N}$, because the condition $a, b \in \mathbb{N}$ does not guarantee that $a - b \in \mathbb{N}$. Determine the smallest set S satisfying $\mathbb{N} \subset S \subseteq \mathbb{R}$ such that the restriction of subtraction to $S \times S$ is an operation on S.

7. Let $\dot{\mathbb{R}}$ denote the set of nonzero real numbers. Show that the division operation on $\dot{\mathbb{R}}$ has no identity element.

8. If an operation $*$ on a finite set S is defined by a table, how can we learn from the table whether there is an identity element for $*$?

9. Suppose $*$ is an operation on the two-element set $\{e, a\}$, and suppose that e is an identity element for $*$. Prove that $*$ is associative.

10. Let $*$ be an operation on a set S. An element $\lambda \in S$ is a **left identity** for $*$ if $\lambda * a = a$ for all $a \in S$; and $\rho \in S$ is a **right identity** for $*$ if $a * \rho = a$ for all $a \in S$.

    (a) Give an example showing that a *left* identity for $*$ need not be an identity element for $*$.

    (b) Show that if the operation $*$ has both a left identity λ and a right identity ρ, then $*$ has an identity element.

11. Assume S is a finite set with an operation $*$ given by a table. Consider the question, "Does every element of S have an inverse with respect to $*$?" How can we answer this question by studying the table?

12. Show that if $*$ is an associative operation on the set S then

$$((a * b) * c) * d = (a * b) * (c * d) = a * (b * (c * d)), \quad \forall a, b, c, d \in S$$

13. In each case determine whether the given rule describes an operation on S. If it does, determine whether the operation has an identity element and (if so) whether every element has an inverse.
    (a) S is the set of odd integers, $(a, b) \longmapsto ab$.
    (b) S is the set of odd integers, $(a, b) \longmapsto a + b$.
    (c) S is the set of even integers, $(a, b) \longmapsto a + b$.
    (d) S is the set of even integers, $(a, b) \longmapsto ab/2$.
    (e) S is the set of nonzero real numbers, $(a, b) \longmapsto a^2 b$.
    (f) S is the set of rational numbers, $(a, b) \longmapsto a\sqrt{b^2}$.

14. Suppose $*$ is an associative operation on the three-element set $S = \{e, a, b\}$. Suppose further that e is an identity element for $*$ and that every element of S has an inverse. Prove that there is exactly one possibility for $*$, and exhibit its table.

15. Suppose r and s are fixed integers, and an operation $*$ is defined on $\mathbb{Z}$ by

$$a * b = ra + sb \quad \text{for all } a, b \in \mathbb{Z}$$

Under what conditions on r and s does this operation have an identity element?

6.2 The Integers: Operations and Order

We have already used integers in this book for a variety of purposes, and we have assumed a familiarity with the basic facts of arithmetic. Before proceeding into number theory, we'll begin by reviewing some of those facts and pointing out some others, mostly without proof. (In fact, in many cases the proofs are surprisingly difficult.)

Addition and multiplication are associative and commutative operations on $\mathbb{Z}$, and each has its own identity: 0 for addition and 1 for multiplication. (Note: By Theorem 6.4 these are the *only* identities for addition and multiplication.) Additive inverses exist; but with respect to multiplication, integers other than 1 and -1 have no inverses.

The operations on $\mathbb{Z}$ not only coexist, they *interact* via the **distributive laws**:

$$(6.7) \qquad a(b + c) = ab + ac \qquad \text{and} \qquad (a + b)c = ac + bc$$

for all $a, b, c \in \mathbb{Z}$. Multiplication and addition are further related by the following implication involving the additive identity: for all $a, b \in \mathbb{Z}$,

$$(6.8) \qquad\qquad ab = 0 \quad \Rightarrow \quad a = 0 \text{ or } b = 0$$

Now we will *prove* several other basic facts about $\mathbb{Z}$ using the assumptions we have made. Resist the temptation to declare the assertions obvious.

6.9 Theorem. Let $a, b, c \in \mathbb{Z}$. Then

(a) $0 \cdot a = 0$;
(b) $a \cdot (-b) = -ab$;
(c) **Cancellation law:** If $a \neq 0$ and $ab = ac$, then $b = c$.

PROOF. (a) We have

$$0 \cdot a = (0 + 0) \cdot a = 0 \cdot a + 0 \cdot a$$

Now add $-(0 \cdot a)$ to both sides of this equation. On the left side we get zero, while on the right side we get

$$-(0 \cdot a) + (0 \cdot a + 0 \cdot a)$$

$$= [-(0 \cdot a) + 0 \cdot a] + 0 \cdot a \qquad \text{by associativity of addition}$$

$$= 0 + 0 \cdot a \qquad \text{by definition of } -(0 \cdot a)$$

$$= 0 \cdot a \qquad \text{since 0 is the additive identity}$$

Thus $0 \cdot a = 0$, as desired.

(b) By definition, $-ab$ is the additive inverse of ab, and we know from Theorem 6.6 that there is only one such object. Therefore, to verify the claim it suffices to add $a \cdot (-b)$ to ab and check that the result is zero. But

$$a \cdot (-b) + ab = a(-b + b)$$

$$= a \cdot 0$$

$$= 0 \qquad \text{(by part (a))}$$

(c) Assume the equation $ab = ac$ holds, with $a \neq 0$. Adding $-ac$ to both sides of the assumed equation leads us as follows:

$$0 = ab + (-ac)$$
$$= ab + a \cdot (-c) \qquad \text{by part (b)}$$
$$= a[b + (-c)] \qquad \text{by the distributive law}$$

But since $a \neq 0$, we then infer from 6.8 that $b + (-c) = 0$, and therefore that $b = c$. (Note: Another proof can be obtained by multiplying both sides of the given equation ($ab = ac$) by the rational number $1/a$. But our proof has the philosophical advantage of not relying on the existence of any number outside $\mathbb{Z}$.) □

We have the inclusion $\mathbb{N} \subset \mathbb{Z}$; and for every $n \in \mathbb{Z}$ exactly one of the following holds:

(6.10) $\qquad n \in \mathbb{N}, \qquad n = 0, \quad \text{or} \quad -n \in \mathbb{N}$

Otherwise stated, every integer is either positive, zero, or negative; and the conditions are mutually exclusive. This is called the **trichotomy law**.

We define the order relation "<" on $\mathbb{Z}$ by

(6.11) $\qquad a < b \quad \Leftrightarrow \quad b = a + n \quad \text{for some } n \in \mathbb{N}$

(This is also written $b > a$.)

6.12 Ordering Properties. (a) for all $a, b \in \mathbb{Z}$, exactly one of the following holds:

$$a < b, \qquad a = b, \quad \text{or} \quad a > b$$

(b) For all $a, b, c \in \mathbb{Z}$,

$$a < b \quad \text{and} \quad b < c \quad \Rightarrow \quad a < c \qquad \text{(the transitive law)}$$

The **absolute value function** $||$ on $\mathbb{Z}$ is defined by

$$|n| = \begin{cases} n & \text{if } n \geq 0 \\ -n & \text{if } n < 0 \end{cases}$$

Here are some of its properties:

$$|n| \in \mathbb{N} \cup \{0\}$$

$$|n| = 0 \quad \Leftrightarrow \quad n = 0 \qquad \text{(In particular, if } n \neq 0 \text{ then } |n| \geq 1.)}$$

$$|ab| = |a|\,|b|$$

$$|a + b| \leq |a| + |b| \qquad \text{(the \textbf{triangle inequality})}$$

Exercises

1. Two distributive laws are presented in statement 6.7. Deduce the right-hand law from the left-hand law, using the fact that multiplication is commutative.

2. State 6.9(b) in words, without using any mathematical symbols. (Start like this: "When one integer is multiplied by the additive inverse of . . . .")

3. Prove that the following equations hold for $a, b, c, d \in \mathbb{Z}$.
   (a) $(a + b)(c + d) = ac + bc + ad + bd$
   (b) $(-a)(-b) = ab$

4. The expression $x - y$ is an abbreviation for $x + (-y)$. Use this information to prove the following statement:

   $$a - (b + c) = (a - b) - c \quad \text{for all } a, b, c \in \mathbb{Z}$$

5. A direct proof is given in the text for the fact that $0 \cdot a = 0$ for all $a \in \mathbb{Z}$. Now prove this fact by contradiction.

6. Reprove statement 6.9(c) using multiplication by $1/a$, as suggested by the note in the text.

7. Show that statement 6.12(a) is equivalent to the trichotomy law, 6.10.

8. Show that if $a, b \in \mathbb{Z}$ with $b \geq 0$, then

   $$|a| \leq b \quad \Leftrightarrow \quad a \leq b \text{ and } -a \leq b$$

9. (a) Show that if $a \leq b$ and $c \leq d$ then $a + c \leq b + d$.
   (b) Show that if $0 \leq r < b$ and $0 \leq r_1 < b$, then

   $$0 \leq |r - r_1| < b$$

10. For $a, b \in \mathbb{Z}$, prove the inequality

    $$\big||a| - |b|\big| \leq |a - b|$$

    (Suggestion: Start by writing $a = (a - b) + b$, and then apply the triangle inequality.)

6.3 Divisibility: The Fundamental Theorem of Arithmetic

6.13 Definition. Let $a, b \in \mathbb{Z}$, with $a \neq 0$. We say that a **divides** b, or b is **divisible** by a, or a is a **divisor** or **factor** of b, or b is a **multiple** of a if $b = ac$ for some $c \in \mathbb{Z}$. The statement "a divides b" is written $a \mid b$, and its negation is written $a \nmid b$.

6.14 EXAMPLES. $3 \mid (-12)$, $6 \mid 18$, $17 \mid 0$, $-5 \mid 20$, $-4 \mid 4$, $6 \nmid 1$

Note: Current usage prefers "a is a divisor of b" to "a is a factor of b" for the statement "$a \mid b$." It is now more common to use "factor" for a number appearing in a particular expression of an integer as a product. Thus, 1, 2, 3, 4, 6, and 12 are the positive "divisors" of 12, while 3 and 4 are the "factors" of 12 in the expression $12 = 3 \cdot 4$.

6.15 Theorem. Let $a, b, c \in \mathbb{Z}$.

(a) If $a \mid b$ and $b \neq 0$ then $|a| \leq |b|$.

(b) If $a \mid b$ and $a \mid c$ then $a \mid (b + c)$ and $a \mid (b - c)$.

PROOF. (a) If $a \mid b$ and $b \neq 0$ then $b = ac$ for some $c \in \mathbb{Z}$, with $c \neq 0$. Then $|c| \geq 1$, and so $|b| = |ac| = |a||c| \geq |a|$.

(b) Exercise. $\square$

We defined the notion of *prime number* in Example 1.2(b), and we showed in Theorem 2.74 that every integer $n \geq 2$ is a product of primes. Given this result, it is reasonable to expect that a thorough understanding of the integers will require an understanding of the primes. To this day, the primes remain rather mysterious creatures, but at least we know this: there are a lot of them. The following theorem is one of the most famous in mathematics, due to the strength of its statement and the swiftness with which it is proved. To appreciate the theorem fully, its level of sophistication should be compared with that of other realms of human activity over the years. For example, more than 2,000 years after the theorem was proved, many people still believed (despite substantial evidence to the contrary) in "spontaneous generation"—the theory that certain living creatures grow naturally from nonliving material: frogs from mud, flies from garbage, mice from old rags, and so on.

6.16 Theorem.   (Euclid, ca 300 B.C.) There are infinitely many prime numbers.

PROOF.   We will use induction to prove the theorem in this form: For every positive integer n, there are at least n prime numbers. It is easy to start a list of primes: 2 is prime. Now suppose $p_1, p_2, \ldots, p_k$ are distinct primes, with $k \geq 1$. We must show there is another prime, p_{k+1}. Consider the number $M = (p_1 p_2 \cdots p_k) + 1$; it has a prime divisor p by Theorem 2.74, say $M = pq$. If $p \in \{p_1, \ldots, p_k\}$, then by relabelling (if necessary) we can suppose that $p = p_1$. But then we have

$$1 = M - p_1 p_2 \cdots p_k = p_1 q - p_1 p_2 \cdots p_k = p_1(q - p_2 \cdots p_k)$$

So $p_1 \mid 1$, which is impossible since $p_1 > 1$. Therefore $p \notin \{p_1, \ldots, p_k\}$, and so $\{p_1, \ldots, p_k, p\}$ is a set of $k + 1$ prime numbers.   □

Euclid's theorem gives no *efficient* way to actually produce new primes. It tells us this: given any finite list of primes, the number N obtained by adding 1 to their product will have a prime divisor not on the given list. But if N is large, factoring it into primes may not be a picnic. Furthermore, whatever new primes appear in the factorization of N might be much larger than other primes that have not yet been found. In fact, it was proved by Chebychev in 1852 that if n is any integer greater than 1, there is a prime p satisfying $n < p < 2n$. (This result is known as *Bertrand's postulate*. We leave its proof for a number theory course.) However, there is no reason to expect Euclid's method to yield a new prime that is less than twice the largest previously known prime.

The list of prime numbers includes occasional pairs of the form $\{n, n + 2\}$; for instance,

$$\{3, 5\} \quad \{5, 7\} \quad \{11, 13\} \quad \{17, 19\} \quad \{29, 31\} \quad \{41, 43\}$$

are the first six such pairs. These pairs are called **twin primes**. Inspired by Euclid's theorem, we ask:

Are there infinitely many twin primes?

No one knows the answer, although the question has been around for centuries.

Another famous unsolved problem on primes is known as **Goldbach's conjecture**. In 1742 Goldbach conjectured, but did not prove, the following statement:

Every even integer greater than 2 can be expressed as a sum of two primes. (The primes need not be distinct.)

Evidence in favor of the conjecture:

$$4 = 2 + 2 \qquad 6 = 3 + 3 \qquad 8 = 3 + 5 \qquad 10 = 5 + 5 \qquad 12 = 5 + 7$$

and so on. Write a few more examples. If you can prove the conjecture, your proof will be the first one.

In elementary school we learn an algorithm for dividing one integer by another, obtaining a quotient together with a remainder strictly less than the divisor. For instance, we have

$$
\begin{array}{r}
36 \leftarrow \text{quotient} \\
\text{divisor} \rightarrow 16\overline{)581} \\
\underline{48} \\
101 \\
\underline{96} \\
5 \leftarrow \text{remainder}
\end{array}
$$

Hence $581 = 16 \cdot 36 + 5$. We also learn (to our sorrow) that there is only one correct solution for each example of this kind. Missing from our early education was a *proof* of the existence and uniqueness of this solution, and we will now provide it.

6.17 Theorem (Division Algorithm). Let $a, b \in \mathbb{Z}$, with $b > 0$. Then there are integers q and r such that

$$a = bq + r \qquad \text{and} \qquad 0 \leq r < b$$

Moreover, q and r are uniquely determined by these conditions. (Here q is the **quotient** and r is the **remainder**.)

PROOF. First the intuition. The number a is either a multiple of b or strictly between two multiples of b. In the former case we can write $a = bq$. In the latter case we let r denote the distance from a to the nearest multiple of b below a; then r is less than b.

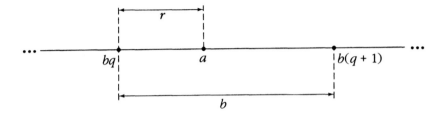

Now for the formal proof.

Existence. Let bq be the largest multiple of b not exceeding a. Then $bq \le a < b(q + 1)$. Define $r = a - bq$. Thus

$$r = a - bq < b(q + 1) - bq = b$$

as desired.

Uniqueness. If $a = bq + r$ and also $a = bq_1 + r_1$, with $0 \le r < b$ and $0 \le r_1 < b$, then subtraction of the second equation from the first yields $b(q - q_1) = r_1 - r$; thus $b \mid (r_1 - r)$. But a manipulation of the inequalities gives $b > |r_1 - r|$. (Check this.) Therefore from 6.15(a) we must have $r_1 - r = 0$; so $r_1 = r$ and therefore $q = q_1$.   □

With the division algorithm in hand, we can give a shorter version of Euclid's proof of the infinity of primes. Here goes. If $p_1, p_2, \ldots, p_k$ are the only primes, then the number $N = p_1 p_2 \cdots p_k + 1$ has a prime divisor, say p_1. Then $N = p_1 q = p_1 q + 0$ for some integer q. But also $N = p_1(p_2 \cdots p_k) + 1$, and this contradicts the uniqueness of the remainder given by the division algorithm. Therefore no finite list $p_1, p_2, \ldots, p_k$ of primes is complete.

6.18 Definition.   Let a and b be integers. An integer $d \ne 0$ is said to be a **common divisor** of a and b if $d \mid a$ and $d \mid b$. A common divisor d of a and b is said to be the **greatest common divisor** if $d > 0$ and if every common divisor of a and b is also a divisor of d.

6.19 EXAMPLE.   (a) The divisors of 12 are ± 1, ± 2, ± 3, ± 4, ± 6, ± 12; the divisors of 16 are ± 1, ± 2, ± 4, ± 8, ± 16. The *common* divisors of 12 and 16 are ± 1, ± 2, ± 4. The *greatest* common divisor is 4.

(b) If $a \in \mathbb{Z}$ and $a \ne 0$, then the greatest common divisor of 0 and a is $|a|$.

6.20 Theorem. If a and b are nonzero integers, then a and b have a unique greatest common divisor.

PROOF. *Existence.* Consider the set

$$L = \{xa + yb \mid x, y \in \mathbb{Z}\}$$

(The members of L are called the **linear combinations** of a and b.) The set L contains positive integers. For example, we can write

$$|a| = (\pm 1) \cdot a + 0 \cdot b$$

and therefore $|a| \in L$. Let d be the *smallest* positive integer in L; say, $d = x_1 a + y_1 b$, with $x_1, y_1 \in \mathbb{Z}$. If we had $d \nmid a$ then, by the division algorithm, there would be integers q and r such that $a = dq + r$, with $0 < r < d$. But then

$$r = a - dq = a - (x_1 a + y_1 b)q = (1 - x_1 q)a + (-y_1 q)b$$

which is a positive linear combination of a and b smaller than d. This contradicts the minimality of d in L, therefore we must have $d \mid a$. A similar argument shows that $d \mid b$, so d is a common divisor of a and b.

Now suppose d' is any common divisor of a and b; say, $a = d'a_1$ and $b = d'b_1$. Then

$$d = x_1 a + y_1 b = x_1 d'a_1 + y_1 d'b_1 = d'(x_1 a_1 + y_1 b_1)$$

and hence $d' \mid d$. Thus d is a greatest common divisor of a and b.

Uniqueness. If d and d_1 are both greatest common divisors for a and b, then $d_1 \mid d$ (since d is a greatest common divisor) and similarly $d \mid d_1$. Therefore, by 6.15(a), we have $|d| = |d_1|$. But d and d_1 are both positive, so the absolute value signs are redundant, and $d = d_1$. □

Notation. The expression "greatest common divisor" is usually abbreviated **gcd**. Following custom, we will use (a, b) for the gcd of a and b. In the mathematical literature, the greatest common divisor is also called the **highest common factor**, and the corresponding abbreviation **hcf** is used.

The fact that (a, b) *is a linear combination of a and b* (see the proof of 6.20) will turn out to be crucial, especially in the proof of Theorem 6.26, which gives a fundamental property of prime numbers. It's worth stating as a separate result:

6.21 Corollary. Let $d = (a, b)$. Then there are integers x and y such that

$$d = ax + by$$

How can we *compute* the greatest common divisor of two nonzero integers a and b? The proof of Theorem 6.20 is of no use for this purpose, since it requires us to scan an infinite set L for its smallest positive element, and in a finite lifetime we're unlikely to know when we have found it. There is an alternate approach, used in Example 6.19: use repeated trials (divide by smaller numbers, see when remainder 0 occurs) to obtain explicit lists of all the divisors of a and b, and then note the largest entry that appears on both lists. But if a and b are large, this can be a long and extraordinarily tedious process. Fortunately, Euclid developed a faster algorithm for computing the gcd, and the following lemma provides the key to this algorithm.

6.22 Lemma. If $a = bq + r$ then $(a, b) = (b, r)$.

PROOF OUTLINE. Let $d = (a, b)$. Check that every divisor of a and b is also a divisor of r; in particular, $d \mid r$ and hence $d \mid (b, r)$. [Apply Definition 6.18 to (b, r).] A similar argument shows that $(b, r) \mid d$, and the desired equality follows. □

It is easily checked that $(a, b) = (|a|, |b|)$ for all $a, b \in \mathbb{Z}$. Therefore, to compute greatest common divisors, it suffices to give an algorithm for the gcd of two *positive* integers.

6.23 Euclid's Algorithm for Computation of (a, b).
In Words. Divide b into a, getting a quotient q and remainder r_1:

$$a = bq + r_1 \quad \text{with } 0 \le r_1 < b$$

If $r_1 = 0$ then $b = (a, b)$; otherwise, divide r_1 into b and get another quotient and remainder r_2 (less than r_1). Continue to divide each new remainder into its predecessor until zero occurs as a remainder. (This must eventually happen since the remainders are successively smaller nonnegative integers.) The last nonzero remainder is (a, b). [To see this, observe that $(a, b) = (b, r_1)$ by Lemma 6.22; and $(b, r_1) = (r_1, r_2)$ for the same reason, so $(a, b) = (r_1, r_2)$. Similar reasoning holds in subsequent steps of the computation. So, if r_k is the last nonzero remainder, we get

$$(a, b) = (r_1, r_2) = (r_2, r_3) = \cdots = (r_k, r_{k+1}) = (r_k, 0) = r_k$$

as claimed.]

Computer Program Format. Here all letters represent nonnegative integers. First observe that if $a = bq + r$, with $0 \le r < b$, then

$$\frac{a}{b} = q + \frac{r}{b} \quad \text{with } 0 \le \frac{r}{b} < 1$$

Therefore $[a/b] = q$, where [ ] denotes the greatest integer function (see Example 3.8(b)). Now we can write Euclid's algorithm in the format of a program. (If you have had programming experience, convert the material presented here into an actual program.)

```
INPUT A,B
DO UNTIL R = 0:
   ┌→LET R = A - B · [A/B]
   │  IF R = 0 THEN GCD = B
   │  LET A REPRESENT WHAT HAS BEEN CALLED B UP TO NOW
   │  LET B REPRESENT WHAT HAS BEEN CALLED R UP TO NOW
   └─ RETURN
END
```

6.24 EXAMPLES. Compute $(2880, 504)$ and $(10374, 2574)$.

SOLUTION. We used repeated division, as instructed by Euclid.

$$
\begin{array}{r}
5 \\
b \rightarrow 504\overline{)2880} \leftarrow a \\
\underline{2520} \quad 1 \\
r_1 \rightarrow 360\overline{)504} \\
\underline{360} \quad 2 \\
r_2 \rightarrow 144\overline{)360} \\
\underline{288} \quad 2 \\
r_3 \rightarrow 72\overline{)144} \\
\underline{144} \\
r_4 \rightarrow 0 \qquad (2880, 504) = 72
\end{array}
$$

$$\begin{array}{r} 4 \\ b \rightarrow 2574\overline{)10374} \leftarrow a \\ \underline{10296} \end{array}$$

$$\begin{array}{r} 33 \\ r_1 \rightarrow 78\overline{)2574} \\ \underline{234} \\ \underline{234} \\ \underline{234} \\ r_2 \rightarrow 0 \end{array} \qquad (10374, 2574) = 78$$

To appreciate the strength of Euclid's algorithm, compare the ease of these computations to the pain of listing all the divisors of each number, as in Example 6.19.

We saw in Corollary 6.21 that the greatest common divisor (a, b) is equal to $ax + by$ for some integers x and y. If we wish, we can *find* x and y by manipulating the data that arises in applying Euclid's algorithm. The following example illustrates the method.

6.25 EXAMPLE.   The first three steps of the computation $(2880, 504) = 72$ in Example 6.24 can be stated as a sequence of equations as follows:

(a) $2880 = 504 \cdot 5 + 360$
(b) $504 = 360 \cdot 1 + 144$
(c) $360 = 144 \cdot 2 + 72$

This yields

$$\begin{aligned} 72 &= 360 + 144 \cdot (-2) & \text{[from (c)]} \\ &= 360 + (504 - 360) \cdot (-2) & \text{[from (b)]} \\ &= 360 \cdot 3 + 504 \cdot (-2) \\ &= (2880 - 504 \cdot 5) \cdot 3 + 504 \cdot (-2) & \text{[from (a)]} \\ &= 2880 \cdot 3 + 504 \cdot (-17) \end{aligned}$$

We proved in Theorem 2.74 that every integer $n \geq 2$ can be expressed as the product of prime factors. Our next goal is to prove that this decomposition into primes is *unique*. This is not obvious. For example, we have

$$24 = 6 \cdot 4 = (3 \cdot 2) \cdot 2^2 = 2^3 \cdot 3 \qquad \text{and} \qquad 24 = 8 \cdot 3 = 2^3 \cdot 3$$

The final results are the same, but the intermediate factorizations are quite different. A theorem is needed to assure us that we are not witnessing a special feature of the number 24.

Notice this: if a product of two integers is divisible by 5, then at least one of the two integers is divisible by 5. You probably believe this, but can you prove it? The following theorem does the job and, in so doing, it gives a special property of prime numbers that we will need in proving the uniqueness result.

6.26 Theorem. Let p be a prime number and let a and b be integers. Then the following implication holds:

$$p \mid ab \quad \Rightarrow \quad p \mid a \text{ or } p \mid b$$

PROOF.   Assume that $p \mid ab$. Our goal is to deduce the truth of "$p \mid a$ or $p \mid b$." For this purpose it suffices to assume (as we now do) that $p \nmid a$ and deduce that $p \mid b$.

Because $p \nmid a$, we know that $(p, a) = 1$, since the only positive divisors of p are 1 and p. Then from Corollary 6.21 there are integers x and y such that $xp + ya = 1$. So

$$b = b \cdot 1 = b(xp + ya) = p(xb) + (ab)y$$

Since $p \mid ab$, both terms on the right side of this equation are divisible by p, and therefore p divides their sum [by 6.15(b)]; that is, $p \mid b$.   □

6.27 Corollary. Let p be prime, and let $a_1, \ldots, a_t \in \mathbb{Z}$. If $p \mid a_1 \cdots a_t$, then $p \mid a_i$ for some i.

PROOF OUTLINE.   The case $t = 1$ is trivial, the case $t = 2$ is Theorem 6.26, and induction on t yields the result for all larger t.   □

It's easy to see that not every integer has the property stated for primes in Theorem 6.26. For example, $6 \mid 3 \cdot 4$, but $6 \nmid 3$ and $6 \nmid 4$. The next corollary shows that the property in Theorem 6.26 actually completely characterizes the primes.

6.28 Corollary. Let m be an integer greater than 1. Then m is prime if and only if the following implication holds for all $a, b \in \mathbb{Z}$:

$$m \mid ab \quad \Rightarrow \quad m \mid a \text{ or } m \mid b$$

PROOF. "Only if" is Theorem 6.26. Conversely, if m is not prime, there are integers a and b, with $1 < a < m$ and $1 < b < m$, such that $m = ab$. Then $m \mid ab$, while $m \nmid a$ and $m \nmid b$. □

Now we can show that the decomposition of an integer $n > 1$ into prime factors is essentially unique.

6.29 The Fundamental Theorem of Arithmetic. Let n be an integer greater than 1. Then there are prime numbers $p_1, \ldots, p_r$ such that $n = p_1 \cdots p_r$. Moreover, this factorization of n is unique in the following sense: if $n = q_1 \cdots q_s$ also, with the q's prime, then the q's are just a rearrangement of the p's. That is, $r = s$ and, if we label the primes so that $p_1 \leq \cdots \leq p_r$ and $q_1 \leq \cdots \leq q_s$, then $p_i = q_i$ for $1 \leq i \leq r$.

PROOF. The existence of a prime factorization was proved in Theorem 2.74, so only the uniqueness requires proof here.

We will argue by induction on n (in the format of 2.73). Suppose $n = p_1 \cdots p_r = q_1 \cdots q_s$, with the p's and q's prime and $p_1 \leq \cdots \leq p_r$. If $n = 2$, then since 2 is prime we have $2 = p_1 = q_1$, and we are done. Now assume that $n > 2$, and assume that the theorem is known for all integers t satisfying $2 \leq t \leq n - 1$. Since $p_1 \cdots p_r = q_1 \cdots q_s$, we have $p_1 \mid q_1 \cdots q_s$, so $p_1 \mid q_i$ for some i (by 6.27). By a change of subscripts on the q's (if necessary), we can suppose $p_1 \mid q_1$. But q_1 is *prime*, and hence $p_1 = q_1$. It follows from the cancellation law (see 6.9(c)) that $p_2 \cdots p_r = q_2 \cdots q_s$. Because $p_2 \cdots p_r < n$, from the induction hypothesis we then know that $r = s$ and, assuming $q_2 \leq \cdots \leq q_r$, we know that $p_i = q_i$ for $2 \leq i \leq r$. □

6.30 Corollary. Let $n \in \mathbb{Z}$, with $|n| \geq 2$. Then n has a unique factorization of the form

$$n = \pm p_1^{\alpha_1} \cdots p_t^{\alpha_t}$$

where $t \geq 1$, the p_i are distinct primes satisfying $p_1 \leq \cdots \leq p_t$, and $\alpha_i \geq 1$ for $1 \leq i \leq t$. (This factorization is called the **standard** or **canonical factorization** of n.)

PROOF OUTLINE. If $n \geq 2$, consider the prime decomposition in Theorem 6.29, and gather together all the prime factors equal to p_1, getting $p_1^{\alpha_1}$. Then repeat the process on the remaining prime factors, if there are any.

If n is negative, use the same procedure on $|n|$. □

The following proposition was known to the Pythagoreans around 400 B.C.

6.31 Theorem. The real number $\sqrt{2}$ is irrational.

PROOF *(by Contradiction).* If $\sqrt{2}$ is rational we can write

(∗)
$$\sqrt{2} = \frac{a}{b}$$

for some integers a and b. By factoring the numerator and denominator into primes and removing any common prime factors, we can assume $(a, b) = 1$. Squaring both sides of equation (∗) yields $2b^2 = a^2$, and so $2 \mid a^2$. Since 2 is prime, it follows from Theorem 6.26 that $2 \mid a$, say $a = 2m$. Thus $2b^2 = 4m^2$, and cancellation gives $b^2 = 2m^2$. Therefore $2 \mid b$, and this contradicts the fact that $(a, b) = 1$. Thus our initial assumption that $\sqrt{2}$ is rational has led to a contradiction, and the proof is complete. □

We have just shown that there is no rational number whose square is 2. How do we know there is a *real* number whose square is 2? In fact, the existence in ℝ of square roots of nonnegative real numbers is guaranteed by the way in which ℝ is constructed. That construction is a complicated matter, and we leave the details for a later course, but we note that Example 3.17 (the divide-and-average method) shows that it is possible to compute a sequence of rational numbers whose squares get closer and closer to 2. The Pythagoreans had further evidence that in a reasonable world $\sqrt{2}$ must exist: in a square with side of length 1, the length d of the diagonal satisfies the equation $d^2 = 1^2 + 1^2 = 2$.

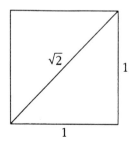

Incidentally, the irrationality of $\sqrt{2}$ has the following intuitive meaning with respect to the picture: given a measuring stick that has been precisely marked to indicate halves, thirds, fourths, fifths, and so on, there is no way to position the stick on the square's diagonal in such a way that the endpoints of the diagonal are both covered by marks on the stick.

If a and b are integers, there are distinct primes $p_1, \ldots, p_t$ and integers $\alpha_i \geq 0$ and $\beta_i \geq 0$, for $1 \leq i \leq t$, such that

(6.32)
$$a = \pm p_1^{\alpha_1} \cdots p_t^{\alpha_t} \quad \text{and} \quad b = \pm p_1^{\beta_1} \cdots p_t^{\beta_t}$$

To see this, start with the standard factorizations of a and b. If there is a prime number occurring in one of these factorization but not in the other, regard it as occurring to the power 0 in the standard factorization in which it does not appear. For instance, if $a = 1386$ and $b = -1275$, we have the standard factorizations

$$1386 = 2 \cdot 3^2 \cdot 7 \cdot 11 \quad \text{and} \quad -1275 = -3 \cdot 5^2 \cdot 17$$

In the format of 6.32, these become

$$1386 = 2 \cdot 3^2 \cdot 5^0 \cdot 7 \cdot 11 \cdot 17^0 \quad \text{and} \quad -1275 = -2^0 \cdot 3 \cdot 5^2 \cdot 7^0 \cdot 11^0 \cdot 17$$

6.33 Exercise. Given integers a and b with factorizations as in 6.32, show that

$$(a, b) = p_1^{\min\{\alpha_1, \beta_1\}} \cdots p_i^{\min\{\alpha_i, \beta_i\}} \cdots p_t^{\min\{\alpha_t, \beta_t\}}$$

where $\min\{\alpha_i, \beta_i\}$ denotes the minimum of α_i and β_i.

Recall from Definition 5.43 that the **least common multiple** of integers a and b is the smallest nonnegative integer that is a multiple of both a and b. We now write this as $[a, b]$. With the factorizations in 6.32, we claim that

(6.34)
$$[a, b] = p_1^{\max\{\alpha_1, \beta_1\}} \cdots p_t^{\max\{\alpha_t, \beta_t\}}$$

To see this, first write R for the expression on the right in 6.34, and observe that R is a positive multiple of a and of b. Therefore $[a, b] \leq R$. On the other hand, since $a \mid [a, b]$ and $b \mid [a, b]$, we know that $p_i^{\alpha_i}$ and $p_i^{\beta_i}$ both divide $[a, b]$, and hence $p_i^{\max\{\alpha_i, \beta_i\}}$ divides $[a, b]$, for $1 \leq i \leq t$. Therefore, in the standard factorization of $[a, b]$, each prime p_i appears at least to the power $\max\{\alpha_i, \beta_i\}$. Hence $R \mid [a, b]$, and so $R \leq [a, b]$, and the claim follows.

6.35 Theorem. If a and b are nonzero integers, then

$$[a, b] = \frac{|ab|}{(a, b)}$$

PROOF *(Proof Outline)*. Write a and b as in 6.32. Then write (a, b) as in 6.33, apply the appropriate law of exponents, and compare the result with 6.34. □

6.36 EXAMPLE. We compute $[-10140, 2600]$. To use 6.34, we first have to factor the given numbers into primes (this can be tedious!), and then we can read off the answer. We have

$$-10140 = -2^2 \cdot 3 \cdot 5 \cdot 13^2$$
$$2600 = 2^3 \cdot 5^2 \cdot 13 = 2^3 \cdot 3^0 \cdot 5^2 \cdot 13$$

This gives $[-10140, 2600] = 2^3 \cdot 3 \cdot 5^2 \cdot 13^2 = 101400$. An alternate approach is to use Euclid's algorithm (6.23) to compute

$$(-10140, 2600) = 260$$

then by 6.35 we get

$$[-10140, 2600] = \frac{(10140)(2600)}{260} = 101400$$

Exercises

1. Show that if $a \mid b$ and $a \mid c$ then $a \mid (mb + nc)$ for all $m, n \in \mathbb{Z}$.
2. Label each of the following *true* or *false*, and justify your answer.
   (a) $8 \mid 0$
   (b) $a \mid b$ and $b \mid c \Rightarrow a \mid c$
   (c) $a \mid b$ and $a \mid c \Rightarrow a \mid bc$
   (d) $a \mid b \Rightarrow -a \mid b$
   (e) $a \mid bc \Rightarrow b \mid a$ or $c \mid a$
   (f) $a \mid b$ and $b \mid a \Rightarrow a = \pm b$
3. Let a and b be integers, with $a \neq 0$. Prove that

$$a \mid b \iff \frac{b}{a} = \left[\frac{b}{a}\right]$$

where $[\ ]$ denotes the greatest integer function.

4. An integer $n \neq 0$ is said to be **composite** if n has a positive divisor other than 1 and $|n|$. (For example, -6 and 15 are composite, while -7, 1, and 13 are not composite.) Show that if n is composite, then n has a prime divisor $p \leq \sqrt{|n|}$.

5. (For students with computer programming experience) Write a computer program that accepts an integer $n > 1$ as input and either tells you that n is prime or lists eac⌐ divisor k of n that satisfies $1 < k < n$. (Suggestion: For each integer k satisfying $2 \leq k \leq \sqrt{n}$, test whether k is a divisor of n by the method of Exercise 3.)

6. Euclid proved that there are infinitely many primes. The key to his proof is in showing that the number $M = p_1 \cdots p_k + 1$ has a prime factor distinct from $p_1, p_2, \ldots, p_k$. It is tempting to conjecture that M must actually be prime. Test this conjecture for $1 \leq k \leq 6$.

7. In this exercise you will use an algorithm, called the *sieve of Eratosthenes*, that isolates prime numbers. (Eratosthenes lived from about 276 to 194 B.C. He was also known for his computation of the circumference of the earth and for his treatises on the theater, moral philosophy, and history.) Here is how it works. List the integers from 2 through n. Circle the number 2, then cross off all the higher multiples of 2 (namely, 4, 6, 8, 10, etc.). Circle 3, which is the first remaining number after 2. Then cross off all the multiples of 3 that have not yet been crossed off. Then circle 5. Et cetera. When you are finished with the repeated sieving operations, only the primes will remain on the list, and they will have been circled for emphasis. The exercise: perform the sieve of Eratosthenes with $n = 120$. As you do this, cross off the multiples of different primes by using different kinds of slashes (slashing in different directions, or using different colors), and provide a key for the reader. By this device the reader will immediately know the smallest prime divisor of each composite number on your list. (In view of Exercise 4, after the multiples of 7 have been crossed off, the remaining numbers will all be prime and can be circled to mark this fact.)

8. Define a **prime triple** to be a set of three prime numbers of the form $\{n, n + 2, n + 4\}$. For example, $\{3, 5, 7\}$ is a prime triple. Are there any others? Either exhibit another or prove there are none. (Suggestion: First observe what happens when any of the twin primes $\{n, n + 2\}$ listed in the text is supplemented with $n + 4$.)

9. Suppose $n = k(k + 1)(k + 2)$ for some $k \in \mathbb{Z}$. Show that n is divisible by 6.

10. Use Euclid's algorithm to compute the following greatest common divisors.

(a) $(56, 104)$

(b) $(462, 3003)$

(c) $(442, -182)$

(d) $(922, 2161)$

11. Show that when Euclid's algorithm is used to compute the greatest common divisor of two integers, it doesn't matter which integer is labelled a and which is labelled b.

12. Let a and b be integers. Show that if $(a, b) = 1$ then $(a, a + b) = 1$.

13. Show that if a, b, c are integers, not all zero, then

$$((a, b), c) = (a, (b, c))$$

Here each ordered pair is understood to represent a greatest common divisor.

14. Write each greatest common divisor computed in Exercise 10 as a linear combination of the given integers.

15. Two nonzero integers are said to be **relatively prime** if their greatest common divisor is 1. Let $a, b, c \in \mathbb{Z}$. Show that if $(a, c) = 1$ and $c \mid ab$, then $c \mid b$. (Hint: Mimic the proof of Theorem 6.26.)

16. In the manner of Example 6.19, list the divisors, the common divisors, and the greatest common divisor of 748 and 1258.

17. Prove that the real number $\sqrt[3]{5}$ is irrational.

18. Suppose $k, n \in \mathbb{N}$. Prove that if n is not the kth power of an integer, then $\sqrt[k]{n}$ is irrational.

19. Give a recursive procedure for constructing a line segment of length $\sqrt{n}$ for each integer $n \geq 2$, using only an unmarked straightedge and a compass. Assume that a line segment of length 1 has been given. (Recall that with a straightedge and compass, we can construct a line perpendicular to a given line at a given point.)

20. (a) Suppose d and n are natural numbers, and $d \mid n$. How does the standard factorization of d relate to the standard factorization of n?

    (b) Use part (a) to show how the standard factorization of n can be used to determine the number of positive divisors of n.

21. Compute the least common multiple $[462, 1574573]$ in two ways:

    (a) by factoring both integers into primes and applying formula 6.34;

    (b) by using Euclid's algorithm to compute the greatest common divisor $(462, 1574573)$ and then applying Theorem 6.35.

22. The fact that there are infinitely many prime numbers, together with the apparent abundance of twin primes, might lead the innocent to suspect that the gaps between consecutive primes are of bounded size. Show that this is *not* the case. (Suggestion: Consider sequences of the form

$$n! + 2, \qquad n! + 3, \qquad n! + 4, \ldots$$

where n is a large positive integer.)

6.4 Congruence; Divisibility Tests

The *congruence* relation, which we are about to define, is an important vehicle for the discussion of divisibility problems in $\mathbb{Z}$. Moreover, by using congruence, certain computational problems with large integers (whose storage and manipulation may be difficult) can be converted to corresponding problems with small integers. (For instance, in this way the hazards of *overflow* in machine calculations can sometimes be eliminated without loss of accuracy.)

Convention: *Throughout this section, all numbers under discussion will be understood to be integers.* For example, the assertion "$m > 0$" will mean "$m \in \mathbb{N}$."

6.37 Definition.   Fix $m > 0$. Numbers a and b are said to be **congruent modulo m** if $a - b$ is divisible by m. Symbolically:

$$a \equiv b \ (\text{mod } m) \quad \text{means} \quad m \mid (a - b)$$

The number m is called the **modulus** of the congruence.

6.38 EXAMPLE. $3 \equiv -5 \ (\text{mod } 4)$, $0 \equiv 15 \ (\text{mod } 5)$, $-7 \equiv 5 \ (\text{mod } 6)$, $5743 \equiv 43 \ (\text{mod } 100)$.

It is often useful to reformulate the congruence relation as follows:

(6.39) $a \equiv b \ (\text{mod } m) \quad \Leftrightarrow \quad a - b = mk \quad$ for some k

$\Leftrightarrow \quad a = b + mk \quad$ for some k

6.40 EXAMPLES.   (a) Your bicycle's odometer (the mileage gauge) returns to zero after 1000 miles, so after you ride 3472 miles the odometer reads 472. The reason, in our present notation: $3472 \equiv 472 \ (\text{mod } 1000)$.

(b) Suppose it is now five o'clock. (Never mind whether it is morning or evening.) Consider how to compute what the time will be after 784 hours have elapsed. Sine it is now 5 hours past twelve o'clock, after the given time interval it will be 789 hours past twelve o'clock. Division by 12 yields the equation $789 = 12 \cdot 65 + 9$. This equation tells us that in 789 hours, a clock's hour hand will complete 65 full revolutions and will then mark off 9 more hours. The result: in 784 hours from now the time will be nine o'clock. More generally, to compute the time t at h hours after time t_0, we use the division algorithm to write

$$t_0 + h = 12q + r$$

with $0 \le r < 12$. Then

$$t = \begin{cases} r & \text{if } r \neq 0, \\ 12 & \text{if } r = 0. \end{cases}$$

(The temptation is to write simply "$t = r$," but we do not speak of "zero o'clock.") In congruence notation, the time t is the number satisfying these two conditions:

$$1 \le t \le 12 \qquad \text{and} \qquad t \equiv t_0 + h \pmod{12}$$

(Remember: we are assuming that all numbers are integers.)

6.41 Theorem. Fix $m > 0$. Then congruence modulo m is an equivalence relation on $\mathbb{Z}$.

PARTIAL PROOF.   There are three things we need to verify.

(i) $a \equiv a \pmod{m}$ for all a

(ii) $a \equiv b \pmod{m} \Rightarrow b \equiv a \pmod{m}$

(iii) $a \equiv b \pmod{m}$ and $b \equiv c \pmod{m} \Rightarrow a \equiv c \pmod{m}$

We leave (i) and (ii) as exercises. As for (iii), the hypothesis gives

$$a = b + mk_1 \qquad \text{and} \qquad b = c + mk_2$$

for some k_1 and k_2 (use 6.39). Then $a = c + m(k_1 + k_2)$, and so $a \equiv c \pmod{m}$.   □

We now show that with a fixed modulus, congruences behave in some ways like equations.

6.42 Theorem. If $a \equiv b$ (mod m) and $c \equiv d$ (mod m), then

$$a + c \equiv b + d \ (\text{mod } m) \quad \text{and} \quad ac \equiv bd \ (\text{mod } m)$$

PROOF.   The hypothesis gives $a = b + mk_1$ and $c = d + mk_2$ for some k_1 and k_2. Then

$$a + c = (b + d) + m(k_1 + k_2)$$

and so $a + c \equiv b + d$ (mod m). Also,

$$ac = bd + m(k_1 d + k_2 b + m k_1 k_2)$$

so $ac \equiv bd$ (mod m).   □

6.43 Corollary.   Suppose there are congruences $a_1 \equiv b_1$ (mod m), $a_2 \equiv b_2$ (mod m), ..., $a_n \equiv b_n$ (mod m). Then

$$\sum_{i=1}^{n} a_i \equiv \sum_{i=1}^{n} b_1 \ (\text{mod } m) \quad \text{and} \quad \prod_{i=1}^{n} a_i \equiv \prod_{i=1}^{n} b_i \ (\text{mod } m)$$

(So congruences mod m can be added or multiplied, like equations.) In particular, if $a \equiv b$ (mod m), then $a^n \equiv b^n$ (mod m) for all $n \geq 1$.

PROOF IDEA.   Argue by induction on n, using Theorem 6.42 to establish the result when $n = 2$.   □

6.44 MAGIC TRICK. Take the last four digits of your telephone number, add your weight, and multiply the resuit by 9. Then write down the sum of the digits of the answer. If your sum has one digit, stop; if your sum has two digits write down *their* sum. Prediction: Your answer is 9. Sample:

$$
\begin{array}{rr}
\text{First four digits of telephone number} & 3785 \\
\text{weight} & +\ 197 \\
\hline
& 3982 \\
& \times 9 \\
\hline
& 35838
\end{array}
$$

$$3 + 5 + 8 + 3 + 8 = 27$$
$$2 + 7 = \ 9$$

An explanation of 6.44 requires a close look at decimal notation. A nonnegative integer n written in base 10 has the form $a_t a_{t-1} \ldots a_1 a_0$, where each a_i satisfies $0 \leq a_i \leq 9$; each a_i is called a **decimal digit** of n. Here the juxtaposition of digits does not mean multiplication; instead, it means this:

$$n = a_t \cdot 10^t + a_{t-1} \cdot 10^{t-1} + \cdots + a_1 \cdot 10 + a_0 = \sum_{i=0}^{t} a_i \cdot 10^i$$

For example, $4708 = 4 \cdot 10^3 + 7 \cdot 10^2 + 8$. The following result is the key to the "magic" displayed in 6.44.

6.45 Theorem. Every nonnegative integer is congruent modulo 9 to the sum of its decimal digits. Symbolically, if $0 \leq a_i \leq 9$ for $0 \leq i \leq t$, then

$$\sum_{i=0}^{t} a_i \cdot 10^i \equiv \sum_{i=0}^{t} a_i \pmod{9}$$

PROOF. Clearly $10 \equiv 1 \pmod 9$. Then three applications of Corollary 6.43 yield the following three statements:

$$10^i \equiv 1 \pmod 9 \qquad \text{for all } i \geq 0$$
$$a_i \cdot 10^i \equiv a_i \pmod 9 \qquad \text{for } 0 \leq i \leq t$$
$$\sum_{i=0}^{t} a_i \cdot 10^i \equiv \sum_{i=0}^{t} a_i \pmod 9 \qquad \square$$

6.46 Corollary (Test for Divisibility by 9). An integer is a multiple of 9 if and only if the sum of its decimal digits is a multiple of 9.

PROOF OUTLINE. First notice that it suffices to check the assertion for *nonnegative* integers. Then verify the following statement:

(6.47) If $a \equiv b \pmod m$, then $m \mid a \Leftrightarrow m \mid b$.

Finally, apply 6.47 to the congruence in the statement of Theorem 6.45, with $m = 9$. $\square$

Now we can understand the idea underlying 6.44. Once we somehow produce a multiple of 9, we know that the sum of its digits is also a multiple of 9, as is each subsequent digital sum. Eventually we reach a one-digit nonzero multiple of 9, and that's 9.

It is a straightforward matter to extend these results on decimal representation of integers to results in other bases, as follows. If $b \geq 2$, writing an integer n **in the base b** means writing $n = a_t a_{t-1} \ldots a_0$ as an abbreviation for

$$n = \sum_{i=0}^{t} a_i b^i \quad \text{with } 0 \leq a_i \leq b - 1$$

Then the congruence in Theorem 6.45 generalizes to

$$\sum_{i=0}^{t} a_i b^i \equiv \sum_{i=0}^{t} a_i \pmod{b - 1}$$

by essentially the same argument. Corollary 6.46 extends to this: An integer is a multiple of $b - 1$ if and only if the sum of its digits in base b representation is a multiple of $b - 1$.

6.48 Theorem (Test for Divisibility by 11).   An integer n with decimal representation $n = a_t a_{t-1} \ldots a_0$ is divisible by 11 if and only if the number $a_t - a_{t-1} + a_{t-2} - \cdots \pm a_0$ is divisible by 11.

PROOF OUTLINE.   We are given that

$$n = \sum_{i=0}^{t} a_i \cdot 10^i$$

Starting with the congruence $10 \equiv -1 \pmod{11}$, we then proceed as in the proof of Theorem 6.45, but this time deducing the congruence

$$(*) \qquad \sum_{i=0}^{t} a_i \cdot 10^i \equiv \sum_{i=0}^{t} (-1)^i a_i \pmod{11}$$

Apply 6.47 (with $m = 11$) to $(*)$, and observe that the number $\sum_{i=0}^{t} (-1)^i a_i$ is equal to $\pm(a_t - a_{t-1} + a_{t-2} - \cdots \pm a_0)$. $\square$

6.49 EXAMPLE. The number 319,245,386,597,518,260 is divisible by 11, because the number

$$3 - 1 + 9 - 2 + 4 - 5 + 3 - 8 + 6 - 5 + 9 - 7 + 5 - 1 + 8 - 2 + 6 - 0 = 22$$

is divisible by 11.

Exercises

1. In each part answer *true* or *false*, without proof.
   (a) $-297 \equiv 533613 \pmod 5$
   (b) $a \equiv b \pmod m$ and $n \mid m \Rightarrow a \equiv b \pmod n$
   (c) $a \equiv b \pmod m$ and $m \mid n \Rightarrow a \equiv b \pmod n$
   (d) $a \equiv b \pmod m \Rightarrow a^2 \equiv b^2 \pmod{m^2}$
   (e) $a \equiv b \pmod m$ and $a \equiv b \pmod n \Rightarrow a \equiv b \pmod{(m, n)}$
   (f) $a \equiv b \pmod m$ and $a \equiv b \pmod n \Rightarrow a \equiv b \pmod{[m, n]}$
   (g) $a \equiv b \pmod m$ and $a \not\equiv b \pmod n \Rightarrow a \equiv b \pmod{mn}$
   (h) $(10^{50} - 1)^{12} \equiv 6 \pmod 3$

2. For which integers a and b is the statement $a \equiv b \pmod 1$ correct?

3. Prove that if n is an odd integer then $n^2 \equiv 1 \pmod 8$.

4. Prove that every integer n satisfies the congruence $n^3 \equiv n \pmod 6$.

5. Consider the integer $n = 12345678910111213 \ldots 100$. (The number is written by listing the positive integers from 1 to 100 without spaces between them.)
   (a) How many digits does n have?
   (b) Is n divisible by 9?

6. Prove statement 6.47.

7. In the country of Zzyzzx the clocks have eight-hour faces. Suppose it is now five o'clock in Zzyzzx. What time will it be in 4725 hours?

8. Suppose it is now 8 A.M. in Boston. What time of day will it be in Boston in 6538 hours? (Be sure to indicate whether the hour will be A.M. or P.M.)

9. An assortment of numbered tiles is assembled on a rack, forming an integer n, and the rack is placed on view in a local gallery. A clumsy visitor overturns the rack. He hurriedly gathers up the tiles and repositions them on the rack, producing an integer n'. Show that the difference between n and n' is divisible by 9.

10. (a) Show that if $(k, m) = 1$ then the following cancellation law holds:
$$ka \equiv kb \pmod m \quad \Rightarrow \quad a \equiv b \pmod m$$
    (b) Is the condition $(k, m) = 1$ in part (a) essential?

11. Let m be a positive integer.

   (a) Show that every integer is congruent modulo m to exactly one of the integers $0, 1, \ldots, m - 1$.

   (b) Suppose $(k, m) = 1$. Show that every integer is congruent modulo m to exactly one of the integers $0, k, 2k, \ldots, (m-1)k$. (Hint: Use Exercise 10(a).)

12. In each part, fill the blank with one or more numbers from the set $\{0, 1, \ldots, 7\}$, using the smallest number of elements that yields a true statement. Then prove the statement.

   (a) If n is the square of an even integer, then $n \equiv$ ____ (mod 8).

   (b) If n is the square of an odd integer, then $n \equiv$ ____ (mod 8).

13. (a) Use the results of Exercise 12 to show that the equation $98765487 = x^2 + y^2$ is not solvable in $\mathbb{Z}$.

   (b) Is the equation $78135 = x^2 + y^2 + z^2$ solvable in $\mathbb{Z}$?

   [*Historical note* (not needed for the solution of this exercise): In the eighteenth century it was shown by J. L. Lagrange that every positive integer can be expressed in the form $x^2 + y^2 + z^2 + w^2$ for some $x, y, z, w \in \mathbb{Z}$.]

14. Suppose n is a positive integer whose digits add to 24. Name a positive divisor of n other than 1 and n, and prove your claim.

15. (a) Let n be a positive integer. Prove that if $2^n - 1$ is prime, then n is prime.

   (b) Write the number $2^n - 1$ in binary (base 2) form.

16. Write the integer 35481 in base 7 notation. (Suggestion: Begin by finding the largest integer t such that $7^t \leq 35481$. Then find $a_t \in \mathbb{N}$ such that $35481 = a_t \cdot 7^t + r$, with $0 \leq r < 7^t$. The number a_t is the leftmost digit of the answer.)

17. (a) Describe a simple procedure for converting a number given in base 2 notation to base 4 notation. Your procedure should go directly from base 2 to base 4, without using decimal notation as an intermediate step.

   (b) Illustrate your method by converting the binary number

$$11101011011001101$$

   to base 4 notation.

18. Consider the following list of numbers:

$$1$$
$$12$$
$$123$$
$$\vdots$$
$$123456789$$
$$1234567891$$
$$12345678912$$
$$123456789123$$
$$\vdots$$

What is the first number on this list that is divisible by 11?

19. Design a simple procedure for testing whether an integer given in binary notation is divisible by 3, and justify your claim.

20. For a positive integer a, let $D(a)$ denote the integer obtained by taking the sum of a's digits, then taking the sum of the digits of *that* number, and continuing this process until a one-digit number is obtained. (We did this sort of thing in 6.44.) Show that

$$D(a + b) = D\big(D(a) + D(b)\big) \qquad \text{and} \qquad D(ab) = D\big(D(a) \cdot D(b)\big)$$

(Hint: Use Theorem 6.45.)

[The results of this exercise can be used to check computations with large integers. For instance, if computation seems to show that $ab = c$, then according to Exercise 20 we must have $D\big(D(a) \cdot D(b)\big) = D(c)$. Checking that this is the case will catch eight errors out of nine. (Think about why this is so.) This procedure of checking computations by replacing each integer by the sum of its digits is called **casting out nines**.]

6.5 Introduction to Euler's Function

Suppose we are given a positive integer m, and we want to determine whether m is prime or composite. How should we proceed? An initial answer might be this: We have to determine whether m is divisible by some positive integer strictly between 1 and m, and for this purpose it is enough to test for divisibility by *primes* up to $\sqrt{m}$. Just by looking at the right-most digit of m, we can see whether m is divisible by 2 or by 5. And m is divisible by 3 if and only if the sum of m's digits is divisible by 3. (The argument for this is the same as for the test for divisibility by 9 given in Corollary 6.46.) In general, if no special trick occurs to us, we can just divide m by larger and larger prime values up to $\sqrt{m}$ in the standard elementary school way, and see if we ever get a remainder of 0. If we never do, then m must be prime.

While the method described in the preceding paragraph is correct, we can easily see that if m is large, say a 50-digit number, then the process might take a *long* time. It turns out that the subject of "primality testing" has much more to it than this simple-minded and tedious process of repeated divisions. One of the goals of this section is to indicate a procedure that can sometimes demonstrate that a given integer is not prime without actually dredging up a prime divisor. For this purpose, we will now discuss a remarkable function that was first introduced by the great mathematician Leonhard Euler in 1760. *Throughout this section, all numbers will be understood to be integers.*

If $m > 0$, consider how many of the numbers $1, 2, \ldots, m$ are relatively prime to m. Let's label this quantity: define

$$\varphi(m) = \#\{k \in \mathbb{N}_m \mid (k, m) = 1\}$$

(Reminder: $\mathbb{N}_m = \{1, 2, \ldots, m\}$.) This function $\varphi \colon \mathbb{N} \to \mathbb{N}$ is known as *Euler's φ-function*. It is also known as the *totient* function. (Incidentally, φ is the Greek letter "phi.")

6.50 EXAMPLES. $\varphi(1) = 1$, $\varphi(p) = p - 1$ if p is prime; $\varphi(6) = 2$, because there are two numbers satisfying $1 \le k \le 6$ and $(k, 6) = 1$, namely, 1 and 5.

Euler's function turns out to be extremely useful, although many of its properties are shrouded in mystery and are the subject of ongoing research. Before confronting the abyss of the unknown, let's develop a few of the known properties of φ, starting with a theorem that is the key to φ's role in primality testing. In Section 6.6 we'll derive a formula for computing $\varphi(n)$ in terms of the standard factorization of n and explore other properties of this intriguing function.

6.51 Lemma.   (i) If $m \mid ab$ and $(a, b) = 1$, then $m \mid b$.

(ii) **(The Cancellation Law)** If $ax \equiv ay \pmod{m}$ and $(a, m) = 1$, then $x \equiv y \pmod{m}$.

PROOF.   (i) Since $m \mid ab$, we can write $ab = mc$. Then, because $(a, m) = 1$, Corollary 6.21 tells us that there are integers x, y such that $ax + my = 1$. So $b = abx + mby = m(cx + by)$, and therefore $m \mid b$ as claimed.

(ii) The condition $ax \equiv ay$ (mod m) yields $m \mid a(x - y)$. Then part (i) gives $m \mid x - y$; that is, $x \equiv y$ (mod m). □

6.52 Euler's Theorem. Suppose m is positive and $(x, m) = 1$. Then

$$x^{\varphi(m)} \equiv 1 \text{ (mod } m)$$

PROOF. Let $S = \{y \mid 1 \leq y \leq m \text{ and } (y, m) = 1\} = \{a_1, \ldots, a_{\varphi(m)}\}$. Then for each i satisfying $1 \leq i \leq \varphi(m)$, we have $(xa_i, m) = 1$. Why? Because from Theorem 6.26, any prime divisor of xa_i must divide either x or a_i, and both of them are given to be relatively prime to m. Also, from the division algorithm we can write $xa_i = mq + r \equiv r$ (mod m) for some r satisfying $0 \leq r < m$. Then, because $(xa_i, m) = 1$, we must have $(r, m) = 1$. (Be sure to check this point. What would happen if r and m had a common divisor bigger than 1?) Thus $r \in S$; that is, $r = a_j$ for some j. No two of the elements $a_1, \ldots, a_{\varphi(m)}$ are congruent mod m. Therefore, from the Cancellation Law (Lemma 6.51(ii)), it follows that if $1 \leq i_1, i_2 \leq \varphi(m)$ and $i_1 \neq i_2$, then $xa_{i_1} \not\equiv xa_{i_2}$ (mod m). (Here we use the hypothesis $(x, m) = 1$.) That is, the integers $xa_1, \ldots, xa_{\varphi(m)}$ are congruent mod m to different elements of S. So we have a system of $\varphi(m)$ congruences:

$$xa_1 \equiv a_{j_1} \text{ (mod } m)$$

$$xa_2 \equiv a_{j_2} \text{ (mod } m)$$

$$\vdots$$

$$xa_{\varphi(m)} \equiv a_{\varphi(m)} \text{ (mod } m)$$

where each $a_i \in S$ appears exactly once on each side of this list of congruences. Then, by Corollary 6.43, the product of all of these congruences is also a congruence, namely

$$x^{\varphi(m)} \cdot \prod_{i=1}^{\varphi(m)} a_i \equiv \prod_{i=1}^{\varphi(m)} a_i \text{ (mod } m)$$

But $\prod_1^{\varphi(m)} a_i$ is relatively prime to m because each a_i is. Therefore (again by the Cancellation Law) we have $x^{\varphi(m)} \equiv 1$ (mod m), as desired. □

6.53 Corollary (Fermat's Theorem). If p is prime and $(a, p) = 1$, then $a^{p-1} \equiv 1$ (mod p).

PROOF. This is the special case of Euler's theorem in which $m = p$, since $\varphi(p) = p - 1$. □

Now suppose we have a large number m whose primality we would like to investigate. In other words, we want to answer this question: *Is m a prime or isn't it?* If m's primality really is a mystery to us, presumably we have already checked (by glancing at its units digit) that m is odd. So Fermat's Theorem tells us that if m were actually prime, then we would have $2^{m-1} \equiv 1$ (mod m). Equivalently (taking the contrapositive): *if* $2^{m-1} \not\equiv 1$ (mod m), *then m is not prime*.

Assume $m > 0$. Then, from the division algorithm, we know that for every x there are unique integers q and r such that $x = mq + r$ and $0 < r \leq m - 1$. That is, there is a unique r such that $0 < r \leq m - 1$ and $x \equiv r$ (mod m). We call this number r the **residue of x modulo m**, sometimes denoted x (mod m). (Just as ashes are a fire's residue, the material left over after the burning has taken place, here the residue is what's left over after the largest multiple of m not exceeding x has been "burned off"—that is, subtracted.) We leave it for the reader to check that two given integers are congruent mod m if and only if they have the same residue mod m. In any congruence mod m, any integer can be replaced by its residue mod m, resulting in a congruence with the same truth value. Incidentally, replacing a number by its residue is often called **reduction mod m**.

Given integers a, b, m, and n, with m and n positive, how should we check the truth value of the congruence $a^n \equiv b$ (mod m) if n is large? First let's consider the special case in which n is a power of 2, say, $n = 2^k$. Then

$$a^n = a^{2^k} = a^{2 \cdot 2 \cdots 2} = (\cdots((a^2)^2)^2 \cdots)^2$$

with k squaring operations. In carrying out this sequence of squarings, whenever a number greater than or equal to m has been obtained, it can be replaced by its residue mod m. This reduction keeps the numbers at a manageable size. Thus, to find the residue 7^{16} (mod 11), we start with 7 and carry out successive couplings of squaring and reducing mod 11 until reaching the residue of 7^{16}:

$$7^2 = 49 \equiv 5 \pmod{11}$$

$$7^4 \equiv 5^2 \equiv 3 \pmod{11}$$

$$7^8 \equiv 3^2 \equiv 9 \pmod{11}$$

$$7^{16} \equiv 9^2 \equiv 4 \pmod{11}$$

So even though 7^{16} is a gigantic number, in computing its residue modulo 11 we never have to handle a number as big as 11^2.

Now if instead we want the residue of 7^{21} (mod 11), we can express the exponent 21 as a sum of powers of 2, getting $21 = 16 + 4 + 1$. Then $7^{21} = 7^{16} \cdot 7^4 \cdot 7$, so the residue of 7^{21} can be obtained by multiplying together the residues of 7^{16}, 7^4, and 7, and then taking the residue of that product.

6.54 EXAMPLE. Is 529 prime? (If you know the answer, pretend you don't.) Consider the congruence $2^{528} \equiv 1$ (mod 529). If we can show this congruence to be false then, by Euler's Theorem, we will have shown that 529 is not prime. We write 528 as a sum of 2-powers: $528 = 512 + 16 = 2^9 + 2^4$. (We get this decomposition by cranking out some powers of 2 and noticing that 512 is the largest 2-power not exceeding 528. Subtraction yields $528 - 512 = 16$, which is a 2-power, so we're done. Had the difference not been a 2-power, we would have found the largest 2-power less than that difference, subtracted, and continued the process.) So $2^{528} = 2^{2^9 + 2^4} = 2^{2^9} \cdot 2^{2^4}$. Recall that $2^{2^k} = (\cdots((2^2)^2)^2 \cdots)^2$, with k squarings. A session with a calculator (not essential, but certainly helpful) now yields

$$2^{2^3} = 256$$

$$2^{2^4} = (256)^2 = 65536 \equiv 469$$

$$2^{2^5} \equiv (469)^2 = 219961 \equiv 426$$

$$2^{2^6} \equiv (426)^2 = 181476 \equiv 29$$

$$2^{2^7} \equiv (29)^2 = 841 \equiv 312$$

$$2^{2^8} \equiv (312)^2 = 97344 \equiv 8$$

$$2^{2^9} \equiv 8^2 = 64$$

where all congruences are mod 529. This gives

$$2^{528} = 2^{2^9} \cdot 2^{2^4} \equiv 64 \cdot 469 = 30016 \equiv 392 \not\equiv 1 \pmod{529}$$

and so 529 is composite.

Some readers will complain, "But I've known for years that $529 = (23)^2$, so who needs all these congruences?" The answer comes by noticing that the approach to proving that m is composite by Euler's theorem uses roughly $\log_2 m$ squaring-and-reducing steps when m is large. But

$$m = 10^{\log_{10} m} = (2^{\log_2 10})^{\log_{10} m} = 2^{(\log_2 10)(\log_{10} m)}$$

Therefore

$$\log_2 m = (\log_2 10)(\log_{10} m)$$

$$\approx 3.32 \log_{10} m$$

$$\approx 3.32 \times (\#\{\text{decimal digits in } m\} - 1)$$

Thus if m has 50 digits, it may be possible to use Euler's Theorem to show that m is composite in about 165 squaring-and-reducing steps, whereas the elementary school approach might require testing m for divisibility by all the primes up to $\sqrt{m} \approx 10^{25}$. In real life, most serious and extensive numerical calculations are done on computers, where 165 squaring-and-reducing procedures can be done practically instantaneously. But 10^{25} operations exceeds the lifetime work expectancy of even the fastest computers.

6.55 Remark. Let's be clear about the logic. We have seen that the condition $2^{m-1} \equiv 1 \pmod{m}$ is *necessary* in order for m to be prime. We have not claimed that it is also *sufficient*. In fact, the statement

$$2^{m-1} \equiv 1 \pmod{m} \quad \Rightarrow \quad m \text{ is prime}$$

is *false*. For example, it can be shown that $2^{340} \equiv 1 \pmod{341}$, yet 341 is not prime: $341 = 11 \cdot 31$.

Exercises

1. (a) Use the *definition* of Euler's function to evaluate $\varphi(9)$, $\varphi(20)$, and $\varphi(37)$.
   (b) If p is prime and $k \geq 1$, determine $\varphi(p^k)$.

2. Assume that $m \in \mathbb{N}$. Call a set $S \subseteq \mathbb{Z}$ a **complete system of residues mod m** if every integer is congruent mod m to exactly one element of S.
   (a) Show that the set $\{0, \ldots, m - 1\}$ is a complete system of residues mod m.
   (b) Show that if S is any complete system of residues mod m, then $\#S = m$.

3. (a) Prove that if $p > 1$ and p is a divisor of $(p - 1)! + 1$, then p is prime. (Suggestion: Argue by contradiction.)
   (b) Do you feel that the result in part (a) yields a valuable method of testing for primes? Explain.

4. (a) Assume that $m \neq 0$. Use Corollary 6.21 to prove that if $(a, m) = 1$, then the congruence $ax \equiv 1 \pmod{m}$ is solvable. (That is, there is an integer x for which the congruence is true.)

   (b) Give a second proof of the result in part (a) using Euler's Theorem.

   (c) Under the conditions in part (a), prove that if $b \in \mathbb{Z}$, then the congruence $ax \equiv b \pmod{m}$ is solvable.

   (d) Prove that if x_1 and x_2 are both solutions of (b), then $x_1 \equiv x_2 \pmod{m}$.

5. Verify the claim (in Remark 6.55) that $2^{340} \equiv 1 \pmod{341}$.

6. (a) Write down the conclusion of Euler's theorem when $x = 12$ and $m = 17$.

   (b) Use the answer to part (a) to determine the residue of $12^{482} \pmod{17}$ using only a very short computation.

7. (a) Write the number 683 as a sum of powers of 2, using the smallest possible number of terms.

   (b) Show that the answer to part (a) immediately yields the binary (i.e., base 2) representation of 683.

8. (a) Prove that if p is prime and $a \in \mathbb{Z}$, then $a^p \equiv a \pmod{p}$.

   (b) Deduce from part (a) that if p is prime and $a, b \in \mathbb{Z}$, then $(a + b)^p \equiv a^p + b^p \pmod{p}$.

9. (a) Prove that if $a \equiv b \pmod{m_1}$ and $a \equiv b \pmod{m_2}$ and $(m_1, m_2) = 1$, then $a \equiv b \pmod{m_1 m_2}$.

   (b) Use Fermat's Theorem, Exercise 8(a), and part (a) of this exercise to prove that every integer x satisfies the congruence $x^5 \equiv x \pmod{10}$.

   (c) What does the result in part (b) say about the decimal representations of x^5 and x?

10. Obtain a formula for $\log_2 3$ in terms of logs to the base 10.

11. Use Fermat's Theorem to prove that if p is an odd prime, then p is a divisor of $2 + 2^{p-1} + \cdots + (p - 1)^{p-1}$.

6.6 The Inclusion–Exclusion Principle, and Further Properties of Euler's Function

Our first goal in this section is to derive a formula for $\varphi(n)$ in terms of the standard factorization of n. Then we'll use this formula to develop further properties of φ. At the end of the section we will state some unsolved research problems involving this important and mysterious function.

As a preliminary step, we first need to extend a counting result from Chapter 4. Given n finite sets $A_1, \ldots, A_n$ of known size, how many elements are in the union $\bigcup_1^n A_i$? We obtained such a formula when $n = 2$ in Corollary 4.16, and that result will be crucial in what follows. Let's first consider the case $n = 3$, and this will suggest the pattern that will hold in general. In what follows, $|X|$ denotes the number of elements in the set X. So in this notation, Corollary 4.16 becomes $|A \cup B| = |A| + |B| - |A \cap B|$. We have

$$\left| \bigcup_{i=1}^{3} A_i \right| = |(A_1 \cup A_2) \cup A_3|$$

$$= |A_1 \cup A_2| + |A_3| - |(A_1 \cup A_2) \cap A_3| \qquad \text{(by application of 4.16)}$$

$$= |A_1 \cup A_2| + |A_3| - |(A_1 \cap A_3) \cup (A_2 \cap A_3)|$$

$$= |A_1| + |A_2| - |A_1 \cap A_2| + |A_3|$$

$$\quad - (|A_1 \cap A_3| + |A_2 \cap A_3| - |A_1 \cap A_2 \cap A_3|)$$

$$\text{(by two more applications of 4.16)}$$

$$= |A_1| + |A_2| + |A_3| - (|A_1 \cap A_2| + |A_1 \cap A_3| + |A_2 \cap A_3|)$$

$$\quad + |A_1 \cap A_2 \cap A_3|$$

$$= \sum_{i=1}^{3} |A_i| - \left(\sum_{1 \le i < j \le 3} |A_i \cap A_j| \right) + |A_1 \cap A_2 \cap A_3|$$

Let's consider the intuition behind this formula. To count the number of elements in the union of three sets, we first add the cardinalities of the individual sets; this is the sum $\sum_{i=1}^{3} |A_i|$. Then, upon realizing that elements appearing simultaneously in two different A_i have been *included* more than once in the total, we subtract $\left(\sum_{i \le i < j \le 3} |A_i \cap A_j| \right)$ to eliminate or *exclude* each such redundancy. Finally, we observe that the elements occurring simultaneously in all three A_i were each included three times in the counting represented by the first part of the formula, then they were excluded three times in the middle part of the formula, so up to here they weren't really counted at all. So we add back in (or *include*) the number of such elements, and that's the expression $|A_1 \cap A_2 \cap A_3|$ added at the end of the formula.

It is now reasonable to hope that when n is unrestricted, the number of elements in the union of n sets can be found by a similar alternation of inclusions and exclusions. In fact, this can be proven by mathematical induction on n. The details are tedious, and we omit them. But just as the result when $n = 3$ follows from the case $n = 2$, the result for $n = k + 1$ follows from the case $n = k$ in the induction argument, with the linkage being the case $n = 2$.

6.56 Theorem. Let $A_1, \ldots, A_n$ be sets. Then

$$\left| \bigcup_{i=1}^{n} A_i \right| = \sum_{i=1}^{n} |A_i| - \left(\sum_{1 \le i_1 < i_2 \le n} |A_{i_1} \cap A_{i_2}| \right) + \left(\sum_{1 \le i_1 < i_2 < i_3 \le n} |A_{i_1} \cap A_{i_2} \cap A_{i_3}| \right)$$

$$- \cdots + (-1)^{n+1} |A_1 \cap \cdots \cap A_n|$$

6.57 Corollary (Inclusion–Exclusion Principle). Let S be a finite set and suppose $A_1, \ldots, A_n$ are subsets of S. Define $S_0 = |S|$ and, for $1 \le k \le n$, define

$$S_k = \sum_{1 \le i_1 < \cdots < i_k \le n} |A_{i_1} \cap \cdots \cap A_{i_k}|$$

Then

$$|A_1' \cap A_2' \cap \cdots \cap A_n'| = \sum_{k=0}^{n} (-1)^k S_k$$

(Recall that A_i' is the complement of A_i in S.)

PROOF OUTLINE. Check that $A_1' \cap A_2' \cap \cdots \cap A_n' = S - \left(\bigcup_{i=1}^{n} A_i \right)$, hence that

$$|A_1' \cap A_2' \cap \cdots \cap A_n'| = |S| - \left| \bigcup_{i=1}^{n} A_i \right|$$

The result now follows from Theorem 6.56. $\square$

6.58 EXAMPLE. A sports club has 54 members. Of those, 34 play tennis, 22 play golf, and 10 play both. Eleven members play handball and, of those, 6 play tennis, 4 play golf, and 2 play all three sports. How many club members participate in *none* of the sports?

SOLUTION. Fix three sets A_i, each consisting of the club members who play one of the three sports. Taking S to be the set of all club members, the inclusion–exclusion principle gives

$$|A_1' \cap A_2' \cap A_3'| = 54 - (34 + 22 + 11) + (10 + 6 + 4) - 2 = 5$$

Thus five members play no sports.

Suggestion. Draw a Venn diagram corresponding to this example, with three interlocking circles, one for each A_i, sitting inside a rectangle (corresponding to the set of all club members); label each region in the diagram with the number of elements in that region.

Now suppose n has standard factorization $n = p_1^{\alpha_1} \cdots p_r^{\alpha_r}$, and let's derive a formula for $\varphi(n)$.

An integer m is relatively prime to n if and only if m is not divisible by any of $p_1, \ldots, p_r$. Let $A_i = \{m \in \mathbb{N}_n \mid p_i \mid m\}$. Then

$$\varphi(n) = |A_1' \cap \cdots \cap A_r'|$$

and this restatement of the value of $\varphi(n)$ virtually *pleads* with us to use the inclusion–exclusion principle. First note that if k is a positive integer and $k \mid n$, then there are precisely n/k positive multiples of k not exceeding n, namely, $k, 2k, 3k, \ldots, n \ (= \frac{n}{k} \cdot k)$. In particular, we have

$$|A_i| = \frac{n}{p_i}$$

$$|A_{i_1} \cap A_{i_2}| = \frac{n}{p_{i_1} p_{i_2}}$$

$$|A_{i_1} \cap A_{i_2} \cap A_{i_3}| = \frac{n}{p_{i_1} p_{i_2} p_{i_3}}$$

and so on. From this the inclusion–exclusion principle gives us

$$\varphi(n) = n - \sum_i \frac{n}{p_i} + \sum_{i_1 < i_2} \frac{n}{p_{i_1} p_{i_2}} - \sum_{i_1 < i_2 < i_3} \frac{n}{p_{i_1} p_{i_2} p_{i_3}} + \cdots + (-1)^r \frac{n}{p_1 \cdots p_r}$$

$$= n \left(1 - \sum_i \frac{1}{p_i} + \sum_{i_1 < i_2} \frac{1}{p_{i_1} p_{i_2}} - \sum_{i_1 < i_2 < i_3} \frac{1}{p_{i_1} p_{i_2} p_{i_3}} + \cdots + (-1)^r \frac{1}{p_1 \cdots p_r} \right)$$

$$= n \left(1 - \frac{1}{p_1} \right) \left(1 - \frac{1}{p_2} \right) \cdots \left(1 - \frac{1}{p_r} \right)$$

(Note: A really careful proof of the last equality requires mathematical induction.)

Let's state this important result, along with an immediate consequence, in the form of a theorem.

6.59 Theorem. If n has standard factorization $p_1^{\alpha_1} \cdots p_r^{\alpha_r}$, then

$$\varphi(n) = n \prod_{1 \leq i \leq r} \left(1 - \frac{1}{p_i}\right) = n \prod_{1 \leq i \leq r} \left(\frac{p_i - 1}{p_i}\right) = \prod_{1 \leq i \leq r} p_i^{\alpha_i - 1} \prod_{1 \leq i \leq r} (p_i - 1)$$

Moreover:

$$\text{If } (m, n) = 1 \text{ then } \varphi(mn) = \varphi(m)\varphi(n).$$

PROOF. The first statement follows from the preceding paragraph and the fact that $n = p_1^{\alpha_1} \cdots p_r^{\alpha_r}$. For the second, suppose $m = q_1^{\beta_1} \cdots q_s^{\beta_s}$. Since $(m, n) = 1$, the primes $p_1, \ldots, p_r, q_1, \ldots, q_s$ are distinct, so the result follows from the first equation in the first statement. $\square$

6.60 Corollary. If p is prime and $k \geq 1$, then $\varphi(p^k) = p^{k-1}(p - 1) = p^k - p^{k-1}$.

6.61 EXAMPLE.

$$\varphi(280500) = \varphi(2^2 \cdot 3 \cdot 5^3 \cdot 11 \cdot 17) = 2 \cdot 3^0 \cdot 5^2 \cdot 11^0 \cdot 17^0 \cdot 1 \cdot 2 \cdot 4 \cdot 10 \cdot 16 = 64000$$

To appreciate our formula for $\varphi(n)$, imagine computing $\varphi(280500)$ directly from the definition of φ: we would have had to factor all the positive integers up to 280500 into primes, eliminate those that share one or more prime divisors with 280500, and, finally, count the numbers that remain. That final list of numbers to be counted would have had 64000 entries!!

Here is a table displaying the first few values of $\varphi(n)$.

n	1	2	3	4	5	6	7	8	9	10	11	12	13	14	15	16	17	18	19	20	21	22
$\varphi(n)$	1	1	2	2	4	2	6	4	6	4	10	4	12	6	8	8	16	6	18	8	12	10

This table suggests a few possible properties of $\varphi(n)$. For example, it appears that $\varphi(n)$ is even when $n > 2$, that every positive even integer is in the range of φ and in fact is equal to $\varphi(n)$ for at least two values of n, and that $\varphi(n)$ tends to grow, though perhaps erratically, as n grows. Let's pursue these thoughts.

6.62 Theorem. If $n > 2$ then $\varphi(n)$ is even.

PROOF. First suppose n is a 2-power (that is, a power of 2). Say $n = 2^k$, with $k \geq 2$. Then $\varphi(n) = 2^k(1 - \frac{1}{2}) = 2^{k-1}$.

If n is not a 2-power then $n = p^k m$ for some odd prime p, with $k \geq 1$ and $(p, m) = 1$. Then

$$\varphi(n) = \varphi(p^k)\varphi(m) = (p^k - p^{k-1})\varphi(m) = p^{k-1}(p - 1)\varphi(m)$$

But this value is even because p is odd.   □

6.63 Theorem. If n is a positive integer, then $\varphi(n) \geq \frac{\sqrt{n}}{2}$. (Hence, in the language of calculus, $\lim_{n \to \infty} \varphi(n) = \infty$.)

PROOF. The result is clear if $n = 1$, and if n is a 2-power it follows from the proof of Theorem 6.62. Now suppose $n > 1$, with n not a 2-power; say n has standard factorization $n = 2^{\alpha_0} p_1^{\alpha_1} \cdots p_r^{\alpha_r}$, with $\alpha_0 \geq 0$ and $\alpha_i \geq 1$ for $1 \leq i \leq r$. Then

$$\begin{aligned}
\varphi(n) &= 2^{\alpha_0 - 1} p_1^{\alpha_1 - 1} \cdots p_r^{\alpha_r - 1}(p_1 - 1) \cdots (p_r - 1) \\
&\geq 2^{\alpha_0 - 1} p_1^{\alpha_1 - \frac{1}{2}} \cdots p_r^{\alpha_r - \frac{1}{2}} \quad \text{(Here use the fact that } p_i - 1 > \sqrt{p_i}.) \\
&\geq 2^{\alpha_0 - 1} p_1^{\frac{1}{2}\alpha_1} \cdots p_r^{\frac{1}{2}\alpha_r} \quad \text{(Because } \alpha_i - \frac{1}{2} \geq \frac{1}{2}\alpha_i.) \\
&\geq 2^{\frac{\alpha_0}{2} - 1} p_1^{\frac{1}{2}\alpha_1} \cdots p_r^{\frac{1}{2}\alpha_r} = \frac{1}{2}\sqrt{n} \quad \square
\end{aligned}$$

Our little table displaying the initial values of φ suggests that every positive even integer is in the range of φ. The following result kills this dream once and for all.

6.64 Theorem. If $m = 2 \cdot 5^{2k}$, with $k \in \mathbb{N}$, then there is no integer n such that $\varphi(n) = m$.

PROOF. Suppose, to the contrary, that there is such an n; and let's suppose that n then has standard factorization $n = p_1^{\alpha_1} \cdots p_r^{\alpha_r}$. So $\varphi(n) = p_1^{\alpha_1 - 1} \cdots p_r^{\alpha_r - 1}(p_1 - 1) \cdots (p_r - 1)$. In this formula, each of the numbers $p_i - 1$ corresponding to an odd prime p_i is even, and hence introduces at least one 2 into the standard factorization of $\varphi(n)$. But the prime 2 occurs just *once* in the standard factorization $\varphi(n) = 2 \cdot 5^{2k}$, so n must have at most one odd prime divisor p. Moreover n cannot be a 2-power, since otherwise $\varphi(n)$ would also be a 2-power by the proof of Theorem 6.62. Thus we can write $n = 2^{\alpha} p^{\beta}$, where $\alpha \in \{0, 1\}$ and $\beta \in \mathbb{N}$. This leads to

$$\varphi(n) = \varphi(2^{\alpha} p^{\beta}) = \varphi(2^{\alpha})\varphi(p^{\beta}) = \varphi(p^{\beta}) = p^{\beta-1}(p - 1) = 2 \cdot 5^{2k}$$

Our proof will be complete if we can show this equation to be an impossibility. First consider the value of β. If $\beta > 1$ then $p = 5$ and hence $p - 1 = 4$, contradicting the equation. Therefore we must have $\beta = 1$ and hence $\varphi(n) = p - 1 = 2 \cdot 5^{2k}$. That is, $p = 1 + 2 \cdot 5^{2k}$. But $5^{2k} = (5^2)^k \equiv 1 \pmod{3}$, so $2 \cdot 5^{2k} \equiv 2 \pmod{3}$. Therefore $p = 1 + 2 \cdot 5^{2k} \equiv 0 \pmod{3}$; in other words, $3 \mid p$. But p is prime, and therefore $p = 3$. Thus $n = 2^{\alpha} \cdot 3$, and so n is either 3 or 6. But this contradicts our assumption that $\varphi(n) = m = 2 \cdot 5^{2k}$. □

We have now scratched the surface of Euler's φ-function, demonstrating some basic properties and indicating its role in primality testing. But there remain mysteries about φ that are the subject of ongoing research. Here, briefly, are some samples. You may enjoy trying your hand at them. Remember: the toys in your playpen were different from everyone else's toys, and so your view of the world is not the same as anyone else's. You may notice something that everyone else has missed. Good luck!

6.65 Research Questions. (1) The bottom row of our table of values for $\varphi(n)$ has a lot of repetition. So, while Theorems 6.62 and 6.64 show that many natural numbers are not in the image of φ, the data suggests that every element in the range of φ has at least two elements in its pre-image. That is, it is reasonable for us to believe that if $\varphi(n) = k$, then also $\varphi(n') = k$ for some $n' \neq n$. (Incidentally, a table of values for $\varphi(n)$ for the first many thousands of values of n supports this belief.) In 1907 the mathematician Robert Carmichael published a paper claiming to have proved this result. Years later a flaw was found in his proof, so that in 1922 Carmichael blushingly published another paper, beginning, "Two correspondents have recently called my attention to the fact that the supposed proof of the following theorem, which I gave some years ago, is not adequate . . . ." So Carmichael's "theorem" was downgraded to Carmichael's *conjecture*. To this day the problem remains open, though in 1947 Victor Klee showed that if there exists an n for which Carmichael's conjecture is false, then $n > 10^{400}$.

(2) Our table for φ shows three values of n for which $\varphi(n) = \varphi(n + 1)$. In fact, it is known that for $n \leq 2 \cdot 10^8$, there are exactly 391 such numbers n. *Question:* Are there infinitely many n for which $\varphi(n) = \varphi(n + 1)$?

(3) If p is prime then $\varphi(p) = p - 1$, and consequently $\varphi(p) \mid p - 1$. *Question:* Are there any *composite* n for which $\varphi(n) \mid n - 1$? (Incidentally, it is known which n have the property that $\varphi(n) \mid n$. These n are the powers of 2 and the numbers of the form $2^r 3^s$, where $r, s \in \mathbb{N}$. This was shown by Sierpiński in 1959.)

Exercises

1. Compute $\varphi(360)$ and $\varphi(7056)$.

2. How many positive integers ≤ 600 are *not* relatively prime to 600?

3. Show that if $m \mid n$ then $\varphi(m) \mid \varphi(n)$.

4. For which integers n is it true that $\varphi(n) = \varphi(2n)$? Prove your claim.

5. A function $f: \mathbb{N} \to \mathbb{N}$ is said to be **multiplicative** if $f(ab) = f(a)f(b)$ whenever $(a, b) = 1$. And f is **completely multiplicative** if $f(ab) = f(a)f(b)$ for all $a, b \in \mathbb{N}$. From Theorem 6.59 we know that φ is multiplicative. Is φ *completely* multiplicative?

6. Suppose every prime divisor of m divides n. Obtain an equation relating $\varphi(n)$ and $\varphi(mn)$.

7. Show that if p is prime then $\sum_{i=0}^{r} \varphi(p^i) = p^r$.

8. Let $f: \mathbb{N} \to \mathbb{N}$ be a multiplicative function. (See the definition in Exercise 5.)

   (a) Show that f is completely determined by the values $f(p^\alpha)$, where p is prime and $\alpha \geq 0$.

   (b) By the notation $\sum_{d \mid n} f(d)$ we will mean the sum of the values of f on the *positive* divisors of n. (This is a standard notation in number theory.) Show that if $n = p_1^{\alpha_1} \cdots p_r^{\alpha_r}$, then

   $$\sum_{d \mid n} f(d) = \prod_{i=1}^{r} \left(\sum_{\beta_i = 0}^{\alpha_i} f(p_i^{\beta_i}) \right)$$

   (Suggestion: Begin by writing out the right-hand expression in complete detail in the case $n = 60$.)

   (c) Verify that $\sum_{d \mid 12} \varphi(d) = 12$.

   (d) Use part (b) to prove that $\sum_{d \mid n} \varphi(d) = n$ for every $n \in \mathbb{N}$. (Suggestion: To make the meaning of this statement concrete, first check it in the explicit case when $n = 12$.)

9. Recall the definition of the **greatest integer function**, from Example 3.8(b).

(a) Suppose $1 \le t \le n$. Show that exactly $[\frac{n}{t}]$ of the numbers in $\mathbb{N}_n$ are divisible by t. (Hint: Start by using the division algorithm to write $n = qt + r$, with $0 \le r \le t$.)

(b) How many integers from the set $\{1, \ldots, 1000\}$ are divisible by *none* of 5, 6, 8? (Hint: For $k \in \{5, 6, 8\}$, let $A_k = \{m \in \mathbb{N}_{100} \mid k \mid n\}$. Then use part (a) and the Inclusion–Exclusion Principle.)

10. A *derangement* of $\{1, \ldots, n\}$ is a permutation of $\sigma \in S_n$ that leaves no element fixed; that is, for all i we have $\sigma(i) \ne i$.

(a) How many derangements are there of the set $\{1, \ldots, 6\}$? (Suggestion: Use Inclusion–Exclusion, with A_i the set of permutations that fix i.)

(b) Obtain a formula for the number of derangements of $\{1, \ldots, n\}$.

HINTS AND PARTIAL SOLUTIONS TO SELECTED ODD-NUMBERED EXERCISES

SECTION 1.1

1. (a) false proposition (b) not a proposition (c) false proposition
   (d) not a proposition (e) not a proposition (f) true proposition

3. *Theorem.* madam
   Proof.   S
             mSm
            maSam
            madam

5. Without further discussion, "hence" is not truth functional. Consider

   (a) *Spinach is a vegetable, hence there is at least one green vegetable.*

   (b) *Spinach is a vegetable, hence Mars is a planet.*

   Both are sentences of the form "*true sentence*, hence *true sentence*." Most people would agree that (a) is true; but they would be reluctant to assign a truth value to (b), since "hence" suggests an evident linkage (missing in this example) between the components it connects.

SECTIONS 1.2 and 1.3

1. (a) $\sim P \wedge \sim Q$: Howard did not fall and Howard did not break his leg.
   $Q \vee \sim P$: Howard broke his leg or Howard did not fall.

3.

P	Q	$P\underline{\vee}Q$
F	F	F
F	T	T
T	F	T
T	T	F

5. The cards with the following markings need not be turned over: C, 2.

7. Let P denote the statement "I go to the movies in the afternoon," and let Q denote "It is rainy."
   (a) $Q \Rightarrow P$ (b) $P \Rightarrow Q$

9. (b) P: Napoleon is President of the United States.
       Q: Boston is a city.

11. (b)

P	$P \Rightarrow P$	$P \Rightarrow (P \Rightarrow P)$
F	T	T
T	T	T

13. 122

15. The new table has eight times as many rows as the old one.

17. $\sim(P \wedge \sim(\sim(Q \wedge \sim(\sim(R \wedge \sim S)))))$

19. The statements are equivalent since they have the same truth value (namely, *false*).

SECTION 1.4

1. Represent the statements "Dracula seizes power," "democracy is lost," "the use of food additives increases," and "mutations can be expected" by the letters P, Q, R, and S, respectively. Since we are given that P and $P \Rightarrow Q$ are both true, it follows by modus ponens that Q is true. From that and the given truth of $Q \Rightarrow R$, modus ponens yields the truth of R. Continue the argument in this way.

3. (c) I must prove that there exist a point P and a line L such that G consists of all the points that are equidistant from P and L.

5. Try a proof by contradiction. If 5 is *not* prime then (by definition of *prime*) 5 can be written in the form $a \cdot b$ for some integers a, b strictly between 1 and 5. Check that that is *not* the case.

7. Compare a side of the diamond to a radius of the circle, and use the fact that all radii of a given circle have the same length.

SECTION 1.5

1. Statement forms (a), (b), and (d) are tautologies, but (c) is not.

3. (a) $\sim((P \wedge Q) \wedge \sim R)$ (b) $\sim(\sim P \wedge \sim Q)$

5. $\sim P$: $P \downarrow P$; $P \wedge Q$: $(P \downarrow Q) \downarrow (P \downarrow Q)$

7. Use the fact that $(R \vee \sim R)$ is a tautology to deduce that the given expression is logically equivalent to $(P \wedge Q) \vee (P \wedge \sim Q)$, then contract this further using a distributive law. Finally, conclude that the given expression is logically equivalent to P.

SECTION 1.6

1. (a)

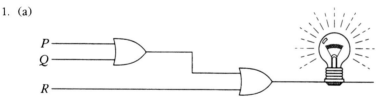

SECTION 2.1

1. yes

3. (a) $\{2, 3, 5\}$ (b) $\{2, 3, 5, 7\}$ (c) $\{1, 2, 3\}$ (d) $\{\pm 1, \pm 2, \pm 3, \pm 4\}$

5. (a) true (b) true (c) false (d) false (e) false (f) false
   (g) true (h) false (i) true (j) false

7. (a) $A = \emptyset$, $B = \{\emptyset\}$, $C = \{\{\emptyset\}\}$
   (b) $A = \emptyset$, $B = \{\emptyset\}$, $C = \{\emptyset, \{\emptyset\}\}$

SECTION 2.3

1. (a) $(\exists x)(x \in \mathbb{N} \wedge x^3 + 15 = 22)$ (c) $\sim(\forall x \in \mathbb{R})(\exists y \in \mathbb{R})(y^2 = x)$
   (e) $(\forall x \in \mathbb{R})(\exists! y \in \mathbb{R})(y^3 = x)$

3. (a) With $A = \emptyset$, statements 2(a) and 2(b) are both true.
   (b) There is no set A for which the *hypothesis* of 2(b) is true, so for every set A, *statement* 2(b) is true.

5. (a) $(\forall \epsilon > 0)(\exists \delta > 0)(|x' - x| < \delta \Rightarrow |f(x') - f(x)| < \epsilon)$

7. P: $x^2 = 5$; Q: $x = 17$

9. (a) true (c) true (e) false (g) true

SECTION 2.4

1. (b) The subsets are $\emptyset$, $\{1\}$, $\{\{2, 3\}\}$, and B.

3. (a) $\{2, -1\}$ (c) $\{2, 7\}$ (e) $S = \{-2, -1, 0, 1, 2, \{1, 2\}\}$

5. Suppose $\{a\} \subseteq S$. Then every member of $\{a\}$ is a member of S. But the only member of $\{a\}$ is a. This shows that $a \in S$, verifying "$\Rightarrow$".

7. (a) The left-hand set is equal to $\{1, 2\}$, and $1 = 2^0$ and $2 = 2^1$.

9. Let $A = \{1\}$ and $B = \{1, \{1\}\}$.

SECTION 2.5

1. (a) $\{1, 2\}$ (c) $\{3, 4, 5\}$ (e) the set of all the even integers except for 4 and 6; in symbols: $\{0, \pm 2, -4, -6, \pm 8, \pm 10, \pm 12, \ldots\}$ (g) the members are 3, 5, and all the even integers: $\{3, 5, 0, \pm 2, \pm 4, \pm 6, \ldots\}$
   (i) $\emptyset$.

3. (a) false (b) true

5. (a) Observe that for any element x the statement $x \in A$ is equivalent to the statement

$$x \in A \vee x \in \emptyset.$$

(c) First note that $A - A = \emptyset$, because no element satisfies "$x \in A \wedge x \notin A$." Then check that $\emptyset - A = \emptyset$.

(e) For every element x, the statements "$x \in A \wedge x \in A$" and "$x \in A$" are equivalent.

7. (a) Every element of $A - B$ is an element of A, but no element of $B - A$ is. Therefore the given intersection contains no elements.

9. Let $z \in Z$. From the hypothesis we then have $z \in X$ and $z \in Y$, as desired.

11. (a) For every element x, the statements

$$x \in A \vee x \in B \quad \text{and} \quad x \in B \vee x \in A$$

are equivalent. Therefore $A \cup B = B \cup A$. This proves that $A + B = B + A$. Proof of $AB = BA$ is similar, using intersection instead of union.

(c) We have $AB = A \iff A \cap B = A \iff B \supseteq A$. Thus the sets B satisfying the given condition are the sets that contain A.

(e) To prove "$\Leftarrow$", check that the statements "$x \in A$" and "$x \in A \vee x \in \emptyset$" have the same truth value. For "$\Rightarrow$", check that if X contains some element w, and A is a set not containing w, then $A + X \neq A$.

SECTION 2.6

1. (a) $\{1, 2, 3, 4, 0, -1\}$ (b) $\{1\}$ (c) $\mathbb{Z} - \{1\}$ (d) $\mathbb{Z} - \{-1, 0, 1, 2, 3, 4\}$

3. Let $x \in \cup A_i$. Then, by definition of union, $x \in A_i$ for some $i \in I$. But A_i is given to be a subset of A_n, so $x \in A_n$. This proves "$\subseteq$". Conversely, if $x \in A_n$ then since $n \in I$, we have that x is a member of $\cup A_i$, from the definition of union.

5. (a) $\mathbb{R}$ (b) $\{0\}$ (c) $[-5, 5]$

7. Proof of "$\subseteq$":

$$x \in A - \cup B_i \implies x \in A \quad \text{and} \quad x \notin \cup B_i$$

$$\implies x \in A \text{ and there is no } i \in I \text{ such that } x \in B_i$$

$$\implies x \in A - B_i \text{ for each } i \in I$$

$$\implies x \in \cap(A - B_i)$$

9. (a) union: $\mathbb{R}$; intersection: $\emptyset$ (b) union: the set of all points in the plane whose horizontal coordinate x satisfies the inequality $-1 \leq x \leq 1$; intersection: $\emptyset$ (d) union: Π; intersection: $\emptyset$

SECTION 2.7

1. (a) $\{\emptyset, \{4\}\}$ (b) $\{\emptyset, \{5\}, \{6\}, \{5, 6\}\}$

3. 127

5. $X \in P(A) \Rightarrow X \subseteq A \Rightarrow X \subseteq A \subseteq B \Rightarrow X \subseteq B \Rightarrow X \in P(B)$. This proves "$\subseteq$".

7. $A \cap B = \emptyset$

SECTION 2.8

1. (a) Associate the ordered pair (t, r) with an incoming call to room r on telephone line t.

   (b) The subset is a collection of four ordered pairs in $T \times R$, no two of which have the same first coordinate or same second coordinate.

3. "⇒". Let $A \times B = \emptyset$. If $A \neq \emptyset$ and $B \neq \emptyset$, let $a \in A$ and $b \in B$. Then $(a, b) \in A \times B$, contradicting the assumption that $A \times B = \emptyset$. Therefore, the assumption "$A \neq \emptyset$ and $B \neq \emptyset$" is false. That is, $A = \emptyset$ or $B = \emptyset$.

5. (a) Let $S = \{(1, 2), (2, 3)\}$. If $S = A \times B$, then $1, 2 \in A$ and $2, 3 \in B$. But then $(1, 3) \in S$, a contradiction.

9. "⊆": Let $P \in (\cup A_i) \times S$. Then $P = (a, b)$ for some $a \in \cup A_i$ and some $b \in S$. Thus $a \in A_i$ for some $i \in I$, by definition of $\cup A_i$, hence $P \in A_i \times S$, and so $P \in \cup (A_i \times S)$.

SECTION 2.9

1. (a) {the set of negative real numbers, the set of nonnegative real numbers}; {the set of nonzero real numbers, $\{0\}$}; {the set of nonnegative rational numbers, the set of negative rational numbers, the set of irrational numbers}

3. (a) false   (b) false   (c) true   (d) false

5. (a) $\Pi_1 = \{\{1\}, \{2\}, \{3\}, \{4\}, \{5, 6\}\}$; $\Pi_2 = \{\{1, 2\}, \{3, 4\}, \{5, 6\}\}$;
   $\Pi_3 = \{\{1, 2, 3, 4\}, \{5, 6\}\}$; $\Pi_4 = \{\{1, 2, 3, 4, 5, 6\}\}$.

7. $R \cup \{(1, 1), (2, 2), (3, 3), (4, 4)\}$

9. $R \cup \{(1, 1), (4, 2), (4, 3), (4, 4)\}$

11. (a) Example 2.53(c), R_1:

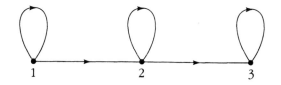

   (b) For each pair of vertices p, q for which there is an edge from p to q, there is also an edge from q to p.

   (d) For each pair of vertices p, q for which there is a path from p to q formed by a succession of directed edges, there is also a single edge leading directly (that is, without passing through any other vertices along the way) from p to q.

15. (b) REFLEXIVE: for each $a \in \mathbb{N}$ we have $a \mid a$, because $a = a \cdot 1$.
   ANTISYMMETRIC: if $a \mid b$ and $b \mid a$, then $b = ac$ and $a = bd$ for some $c, d \in \mathbb{N}$. Then $a = bd = acd$, therefore $cd = 1$, and so $c = d = 1$. This gives $a = b$.
   TRANSITIVE: if $a \mid b$ and $b \mid c$ then $b = ad$ and $c = be$ for some $d, e \in \mathbb{N}$. Then $c = a(de)$, and so $a \mid c$.

17. (a) $(1, 1), (2, 2), (3, 3)$ (b) impossible

19. We know that $A \subseteq A \cup B$ and $B \subseteq A \cup B$. This gives

$$R \subseteq A \times B \subseteq (A \cup B) \times (A \cup B).$$

21. The relation $\{(1, 2), (2, 1), (1, 1), (2, 2)\}$ is symmetric and transitive, but not reflexive.

SECTION 2.10

1. When $n = 1$, both sides of the given expression are equal to 1. Having assumed the result to hold for $n = k$, observe that

   (∗) $$1^2 + 2^2 + \cdots + (k + 1)^2 = (1^2 + 2^2 + \cdots + k^2) + (k + 1)^2.$$

   Now apply the induction hypothesis to expression (∗), and use arithmetic to check that the result is equal to

   $$\frac{(k + 1)[(k + 1) + 1][2(k + 1) + 1]}{6}.$$

3. If $n \le 0$ the result follows from the fact that squares are nonnegative. So it is enough to prove the statement when $n \ge 1$, and for this we use induction. For $n = 1$ the statement is clearly correct. Now suppose we know that $k^2 \ge k$ for some positive integer k. Then we have

   $$(k + 1)^2 = k^2 + 2k + 1 \ge 3k + 1 \ge k + 1,$$

   and this completes the proof.

5. Use the fact that $3k + 3 = 3(k + 1)$.

7. For $n = 10$: $1024 > 1000$. Now assume that $2^k > k^3$ for some $k \ge 10$; it must be shown that $2^{k+1} > (k + 1)^3$. But $2^{k+1} = 2(2^k) > 2k^3$, so it will suffice to verify the inequality $2k^3 > k^3 + 3k^2 + 3k + 1$, or, equivalently, $k^3 - 3k^2 - 3k - 1 > 0$. This can be done in a variety of ways. For instance, the given inequality is equivalent to the inequality $k(k^2 - 3k - 3) > 1$, so it is enough to show that $k^2 - 3k - 3 > 0$ when $k > 10$.

9. Consider whether the argument is legitimate when $k = 1$.

11. Let A be as in the suggestion given with the problem, and let k be the smallest element of A. (Such a k exists by the well-ordering principle.) So k is the smallest positive integer for which $P(k)$ is false. Hence $P(k - 1)$ is true. But then, by 2.67(b), statement $P(k)$ must be true. [Remember: $k = (k - 1) + 1$.] CONTRADICTION. Therefore we must have $A = \emptyset$. So $P(n)$ is true for all $n \in \mathbb{N}$.

13. If $n = 1$, then both sides of the equation being checked are equal to a^{b_1}. Now suppose $P(k)$ is true for some $k \ge 1$. That is, $\prod_{i=1}^{k} a^{b_i} = a^{\sum_{i=1}^{k} b_i}$. Then, by the laws of exponents and the induction hypothesis, we have

$$\prod_{i=1}^{k+1} a^{b_i} = \left(\prod_{i=1}^{k} a^{b_i} \right) \cdot a^{b_{k+1}} = a^{\left(\sum_{i=1}^{k} b_i \right)} \cdot a^{b_{k+1}} = a^{\left(\sum_{i=1}^{k} b_i \right) + b_{k+1}} = a^{\sum_{i=1}^{k+1} b_i}.$$

This completes the induction.

SECTION 3.1

1. Sets f and g are functions from A to B, but h is not a function; j is not a function from A to B, but j is a function from $\{2, 3\}$ to B.

3. If $x \in X$ and $y_1, y_2 \in Y$, then $(x, y_1), (x, y_2) \in X \times Y$. Consider the consequences if $y_1 \ne y_2$.

5. 27

7. (a) $\chi_\emptyset(x) = 0 \quad \forall x \in A$

   (c) "⇐": Assume that $\chi_A = \chi_B$, and let $x \in A$. To show that $x \in B$, it suffices to check that $\chi_B(x) = 1$. But $\chi_B(x) = \chi_A(x) = 1$. (Here the first equality follows from the hypothesis $\chi_A = \chi_B$, and the second equality holds because $x \in A$.) This shows that $A \subseteq B$, and a similar argument shows that $A \supseteq B$.

9. (a) The answer is 0 if $\alpha \in \mathbb{Z}$, and otherwise the answer is -1.

   (b) If $m \le \alpha < m + 1$, with $m \in \mathbb{Z}$, then $n + m \le n + \alpha < n + m + 1$; so $\lfloor \alpha \rfloor = m$ and $[n + \alpha] = n + m = n + [\alpha]$.

   (c) Choose β to satisfy the inequality $(1 + 1/[\alpha]) < \beta < 2$.

   (d) First consider the case $m \ge n$, then the case $m < n$.

11. (a) $\{(1, 1), (2, 1)\}, \quad \{(1, 1), (2, 2)\}, \quad \{(1, 2), (2, 1)\}, \quad \{(1, 2), (2, 2)\}$

    (b) Let $f \in A^C$. That is, $f \subseteq C \times A$, and $\forall c \in C$ there is a unique $a \in A$ such that $f(c) = a$. But $A \subseteq B$, so $a \in B$ and $C \times A \subseteq C \times B$. Thus $f \subseteq C \times B$, and $\forall c \in C$ there is a unique $a \in B$ such that $f(c) = a$. That is, $f \in B^C$; this proves the result.

    (c) Each member of $\{1, 2\}^{\{1,2,3\}}$ is a set of ordered pairs, and one of those pairs has 3 as its first coordinate. Consider whether the same can be said about the members of $\{1, 2\}^{\{1,2\}}$.

SECTION 3.2

1. (a) $\operatorname{im} f = \operatorname{im} g = \{1\}$ (c) the set of nonnegative real numbers   (e) $\operatorname{im} f$ is the set of nonnegative real numbers; $\operatorname{im} g$ is smaller, consisting of just the set of squares of rational numbers. Thus we can write

$$\operatorname{im} g = \{a^2/b^2 \mid a, b \in \mathbb{Z}, \ b \ne 0\}.$$

3. (a) injective only   (c) neither injective nor surjective

5. (a) $g^{-1} = \{(5, 1), (-2, 2), (6, 3)\}$ (b) If $f : A \to B$ is not injective, then there exist distinct elements $a_1, a_2 \in A$ and an element $b \in B$ such that $(a_1, b), (a_2, b) \in f$. But then $(b, a_1), (b, a_2) \in f^{-1}$, and hence f^{-1} is not a function.

7. The only available representatives of $\{1\}$ and $\{6\}$ are 1 and 6, respectively. So the representative of $\{3, 6\}$ must be 3, and therefore the representatives of $\{3, 4\}$ and $\{1, 2, 3\}$ must be 4 and 2, respectively. This forces 5 and 7 to be the respective representatives of $\{2, 4, 5\}$ and $\{1, 4, 7\}$.

9. (a) The function f is a bijection if and only if $a \ne 0$.   (b) The necessary and sufficient condition is that $a = \pm 1$.

13. Parts (a) and (b) follow from the fact that the absolute value of any number is nonnegative, and it is zero if and only if the number itself is zero.

15. Compare the current estimate with the preceding one or, if necessary, with the following one. If the current answer agrees with either of those through n decimal places, then it has the desired degree of accuracy.

17. The idea is to obtain a function h such that $h(1) = f(1)$, $h(2) = g(1)$, $h(3) = f(2)$, $h(4) = g(2)$, and so on. Such a function h will take the odd positive integers onto

im $f = A$ and the even positive integers onto im $g = B$. Explicitly, define h by

$$h(x) = \begin{cases} f\left(\dfrac{x+1}{2}\right) & \text{if } x \text{ is odd,} \\ g\left(\dfrac{x}{2}\right) & \text{if } x \text{ is even.} \end{cases}$$

Then check that this function works.

19. Go from $(1, 1)$ to $(2, 1)$ to $(2, 2)$ to $(1, 2)$, and continue.

21. Spiral out from the origin.

SECTION 3.3

1. (a) $\mathbb{R}$; (c) $\mathbb{R} - \{n\pi \mid n \in \mathbb{Z}\}$.

3. (a) If $f(x) = x + 1$ and $g(x) = x/2$, then $(f \circ g)(3) = \frac{5}{2} \neq (g \circ f)(3) = 2$.

7. (b) Let $c \in C$. Because $g \circ f$ is surjective, there exists $a \in A$ such that $(g \circ f)(a) = c$. That is, $g(f(a)) = c$. Thus we have found an element (namely, $f(a)$) of B that is taken to c by g.

9. Consider a function f defined by

$$f(x) = \begin{cases} x + 5 & \text{if } x \geq 0, \\ x & \text{if } x < 0. \end{cases}$$

This function "tears a hole" in $\mathbb{Z}$. Now try to patch the hole with a suitable function g.

11. The given function *is* a bijection.

13. (a) Suppose $A = \{1, 2\}$ and $C = \{3, 4\}$. Then, because im $f^{-1} = A$ and dom $g^{-1} = C$, it follows that $g^{-1} \circ f^{-1}$ is meaningless, though $(g \circ f)^{-1}$ has meaning.

15. To get the left cancellation law, notice that from the hypothesis we have

$$f^{-1} \circ (f \circ g) = f^{-1}(f \circ h),$$

and proceed from there.

SECTION 4.1

1. (b) We think of two collections as being the same "size" if each object in one can be paired with an object in the other so that when we're done there is nothing left over in either collection. (Demonstrate with a few pears and apples, say.) The statement says that if a first collection and a second collection have the same size in this sense, and also the second collection and a third collection have the same size, then the first and third collections have the same size. (Again demonstrate with actual objects, showing how the pairings for the first and second sets and the pairings for the second and third sets lead naturally to pairings of the elements of the first set with the elements of the third set.)

3. (a) Consider the mapping given by $n \mapsto 5n + 2$.

5. (a) Define $f : [0, 1] \to [2, 7]$ by $f(x) = 2 + 5x$.

   (b) Define $f : \mathbb{Z} \to \{\text{positive evens}\}$ by

$$f(n) = \begin{cases} 4n & \text{if } n > 0 \\ 4|n| + 2 & \text{if } n \leq 0 \end{cases}$$

7. Use differentiation to show that the function is increasing, and hence one-to-one. To show surjectivity it suffices to show that the function is unbounded from above and therefore (why?) also from below.

11. For $n = 1$ there is really nothing to prove, since both sides are equal to $\#A_1$. Corollary 4.16 does the job for $n = 2$. Then rewrite $\bigcup_{i=1}^{k+1} A_i$ in the form $(\bigcup_{i=1}^{k} A_i) \cup A_{k+1}$, and use the case $n = 2$ to complete the induction step.

13. According to the definition of "+" in Exercise 10, the job here is to show that if $X \approx (B - A)$ and $Y \approx A$, where $X \cap Y = \emptyset$, then $X \cup Y \approx B$.

15. (a) Apply the pigeonhole principle (4.9) to a function from a given set of eight people to the set of days of the week.

17. (a) Use the product rule (4.22).

   (b) Once the activities have been chosen as in part (a), there remains the choice of *order* for the activities, and the number of possibilities for that is equal to the number of ways of listing the elements of the set {snack, movie, art}. Having determined that number, invoke the product rule.

19. Be careful not to count a given handshake more than once.

21. (a) Each of the n elements of B has m candidates in A that it might be paired with. In all, there are n choices to be made, with m possibilities for each. Invoke the product rule.

   (b) The hint gives the number of subsets of A that can serve as the function's image and, for each of those, part (a) gives the number of functions with domain B that have that image. Use the product rule.

SECTION 4.2

1. (a) "$\Leftarrow$": Assume $A = \emptyset$. The conditional statement

$$\text{If } x \in \emptyset \text{ then there exists } y \in \emptyset \text{ such that } \emptyset(y) = x.$$

   is true, because its hypothesis is false. Therefore $\emptyset$ is surjective.

3. This proof is a clone of the proof of the first part of the theorem.

5. (a) The mapping $x \longmapsto x$ is an injection from $A - B$ to A.

   (b) Consider the consequences if $\#A > \#B$ and $A \cap B = \emptyset$.

7. A typical element of the square has the form

$$(.a_1 a_2 a_3 \ldots, .b_1 b_2 b_3 \ldots).$$

Now follow the given suggestion.

SECTION 4.3

1. $\mathbb{Z} = \mathbb{N} \cup A \cup B$, where $A = \{n \in \mathbb{Z} \mid n \leq 0 \text{ and } n \text{ is even}\}$ and B is the set of odd negative integers

3. (a) By Corollary 4.15, at least one of the blocks must be infinite. Now apply Theorem 4.36(a).

5. Check that the mapping given by $n \longmapsto 7n + 3$ is a bijection from $\mathbb{Z}$ to the given set. Then apply Example 4.34.

7. (a) Show that $\mathbb{N} \times \mathbb{N} = \bigcup_{i \in \mathbb{N}}(\mathbb{N} \times \{i\})$.

   (b) Theorem 4.39(a) will be useful.

9. First check that for each $q \in \mathbb{Q}$, the collection of all intervals having rational endpoints and right endpoint q is a countable set. Then use the result of Exercise 8.

11. INJECTIVITY: Suppose $g(m, n) = g(r, s)$. That is, $2^{m-1}(2n - 1) = 2^{r-1}(2s - 1)$. Since $2n-1$ and $2s-1$ are both odd it follows (from the Fundamental Theorem of Arithmetic) that $2^{m-1} = 2^{r-1}$ (and hence $m = r$), since both numbers represent the power of 2 in the standard factorization of $g(m, n)$. Therefore $2n - 1 = 2s - 1$, and so $n = s$. This proves that g is injective.

    SURJECTIVITY: Let $k \in \mathbb{N}$; say $k = 2^t \cdot q$, with q odd and $t \geq 0$. Then $k = g(t + 1, \frac{q+1}{2})$; so g is surjective.

13. Bet that neither coordinate will be rational.

SECTION 4.5

1. View x and y as functions from $\mathbb{N}_m$ and $\mathbb{N}_n$ (respectively) into Σ. Then xy is the function from $\mathbb{N}_{m+n}$ into Σ given by

$$(xy)(i) = \begin{cases} x(i) & \text{if } 1 \leq i \leq m, \\ y(i - m) & \text{if } m < i \leq m + n. \end{cases}$$

3. (a) This consists of the set of all words of the form $w\,w$ with $w \in L$.

   (b) Any language containing the empty word ϵ will do.

5. The languages $L(M)$ and $L(N)$ are the same.

7. Let's say that the initial states of M_1 and M_2 are q_0 and q_0', respectively. Erase the arc starting at q_0 that is labelled b, and erase the arc starting at q_0' that is labelled a. Then drag the diagram for M_1 over to the diagram for M_2 in such a way that q_0 and q_0' become superimposed, but so that no other vertices of the two graphs come into contact. The result is the graph of the desired automaton. The point obtained from merging q_0 and q_0' represents the initial vertex of the new automaton, and the new collection of final states is the union of the final state sets of M_1 and M_2. It remains to check that this construction works.

9. (a)

(c)

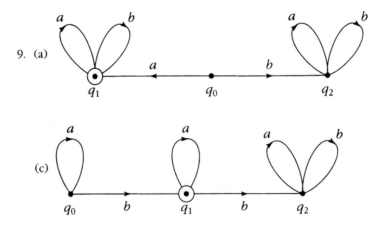

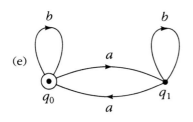

SECTION 5.2

3. (a) 360

   (b) 144 [First determine how many positive divisors *are* divisible by 10, then apply part (a).]

5. 1320

SECTION 5.3

1. (a) a permutation   (c) not a permutation   (e) a permutation

3. There are 24 members altogether.

5. (a) Given $\lambda \in S_m$, extend λ to an element $\lambda \in S_n$ by the formula

$$\lambda(x) = \begin{cases} \lambda(x) & \text{if } 1 \le x \le m, \\ x & \text{if } m + 1 \le x \le n. \end{cases}$$

7. (a) $\begin{pmatrix} 1 & 2 & 3 & 4 & 5 \\ 4 & 2 & 3 & 1 & 5 \end{pmatrix}$ (c) $\begin{pmatrix} 1 & 2 & 3 & 4 & 5 \\ 1 & 3 & 2 & 5 & 4 \end{pmatrix}$

9. Begin by noticing that the sets of elements moved by the given permutations are disjoint.

11. $8! = 40320$

13. (a) 10!   (b) $2 \cdot 3! \cdot 7!$ (c) $7 \cdot 3! \cdot 7!$ (d) Arrange the 7 dogs in a line. There are 7! ways to do this. Each cat will go between two dogs or at an end location. So there are 8 positions in line available for cats. Pick a cat. For it there are 8 possible locations. Having put it in place, there are 7 possible locations for the next cat and 6 possibilities for the third. Final answer: $7! \cdot 8 \cdot 7 \cdot 6$.   (e) $7 \cdot 6 \cdot 8!$

15. (a) If in a move the cup in position i goes to position j, associate $\sigma \in S_5$ such that $\sigma(i) = j$.

   (b) $\frac{5 \cdot 4}{2} = 10$ (c) 5!

   (d) 4! (We know where the left-most cup goes. So it's just a matter of counting the repositions of the remaining 4 cups.)

17. $\frac{7!}{2}$

SECTION 5.4

1. Suppose the triangle's vertices are A, B, C, and let s be a symmetry. Show that if $s(A) = B$ then $s(B) = A$, and therefore $s(C) = C$. Then use this to obtain a contradiction.

3. (a) There are eight members.

   (b) Inscribe a regular triangle in a regular hexagon, and proceed from there.

5. (a) ten symmetries (c) one symmetry (e) four symmetries
   (g) one symmetry (i) the collection of symmetries is countably infinite
   (k) the collection of symmetries is uncountably infinite

7. (a) If $P = Q$ then $R_Q(P) = P$. If $P = (c, d) \neq Q$, then obtain the equation of the line through P and Q and the equation of the circle centered at Q with radius PQ. The intersection of the two geometric figures is obtained by solving these equations simultaneously, and the solution set is $\{P, R_Q(P)\}$.

   (b) Use the formula obtained in (a) to show that for any two points P_1, P_2, the distance between $R_Q(P_1)$ and $R_Q(P_2)$ is equal to the distance between P_1 and P_2.

SECTION 5.5

1. (a) $\begin{pmatrix} 1 & 2 & 3 & 4 & 5 & 6 & 7 \\ 2 & 7 & 1 & 4 & 6 & 5 & 3 \end{pmatrix}$ (c) $\begin{pmatrix} 1 & 2 & 3 & 4 \\ 3 & 1 & 4 & 2 \end{pmatrix}$

3. (a) First notice that once σ^2 has been computed, only one more multiplication is required in order to compute σ^4.

5. They look the same, except that the edge directions are all reversed.

7. (a) The notation tells us that the listed elements are moved cyclically by σ, and that no other elements are moved by σ, but it does not tell us the whole domain.

   (b) $\begin{pmatrix} 1 & 2 & 3 & 4 & 5 & 6 & 7 \\ 5 & 3 & 4 & 2 & 7 & 1 & 6 \end{pmatrix}$

9. (a) $(1 \ \ 5 \ \ 3)(2 \ \ 6 \ \ 7)$ (b) $(1 \ \ 3 \ \ 4 \ \ 5 \ \ 6 \ \ 2)$ (c) $(2 \ \ 4 \ \ 3)$

11. Consider the products $(\sigma\tau)(\tau^{-1}\sigma^{-1})$ and $(\tau^{-1}\sigma^{-1})(\sigma\tau)$.

13. If α satisfies the given equation, it follows that $\alpha = \sigma (2 \ \ 1 \ \ 4)\lambda^{-1}$.

15. Notice that once *some* n is obtained for which S_n contains a non-cycle, then the same is true for all larger values of n.

SECTION 5.6

3. Use the method of Example 5.42.

5. Begin by factoring 2520 into primes, and then use this data to obtain a set of integers whose sum is 30 and whose least common multiple is 2520. Then apply Theorem 5.45.

7. (b) Every element of S_m has a natural extension to an element of S_n. See Exercise 5 in Section 5.3.

9. 18 (Use the method of Example 5.47.)

SECTION 5.7

1. (a) $(1 \ \ 2)(1 \ \ 5)(1 \ \ 4)(1 \ \ 6)(1 \ \ 8)(1 \ \ 7)(1 \ \ 3)$ (c) $(1 \ \ 2)(3 \ \ 4)$

3. (a) two reversals (b) four reversals

5. Show that the permutation

$$\begin{pmatrix} 1 & 2 & 3 & \cdots & n-1 & n \\ n & n-1 & n-2 & \cdots & 2 & 1 \end{pmatrix}$$

has the desired property.

7. Use Theorem 5.54.

9. Use Corollary 5.36, together with the fact that s moves exactly four elements.

11. (a) -1 (b) 1 (c) -1

13. (a) Observe that a shift of the puzzle pieces to the indicated configuration is associated with the permutation $(1 \quad 2 \quad 6 \quad 7 \quad 11 \quad 12 \quad 16)$, an even permutation.

15. Check each of the cases from $n = 1$ through $n = 5$ to get the idea.

SECTION 5.8

1. (a) 9863 (c) 1001 (e) 39711 (g) 1

5. (a) 336 (b) 231 (c) 2398

7. Use the binomial theorem.

11. Check the cases $n = 1, 2, 3$ individually. For $n \geq 4$, use Theorem 5.64.

13. (a) 1120 (b) 1883

15. $\frac{13 \cdot 48}{\binom{52}{5}} = \frac{1}{4165}$

17. (a) $\frac{35}{128}$ (b) $\frac{35}{64}$

19. If a set of n objects is to be assembled in sequence, with only two types of object in the set, consider the consequence of specifying the locations of one of the types.

21. 2,522,520

23. (a) 3,628,800 (b) 30,240 (c) 252

25. -280

SECTION 6.1

1. (a) The left side of the rule becomes $\cdot((a, +((b, c))))$.

3. n^3

5. The case $n = 3$: define a 3-ary (more commonly, *ternary*) operation $*_3 : S^3 \rightarrow S$ by

$$*_3((s_1, s_2, s_3)) = (s_1 * s_2) * s_3.$$

7. Suppose there *is* an identity element; call it e. Then for each $a \in \mathbb{R}$, the equation $a \div e = a$ holds. But this implies that $e = 1$. (Why?) Check that in fact 1 is *not* an identity element for $\div$.

9. The statement $(x*y)*z = z*(y*z)$ must be checked for each substitution of elements from the set $\{e, a\}$ in place of the symbols x, y, z. There are eight statements to check altogether.

11. First explain how to check the table to see if there is an identity element e for the operation. (If there is none, then no inverses exist.) Assuming that e exists, the element e must appear in every row of the table for inverses to exist. Having checked that, it remains to carry out an appropriate check of the *columns* of the table.

13. (a) yes, yes, no (c) yes, yes, yes (e) yes, no, no

15. If e is an identity for $*$, then

$$ra + se = a * e = e * a = re + sa, \quad \forall a \in \mathbb{Z}.$$

Consider the consequences when $a \neq e$.

SECTION 6.2

1.
$$(a + b)c = c(a + b) \quad \text{since multiplication is commutative}$$
$$= ca + cb \quad \text{by the left-hand rule in (6.7)}$$
$$= ac + bc \quad \text{since multiplication is commutative.}$$

3. (a) By using the distributive laws we obtain
$$(a + b)(c + d) = (a + b)c + (a + b)d = ac + bc + ad + bd.$$

5. Suppose that for some $a \in \mathbb{Z}$ we have $0 \cdot a = b \neq 0$. Then, from the properties discussed in the text, we deduce that
$$a = 1 \cdot a = (1 + 0) \cdot a = 1 \cdot a + 0 \cdot a = a + b.$$

Now add $-a$ to both sides of this equation to get a contradiction.

7. Use 6.11.

9. Define "$\leq$" in a way modelled after the definition of "$<$" in 6.11.

SECTION 6.3

1. From the hypothesis, we have $b = ax$ and $c = ay$ for some $x, y \in \mathbb{Z}$. This observation will lead to the result.

3. Notice that if $x \in \mathbb{R}$, then
$$[x] = x \quad \Leftrightarrow \quad x \in \mathbb{Z}.$$

7. After the sieving procedure is complete, thirty primes should remain on your list of integers.

9. It suffices to show that n is divisible by 2 and by 3. Achieve these goals one at a time. (The division algorithm (6.17) will be helpful for this purpose, with $k = a$.)

13. The expression on each side of the alleged equation represents a positive integer. It is enough to check that each of these is a divisor of the other.

17. Refer to the proof of Theorem 6.31 for the strategy.

19. Remember Pythagoras!

21. The least common multiple is 9,447,438.

SECTION 6.4

1. (a) true (c) false (e) true (g) false

3. Write n in the form $2k + 1$ for some integer k.

5. (b) Recall the formula $1 + 2 + 3 + \cdots + k = k(k + 1)/2$, and use the test (6.46) for divisibility by 9.

7. Refer to Example 6.40(a).

9. Use Theorem 6.45.

11. (b) As part of the solution, show that if $x, y \in \{0, k, 2k, \ldots, (m - 1)k\}$ and $x \equiv y \pmod{m}$, then $x = y$. Next apply part (a) to each element of the set $\{0, k, 2k, \ldots, (m - 1)k\}$.

15. Use a proof by contradiction. The equation $2^{ab} = (2^a)^b$ will be helpful.

17. (b) 131123031

19. Use Theorem 6.48 as a guide.

SECTION 6.5

1. (a) $\varphi(9) = 6$, $\varphi(20) = 8$, $\varphi(37) = 36$.

   (b) The numbers *not* relatively prime to p^k are $p, 2p, 3p, \ldots, p^{k-1}p$; therefore $\varphi(p^k) = p^k - p^{k-1}$.

3. (a) If $p = ab$, with $1 < a \leq p - 1$, then $a \mid (p - 1)!$; and also (from the hypothesis) we have $a \mid ((p - 1)! + 1)$. Therefore, $a \mid (((p - 1)! + 1) - (p - 1)!)$; that is, $a \mid 1$, contradicting the fact that $a > 1$.

5. We have $2^{340} = 2^{256+64+16+4} = 2^{256} \cdot 2^{64} \cdot 2^{16} \cdot 2^4$. But

$$2^4 = 16$$

$$2^{16} = 65536 \equiv 64 \pmod{341}$$

$$2^{32} \equiv 64^2 \equiv 4 \pmod{341}$$

$$2^{64} \equiv 4^2 \equiv 16 \pmod{341}$$

$$2^{128} \equiv 256 \pmod{341}$$

$$2^{256} \equiv 65536 \equiv 64 \pmod{341}$$

Therefore, $2^{340} \equiv 64 \cdot 16 \cdot 64 \cdot 16 = 1048576 \equiv 1 \pmod{341}$.

7. (a) $683 = 512 + 128 + 32 + 8 + 2 + 1$ $(= 2^9 + 2^7 + 2^5 + 2^3 + 2^1 + 2^0)$

   (b) 683 in binary: 1010101011

9. (a) We can write $m_1 = p_1^{\alpha_1} \cdots p_r^{\alpha_r}$, $m_2 = p_{r+1}^{\alpha_{r+1}} \cdots p_n^{\alpha_n}$, with the p_i's distinct, since $(m_1, m_2) = 1$. The hypothesis gives that $m_1 \mid a - b$ and $m_2 \mid a - b$, hence $p_i^{\alpha_i} \mid a - b$ for all i. Therefore p_i appears to some power $\geq \alpha_i$ in the standard factorization of $a - b$. Thus $\left(\prod_{i=1}^n p_i^{\alpha_i}\right) \mid a - b$. That is, $a \equiv b \pmod{m_1 m_2}$.

   (b) Let $x \in \mathbb{Z}$. By part (a) it suffices to check the congruences $x^5 \equiv x \pmod{2}$ and $x^5 \equiv x \pmod{5}$.

SECTION 6.6

1. (a) $\varphi(360) = \varphi(2^3 \cdot 3^2 \cdot 5) = 360 \cdot \frac{1}{2} \cdot \frac{2}{3} \cdot \frac{4}{5} = 96$.

3. Write $m = p_1^{\alpha_1} \cdots p_r^{\alpha_r}$ and $n = mk = p_1^{\beta_1} \cdots p_r^{\beta_r} p_{r+1}^{\beta_{r+1}} \cdots p_t^{\beta_t}$, with $\alpha_i \leq \beta_i$ for $1 \leq\leq r$. Then

$$\varphi(m) = m \prod_{i=1}^r \left(1 - \frac{1}{p_i}\right) \quad \text{and} \quad \varphi(n) = n \prod_{i=1}^t \left(1 - \frac{1}{p_i}\right) = \varphi(m) \cdot \left(k \prod_{i=r+1}^t \left(1 - \frac{1}{p_i}\right)\right)$$

5. $\varphi(8) \neq \varphi(4) \cdot \varphi(2)$

7. $\sum_{i=0}^r \varphi(p^i) = 1 + \sum_{i=1}^r \varphi(p^i) = 1 + \sum_{i=1}^r (p^i - p^{i-1}) = p^r$. (The sum "telescopes.")

9. (a) Since $n = qt + r$, there are q numbers in $\mathbb{N}_n$ that are divisible by t, namely $t, 2t, \ldots, qt$. But $[\frac{n}{t}] = [q + \frac{r}{t}] = q$, since $0 \leq r < q$.

(b) From part (a), we have $|A_5| = 200$, $|A_6| = 166$, and $|A_8| = 125$. Moreover $|A_5 \cap A_6| = |A_{30}| = 33$, $|A_5 \cap A_8| = |A_{40}| = 25$, $|A_6 \cap A_8| = |A_{24}| = 41$, and $|A_5 \cap A_6 \cap A_8| = |A_{120}| = 8$. Then

$$|\overline{A_5} \cap \overline{A_6} \cap \overline{A_8}| = 1000 - \left(|A_5| + |A_6| + |A_8| \right)$$

$$+ \left(|A_5 \cap A_6| + |A_5 \cap A_8| + |A_6 \cap A_8| \right) - |A_5 \cap A_6 \cap A_8|$$

$$= 1000 - (200 + 166 + 125) + (33 + 25 + 41) - 8 = 600.$$

INDEX

Lightning Source UK Ltd.
Milton Keynes UK
13 September 2009

143624UK00001B/17/A